The After-Death Room
Journey Into Spiritual Activism

The After-Death Room

Journey Into Spiritual Activism

by Michael McColly

Transition Books

an imprint of Soft Skull Press

Cambridge, MA | Brooklyn, NY

2006

cover photo: Jide Adeniyi-Jones*
book design: Luke Gerwe

Published by Soft Skull Press
55 Washington Street, Suite 804
Brooklyn, NY 11201
www.softskull.com

Distributed by Publishers Group West
800 788 3123 | www.pgw.com

Printed in Canada

ISBN: 1-932360-92-1
ISBN-13: 978-1-932360-92-9

Library of Congress Cataloging-in-Publication Data for this title available from
the Library of Congress.

Some names in this text have been changed.

* Jide Adeniyi-Jones's photograph comes from a series called *HIV In Nigeria: Living On The Edge*. In this series, Adeniyi-Jones provides the following caption: "At the village clinic, Dr. Ofoedu says: 'There are many people here with HIV but the stigma is very strong and there is a lot of ignorance. We can get to them but we must have some help to offer.'" Please visit his website: www.adeniyi-jones.net

To my parents,
who taught me to travel outside of myself,
and my teachers,
who taught me to travel within.

"Not by avoiding actions does a man gain freedom from action."
Bhagavad Gita

Contents

Prologue

"To deny one's own experience is to put a lie into the lips of one's own life."
—Oscar Wilde

If AIDS had never come into this world, if it had never spilled into the blood of that first soul, I would have remembered that June of 1982 as the month that I fell in love with a half-Irish, half-Sicilian woman from Connecticut. But that month marks the beginning of another journey, one I would spend the next nineteen years refusing to take.

I can still hear the voice coming from my short wave radio: *Doctors in Los Angeles have reported a mysterious virus that has caused the death of several men who* . . . That morning was like any other in my life as a Peace Corps volunteer, living among the Wolof and Mandinka twenty miles from the Gambia River. I made my Nescafé. I wrote my letters. I ate my millet porridge with the village chief.

The rainy season had begun, and the farmers were in the fields planting peanuts, seed by seed, row by row, walking behind a plow and a pair of yoked oxen. Women clustered at the well, talking and telling stories, as hand over hand they pulled up water in black bags made of used tire tubing. Outside my hut children waited for the Koranic school to start, throwing stones at the baobab fruit hoping to knock down a treat. Over their excited voices, I listened to the man in London as if he were standing behind me in my little mud-brick hut: *The virus, which doctors say destroys the immune system, has been detected in homosexual and bisexual men* . . .

I attempted to go about my work with the village women as we tried to grow tomatoes and carrots in the heat and the sand, but those words "mysterious virus" and "homosexual" and "death" fused with images I'd believed I'd erased from my memory when I'd crossed the Atlantic and joined the Peace Corps. Though I had no idea what this disease doctors were calling GRID (gay-related immune disease) would eventually mean for the world, I felt in those newscaster's words a terrible truth had been released upon me and the world.

I'd been caught, finally, at the far end of the world in a Muslim village of black Africans, the boy, the fugitive, who'd been running ever since that day that he'd reached out and touched the mirror image of himself in the trembling body of his friend in the barn behind his house.

Each time I heard the news repeated on my short-wave radio that day, images of my sexual history returned with increasing intensity and vividness: I saw myself as a boy take my mother's clothes out of the clothes

1

hamper and slip them on before the bathroom mirror; I saw myself tip-toe through the darkness, kick off my pajamas and run naked, even in the snow, into the fields behind our house; I saw myself staring at the soapy torsos of my teammates in the showers in high school; I saw myself sucking on the tongues of black men in the blue light of video booths on Halsted Street in Chicago. I'd hoped these episodes would one day be absolved by words, by love, by the body of a woman.

The finality of the announcer's voice kept ringing inside me, bringing me back, again and again, to these scenes, dredging up fragments of voices and emotions, until my memory settled on that summer day in my youth on a camping trip with my family in Maine, when my father overheard me confess "my secret" to my sister. The sorrow in the announcer's words had the same tone of truth I'd heard in my father in his speech on the "facts of life." Both men knew of the penalty men must serve for this "secret": sex would become loss—an act that instead of connecting me to the world, would forever sever me from it.

That day in the woods in Maine, my father led me to a great pile of logs, slashed and sawed, and chaotically stacked to be dragged away. We sat on stumps and stared at the wood chips at our feet. I sobbed before he could open his mouth. Over and over I pleaded for him to stop: "I know, I know, I know . . ." But my father dutifully carried on, explaining each biological stage, each effort at calming me having the opposite effect. No matter how softly spoken, each word fell like an axe on my innocence. In silence, we walked back in the sour piney heat of mid afternoon. Refusing his touch, I drifted further behind, wincing at each branch he snapped with his heavy shoes.

As a boy, I had learned in times of emotional chaos to take my body into the stillness of distance, outside and away from people and the things they made. One of my first memories as a child is riding a tricycle to the end of the subdivision where we lived. I was headed for the highway. And that is where neighbors stopped me and took me home. I think I was three. I have no memory of why I left or where I thought I might go. But I remember how good it felt to be pedaling, pedaling past all the houses, traveling further and further away.

So that day in Senegal when I heard the news, I knew I had to escape from the claustrophobia of my emotions and the reminder of my shame in every villager's face who came before me. And though it was midday and so bright you could almost see through your eyelids, I fled into the mirage of distance, desperate for the solace of the savannah. I hiked past the peanut fields and into the forest with its ancient baobab and ten-foot termite mounds. I found a wide-branched acacia and sat leaning against its trunk and watched dung beetles, like Sisyphus, roll ball after ball of goat shit in the sand.

Jokingly, the villagers nicknamed me "Tukkikat"—one who loves to travel, or, as an old man once explained the Wolof word: "a man always on his way someplace else." To the Senegalese, isolating oneself was a sign of spiritual sickness, and so the women, worried by this trait of mine to steal away into the bush, would send their sons to watch over me. Sure enough, my spiritual bodyguards had followed me through the peanut fields. "Mustapha, what are you doing out here?"

A few days after I'd heard the radio report, I left the village to meet my colleagues in the city of Kaolack. There in the courtyard of the Peace Corps house, my American compatriots sat under the neem tree drinking beer and smoking the local ganja, recounting stories of the past week in their villages. On the table I could see the cover of that week's international *Newsweek*. A syringe dripped blood, with a headline that read: "AIDS: The New Hidden Killer."

Almost immediately the subject surfaced. When someone raised the question of how this new disease spread, my worldly, well-educated friends snickered, and I disappeared into the kitchen to get another beer, though I already had one in my hand. When I came back, I caught the eyes of Elizabeth. They were as wide open as they were that first night on the rooftop of the Kaolack house, stunned that I'd entered her, as we lay wrapped in a single sheet under the stars, our colleagues sleeping only feet away.

"Have you read the article?" she asked later that night in the cocoon of our mosquito netting. Brushing away her brunette hair so that I had to confront each olive eye, she pleaded with me to look at the article she had with her in our bed: "There's a guy in the article from Chicago, a man who has *it*—he's in theater, too. Maybe you—you, like *know* him?"

"I'll read it later," I mumbled, rolling away, afraid and drunk from drinking all day.

Two months before, when we first met, I told her that I'd slept with men. It was a relief to tell her, to tell someone what I'd never told anyone before. When I told her what it felt like to be with a man and why I did it, we both heard something more than a confession. We stayed up the whole night telling stories about family and childhood, about friends and lovers, our stories came gushing out, fears mixed with dreams mixed with desire. When the sun came up, I wanted to follow her into the bathroom; I didn't want to ever let her out of my sight.

I stared at the wall until she turned out the lights. I understood why she was concerned, but that tone in her voice terrified me: *He lives in Chicago. He was in theater—like you.* When I was sure she was asleep, I got up, but she stopped me at the door: "Mike, where are you going?"

"I'm going to smoke a cigarette. Is that okay?"

In the dark, I wandered into the main room in our Peace Corps house. This room had become a kind of shrine to those volunteers who'd come and gone since the late sixties. I turned on a light. There, under a torn poster of Che Guevara, lying on a bookshelf holding twenty years of paperback classics, I found the *Newsweek*. I picked it up, sank into a chair, lit a cigarette and never took a drag.

For a while I stared at the first page, not really reading but absorbing words and photos. I turned the last page of the article, and there he was: the guy from Chicago who *had it*—John on his porch with his dog in Lincoln Park.

John was the stage manager at The Goodman Theatre where I had briefly worked as a stagehand on Tennessee Williams's last play. It was John who had invited me to meet the great playwright on opening night. I'd read every one of Williams's plays in high school, hearing in his characters a voice of sadness and longing that I believed only I possessed. That night, a drunken ghost in a fur coat scribbled *Tennessee* in an old paperback of *Cat On A Hot Tin Roof*. A few months later Williams was dead. He would be spared the horrors that would consume his friends and lovers in the years to follow.

In the photograph, John looked as I remembered him, confident, relaxed, smiling, but when I looked closer at the image, I noticed that his hand wasn't petting his dog; his hand was clutching the dog to his side.

I considered not going back to bed, knowing I would have to tell Elizabeth and arouse her fears of my bisexuality. But I had to tell her John was not a lover but only my boss. The next morning I did, but she kept asking questions as if I were lying to her about him and everything I'd told her about my past. Looking back, I don't blame her. She was scared, and so was I.

Lying in bed that night, I watched her as she slept, her breath lifting the sheet over her naked shoulder. I'd never been in love before, never known the comfort of waking up to someone sleeping next to me, never known the fear of love's loss. Looking at her body beside me, I became angrier and angrier knowing that under her sweetness and concern that she, too, now doubted me. It was her lack of doubt that I had clung to when we came together every other week from our posts.

However, desperate for the promise of love, Elizabeth and I continued our fairy-tale life for the next year, trying to teach African farmers twice our age things we didn't really know. I played the part in the romance we both wanted. I was the smiling, blond-haired hero doing good deeds to educate the backward Senegalese. I came to her village where we listened to the elders tell stories of the old times when they killed lions and fought Hitler and the Germans in North Africa with their weapons and sacred medicine.[1] Then we retired to her hut and drank wine and made love on the dirt floor, biting our arms and shoulders to keep from being heard. Together we dreamed grand dreams. We would go home to get married, return with graduate degrees, and devote our lives to the Senegalese.

Toward the end of my second year, her parents and mine visited at the same time. I made the same grand speeches, professing my love and plans to stay a third year so that we could be together and continue our work. My parents, once so troubled when I'd gone to New York and Chicago to act, now looked at me as the man they'd hoped I'd become. The happy ending was a foregone conclusion.

After the dinner, Elizabeth and I snuck out of our parent's rooms in a seaside hotel to take a romantic swim. But I was too drunk to offer much affection, so I took off my clothes and jumped in to sober up. I swam as hard as I could and then stopped. I could hear her calling my name, but the salty water felt so good on my body that I swam further and further until the lights of the hotel became a blur.

When I came back, she stood hands on hips, up to her knees in the surf: "Why did you do that? Why did you scare me? Why tonight?"

I had no answer to that question or why the next month I changed my mind and decided to go home after all. I thought I was losing my mind and so did everyone else, my colleagues and the villagers, who were already planning projects with me for the next year. Elizabeth was heartbroken and humiliated. I tried to explain, pleading with her to come back with me and get on with our lives and leave this playacting of the Peace Corps. She'd been sick for months with hepatitis and dysentery. I begged her to return with me for her own health. But my about-face had confirmed her doubts. Then she got a letter from her sister in San Francisco. I saw it lying on the bed with my name sprinkled throughout, so I read it: "I know what *these guys* are like. You will never be able to satisfy him. Drop him before it's too late!"

My flight was in the middle of the night, so Elizabeth and I went out to eat and I drank as much as I could possibly get down. Back at our cheap hotel, we undressed and lay on a thin mattress supported by a slab of cement. A single light bulb dangled over our naked bodies. Wolof sex workers cackled in the hallway. Mosquitoes bore into the backs of our thighs. She turned her head away and cried.

At the airport, when my flight was announced, I got sick, ruining the shirt she'd given me as a going-away gift. With my romantic dreams and big plans stuffed into a duffle bag, I staggered up the steps of the plane, leaving behind the hopes of two villages and Elizabeth, who stood there on the tarmac, holding a shirt stained with cheap wine and vomit.

❊

I returned to Chicago and enrolled in divinity school, hiding in the only place I knew I could—my head. And there was no better place to do that than the stone fortress on Chicago's South Side, The University of Chicago. Like many Peace Corps volunteers, I came home to discover that there no longer existed a place called *home*. In the two years I'd been gone, America and I had traveled in opposite directions. The Reagan era was in full bloom and the Peace Corps was earmarked for extinction. AIDS was a punch line in an office joke, a judgment from an angry God, a way to rid the world of fags, junkies, and black immigrants who swam ashore from a sinking ship called Haiti.

The HIV virus was quietly spreading across Chicago, too, sweeping through the gay ghetto of Lakeview and north into the Uptown slums, where the city corralled its misfits: refugees from Vietnam and Eritrea, Native Americans from the plains, pale-skinned miners' wives from West Virginia, drug-users, Vietnam vets, and schizophrenics. And on the South Side, where I now lived, AIDS spilled into the black and Latino gay and bisexual underworld, coursed through the drug culture, the gangs, and sex workers, and seeped into the cells of Cook County Jail.

I spent time drifting away from the troubles of the world that surrounded the ivy-walled campus created from the wealth of Rockefeller. It was 1983 and Liberation theology was all the rage. I sat in seminars and discussed the political priests in Latin America. I espoused their iconoclastic beliefs that the historical Jesus of Nazareth was a fearless radical bent on turning the world upside down, as he had the tables of the money changers. I was eager to show my scars fresh from the front. But the Wolof farmers and their families refused to conform to dinner party anecdotes or serve as examples for theological theories. Instead they sent letters painstakingly written in French by market scribes, letters which begged for help in buying sewing machines or medicines for children. I spent whole days in the library deciphering passages from Kierkegaard and Eliade, writing essays on Meister Eckhart and William James, burrowing into the thoughts of others in hopes of forgetting my own. But I couldn't forget the people of Darou Mouniaguene and Elizabeth. Seeing a map of Africa or a woman with black hair cut like hers was enough to spin me into a spell of sadness that lasted for days. It was impossible to study. So, as I had in Senegal, I took to my feet, hiking about Hyde Park and climbing on buses and trains to free myself from the thought that maybe I'd made a mistake. Everywhere I went, however, I seemed to manifest the fears and doubts that animated my despair. Thinking I'd discovered a quiet, wooded reserve near the Lake where I could be alone and watch birds, I discovered I'd stumbled into one of the main cruising spots for black gay and bisexual men in Jackson Park. It didn't take me long to realize, either, that the majority of black residents, who lived in and around Hyde Park, didn't share the welcoming traits of their ancestral relatives, the Wolofs. But then what could you expect from a community that had its businesses and bars closed, its houses bulldozed, and its streets patrolled by an occupying army of university and city police. In Senegal, sometimes old women cried to Allah for protection from my blond hair and blue eyes, but here, in Hyde Park, in one of the largest concentrations of blacks in North America, I represented not only the evil of segregation and racism but the hypocrisy on which this university was built.

But I refused to stay within the unspoken boundaries that kept "us" in and "them" out. I purposely took the wrong buses that passed through the wrong neighborhoods when I traveled to the Loop or North Side. Naïvely, I believed my education and experiences in Africa made me immune from the anger and distrust that African-Americans held toward the university and all who were associated with it. As I traveled back from the North Side one evening on a bus full of people coming home from work, a homeless woman with a purple hat and matching fingernails finally put me in my place. Grabbing my chin, she raised my face out of a book by Heidegger, and shattered the late afternoon silence: "See that telephone pole? We gonna string you up. We gonna crucify your ass, book boy!"

❊

In my second year of divinity school, I began to recover from Elizabeth and Africa. My studies inspired interests in comparative religion and I took up a practice of Kundalini yoga. As a part of a group of seminarians and clergy, I volunteered to work with Eritrean and Cambodian refugees. And I met Naomi, a woman who worked in my neighborhood at a health food store. She told me she'd once been married to an Ethiopian prince and lived in Israel, which explained the unusual religious sect she followed—a combination of Ethiopian Judaism, Rastafarianism, Black Nationalism, and the political philosophy of Pan-Africanism. I liked her radical spirit, her overflowing Rasta locks, her hand-sewn African print clothes, and the taste of her skin on the back of her neck. She reminded me of the poised women of Dakar who nearly blew me over when they sailed through the streets, their flowing gowns ablaze in color. I'm not sure what she saw in me, other than another way to outrage her mother, a jazz singer she had me meet almost as soon as we began to date. She was also amused by my stories of Senegal and my mix of international politics and whatever world religion I was studying at the time. But there was always a tension that went beyond our racial difference. One evening at her apartment, she began talking about homosexuality. "I mean, don't you think it's nasty? Putting their things in each other's booties? Why would anyone want to do that, huh?" She went on, waiting for me to chime in, but I had a suspicion that she was testing me. When I refused either to condemn or condone homosexuality, citing that line by Margaret Mead explaining bisexuality as normal and homosexuality and heterosexuality as abnormal, she burst into laughter: "You're a fag aren't you? That's it! I knew there was something that made you—you act the way you do with your books and bullshit about Africa." Her laughter made me feel as if I were a mouse she'd finally trapped behind the refrigerator with her broom. I quickly left without even defending myself, and I never saw her again.

I dated other women that year, but after that episode with Naomi, I began to experience deeper and deeper spells of depression. My interest in grad school, never that strong, soured and I finally dropped out. I worried that perhaps Naomi was right. For the first time, I tried therapy, but my therapist was no help, counseling self-control or telling long stories about her own struggles with drugs. I quit her, too, and comforted myself, as I learned to do as a child, with my imagination, writing pages and pages of bad poetry under the influence of bad wine. Outside of school, I drifted, spending days without talking to anyone except a fellow classmate, a Blackfoot Indian, who was struggling with drug addiction, though I didn't know it at the time. We drank and talked for hours about theology and politics. We knew we were both being eaten alive by our secrets and shame, but we were too afraid to confess them.

It was during that time that I began to secretly return to the gay demimonde on the North Side. Here, with heavy doses of alcohol and whatever drugs were available, I became anonymous, free from the persona that increasingly seemed false and exhausting to maintain. Yet, I was conflicted as I walked and walked the streets, entering and leaving bars, downing drink after drink, one moment wanting to be seduced, the next wanting to flee. I was disgusted and relieved all at once. I savored the darkness dancing around me and at the same time scorned the frivolity and self-absorption. I positioned myself in a dark corner and watched, a voyeur to these nightly tribal rituals of drink and dance that brought men closer and closer until hands and thighs, mouths and hair seemed to belong to everyone. Sometimes it was enough to just enter a bar and know it was there. Other times, I searched for that pair of eyes which, like me, preferred the margins: the foreigner, the bisexual, the married man, but mostly those men of color, who drifted in late. As soon as we touched, I could feel that they needed my body as badly as I needed theirs. Taste created taste. The fierceness of their grip instantly sobered me, making me feel both acute fear and sick with desire.

With them, with drugs, twisting and tunneling into the darkest hour of the night, our bodies pulled and pried each other open. Fucking often felt like we were trying to peel away our skin, desperate as we were to be freed from all that constrained the flesh. It was more like a lifeguard saving a drowning man, and the drowning man was almost always me. Stroke after stroke, I struggled all the way back to shore and then when we arrived, I felt ashamed and wanted to grab my clothes and run. Often on these nights, I left without even remembering their names. I'd wait until they were asleep, pull their heavy arm off my back, feel around in the dark for my pants, and slip out.

❀

Like most people who find themselves attracted to both sexes, I can't explain how or why I have chosen this fate or it has chosen me. Nor can I fully explain the role black men have played in my sexual life. I have no theories, only experiences. But I think it has something to do with growing up in a racially-mixed neighborhood and living on a basketball court for most of my adolescence.

My parents moved to Marion, Indiana, in 1963 when my father got hired to coach basketball and baseball at the high school there. Marion was known for four things: automotive plants, James Dean, high school basketball, and a mob lynching of two black teenagers in 1930.[2] Like many other cities in the rust belt, Marion was a mix of whites and blacks who'd moved from farms and up from the South to work in factories after World War II. We lived in a working-class neighborhood on what was known as the black side of town, though Marion was really too small to be truly segregated. So when my father erected a hoop and paved our gravel drive, our house became the place where the neighbor kids, black and white, came to play basketball.

Because I had the hoop, a good jump shot, and a father who was respected in the black community as a fair man and a good coach, I began to have a lot of black friends. That I had blond hair and blue eyes and was a know-it-all in school, they let slide. This was Indiana. This was the sixties. This was when a black and white town like Marion came together to roar and chant like hysterical Christians at a revival in praise of their seventeen-year-old sons. Basketball was everything for my home-town, and for me and my father, and the black kids who came from across the field behind my house.

One of the kids who began coming over to my house was a tall, shy, black kid named Lawrence. Lawrence and I battled for every athletic accolade from grammar school until we entered high school. I envied Lawrence. He seemed never to get angry or raise his voice. Effortlessly, he threw a football the length of our side yard, pitched a fast ball so hard, all you could see was his white teeth when he struck you out. As we matured, I remained skinny while his body turned almost overnight into that of a man's, his biceps rising under his shirt even when he lifted a glass of Kool-Aid. My father called him "a natural," and when we shot around, my father would come out of the house to show Lawrence how to perfect his jump shot. Fatherless, Lawrence spent almost every day at our house in the summers, eating with us and often spending the night. When he did, I would have a hard time falling asleep and would lie awake, marveling at his Adam's apple and long fingers—miniature bodies themselves, perfect and sleek like him. In the morning after he left, I would find his hairs—tiny black O's left on the white sheets—and quickly brush them to the floor.

My admiration for Lawrence was more than envy. In that self-absorbed world of adolescence, controlling the body became an all-consuming attempt to manage a confusing and chaotic world. Both at home and on the TV every night the world was falling apart: Vietnam, the Nixon administration, the riots in Detroit, the firebombs and fights at school. My parents too were at war, it seemed, over my father's off-again on-again drinking. As a former athlete, my father could still hit thirty-foot set shots from the end of the driveway and belt baseballs over our house. I idolized his athleticism and strength and the way every male teenager in town respected him. During games, I watched him cajole and console his players, the heroes of our hometown. But as is so often the case with men who are successful and well-liked in the eyes of those with whom they work and socialize, at home, my father seemed uneasy and uncomfortable in his paternal role. He'd never had a father himself, which he would tell my sisters and me sometimes when he was drunk. Underneath the bravado and good times, my father was sad, like my mother, who'd grown up with an Irish man's man, a copy of my father, a sportsman, who fished and played pool, and owned a tavern in the next town over.

As a coach's son, I learned early on that acceptance and masculinity depended on the successful performance of my body in competitive sports. I wanted nothing more than to become the champion in all sports, but particularly basketball. For hours I shot foul shots in the rain or during the coldest days of winter, until my mother, worried I would get sick, begged me to come inside. But I clung to the pursuit of perfection to prove to myself that even though I had broken the male taboo of taboos, on the court I could compete with anyone and often beat them.

Thirty-eighth Street Park was two blocks from my house, and it was here that the best basketball was played in town. It was known as the "black court," and few white kids or men felt comfortable playing there. In summers, my father used to sit in our car across the street from the park and watch games, checking on his players and future talent. When I became old enough, he told me that if I really wanted to learn how to play, I should "get down there and watch how the black guys played," and if I was lucky maybe they'd let me play. So I watched and waited for my chance, sitting beside the court, retrieving errant balls and going for Cokes at the drugstore if asked. Saturdays and Sundays black men came from all over town and the nearby cities of Muncie and Kokomo, driving up in their fat Buicks and purple Lincoln Continentals blaring the Motown sound from their 8-tracks. The first game I played with older men was when Lawrence sprained his ankle and hobbled off, and, eager to keep the game going, they accepted his plea to let me take his place.

During those summers of the early seventies, I lived at Thirty-eighth Street Park. It was like I'd traveled to another country, a place that had different rules, where people wore different clothes and listened to different music. Here another language was spoken, one not bound by words but extending into symbolic movements of the body. Stepping on court was not done with haste or without style; men used special slaps and handshakes or nodded upward with their chins. The bar was set high for flare, drama, and attention to detail. Players dribbled the ball through their legs and yours and pulled up for a jump shot and "pissed in your eye," scooting backwards down court with that smile that demanded that you match the skill and aesthetic of their game. This was not the white game of passing and working the ball to the open man underneath; this was a faster, meaner, more expressionistic game, where rules were broken and new ones created. This was a game of honor, where anyone could rise to momentary glory with a coast-to-coast weave, gliding up and over a sprawling opponent to the rusting rim. The point was to transcend the gravity-bound world that existed off court. In full display of the street, basketball became a theater where I learned to perform.

I studied the game of the older guys: watched how they flicked their wrists at the top of a shot; listened for phrases they used to play with your head; copied the way they tore their sleeveless sweatshirts. I yearned for their age and strength, their oiled revolver-colored backs, their long-legged speed. Off court, too, I tried to model myself on their style, mimicking their dress and slang, practicing their pimp walk swagger in the mirror before school. But more than their strength and style, I was drawn to what seemed down deep to animate them—their rage. I wanted whatever it was that made them mock the police and the ways of the white world. When these guys fought over some foul or some disrespect to their character, it was as if they'd awakened in me a terrifying energy and knowledge. I'd been brought up never to fight; no matter what, I was told to walk away. When anger was leveled at me, for blocking out too well or for shoving them as hard as they did me, guys would trip me to the asphalt, screaming epithets that always ended in "you mother-fucking white punk." But I never said a thing or lifted a finger. I was too terrified. And then once, a teammate got so angry at me for not saying anything after a guy cussed me out for blocking his shot, that he passed the ball so hard at me that he broke my middle finger. That night I wore my bloodied t-shirt and deformed finger like a badge, proudly telling my father and our doctor where it had happened.

As a white teenage boy, with the deck stacked in my favor, I had no conception of the psychological roots of their rage toward me or the world I represented. But as a young man aware that my sexual desire secretly segregated me from the male-dominated mass, I studied how they used this rage to infuse their spirit and protect themselves against the fears of white America, which refused to accept that its identity, as James Baldwin once said, was forever linked to those who came in chains from the African coast.

❊

I lived between the straight and gay world for some time, escaping and returning, returning and escaping, until that spring day of 1996, at the age of thirty-eight I found myself with a baseball cap over my eyes in a public health clinic on Chicago's near South Side. Surrounded by young black and Latino men, I sat in a plastic chair, waiting for results from a test that nobody wants to take.

"You didn't expect this did you?" the Latina social worker asked frowning, exhausted already at 10 a.m. with who knows how many more "death slips" she had to hand out before she got to go home.

I don't remember what I said. I remember only staring at my name on that piece of paper, studying it like a traitor, entertaining the thought that perhaps after all these years it wasn't really mine.

I got into my car and drove around for a while, not sure where to go, landing at a sporting goods store, where I sat in a parking garage and stared at trash twirling in the wind. Keep moving, keep moving, I heard some voice inside urge. I walked in to the store and sat on a bench between two stacks of tennis shoes, sinking deeper and deeper into the reality of what that piece of paper meant.

I looked at the shoes and the bright athletic pants, the baseball mitts and caps, the tents and sleeping bags and the life-sized, cardboard Michael Jordan palming a ball. Buying shoes always reminded me of my mother taking my sisters and me to the shoe store every August before the start of the school year. The boxes and the tissue, the rubber, and the newness all smelled of the year ahead, gym class, recess, the sixth grade team. An employee in a referee's shirt came to my rescue, the first voice to speak to me in my new life: "Sir, can I help you?"

This teenager's face, full of wanting to do right, full of all the life that would bloom before her in the decades ahead, looked at me as if she were peering down into a well. I had to hold my arms down on the bench to keep myself from reaching out and grabbing her legs. I looked up, and forced a smile. "No, not now, thanks."

❊

But I didn't have time to freak out. That afternoon, I began rehearsal for a monologue, a one-person play, to go up in a month. I'd been acting off and on in small productions and doing short dramatic readings at open mics around town more and more. For years I'd wanted to perform my own work, and now I had my chance to make fun of myself and the Peace Corps with a little theater group in Wicker Park.

Denial and anger carried me until the first week of performances. The first night I struggled, skipping large passages from my script. But the play was the least of my problems. I had to start telling friends and family not only that I had been diagnosed with AIDS, but also that for twenty-five years I had not been honest about my sexual life. Worse, I had to tell women I had dated and those men for whom I actually had a name and telephone number. My immune system was a tenth of what it once had been and was fading fast. I woke many nights freezing from sheets drenched in sweat. The doctors promised new treatment, but in the waiting room there were no promises in the eyes of the thirty-year-old bodies leaning on canes and coughing under coats that had become suddenly too big for them.

In the middle of my third performance, I opened my mouth and nothing came out. Not a stuttering paraphrase, not a sound: silence. These were lines I had painstakingly written and rewritten. These were lines that described my own life, lines that drew upon memories and stories of Senegal I'd retold scores of times to friends. But I couldn't retrieve them. It was as if I'd come to the end of speech. I looked into the stage lights begging to be blinded. Standing there in the silence, I felt a kind of perverse pleasure in fucking up. If I never uttered another word again, so be it. My time was up, I thought, what difference did it make now.

But my old friend Paul, who was the first person I told of my diagnosis, jumped out of the lighting booth and up on stage to hand me my dog-eared script. "Just read it, Mike. It'll be alright."

I tried, but I was so humiliated I could barely move my lips. When people, trying to encourage me, chuckled at my comic lines, I became enraged. All I could think about was the window back stage that dropped twenty feet to the street. I could be out to my car in a few minutes, I thought. From there it would take only a couple of hours to get to Michigan. I'd had it all worked out before I'd gotten my diagnosis. I would drive there and buy a gun, rent a boat, and take it out into the middle of a lake. I'd even looked at a map and picked a few lakes. I would wait till dark. Drink myself into proper numbness. Sit on the bow and hope the blast would carry my body overboard.

I made it through that theatrical nightmare but didn't know how I'd ever finish the run. I couldn't call it off. People were coming from out of town, including my parents and sisters. Critics were scheduled. My director had spent weeks on the performance along with her fledgling theater company's money.

The first night of the next week's run, I got to the theater early and lay on the floor trying to calm down, but I kept thinking about where in the show I'd blank out. I'd hidden a bottle of Jameson's back stage and sat down on a folding chair to wait out the inevitable, pouring shots into lemon tea. The voices of the audience as they filed to their seats made me shrink. It was a small theater, but they were expecting a full house.

I closed my eyes. The music began, and as it did I felt the cold hand of panic reach under my ribs and squeeze my lungs of breath. I took another quick swig and grabbed a hold of my chair. My director had chosen Senegalese music for the show: Youssou N'dour, Baaba Maal, Cheikh Lo. I reached down for my script one more time, wanting to know it was there so I could get it myself this time. There was nothing I could do now. So I began to meditate. Within seconds the sound of my breath gave way to the voice of Youssou N'dour, a voice I'd first listened to on homemade tapes anyone could buy for fifty cents in Dakar. I'd listened to his music hundreds of times, but I realized I'd never really heard the emotion, the sadness, the longing in his voice. As I listened to him, I began to feel as if his voice were vibrating inside me. Then out of the voices and the drums and electric guitars came the faces of the people from my village: the children, the Chief's sons, El Hadj—the village Chief, his wives—Amina Ba, Ome Lo, Isitu Cissay, old Loum, the prayer caller, and Babacar Jeng, the healer. Face after face, they all came before my eyes. When I could no longer think of anyone else in the village, I began to conjure up the faces of my friends and sisters, Elizabeth, my old girlfriends and lovers, my mother and father, and my dead grandparents. Then the music stopped, the lights went out, and I walked out on stage.

The run ended without any further incident. Afterward, my doctor and therapist suggested I attend a support group. So every Wednesday night, I sat in a church basement on old couches and listened to rambling rages about failing bodies, ineffective drugs and T cells. Arms crossed, I rarely spoke. Then one night, I looked around and saw an empty seat where a funny but very sick man used to sit. After that night I never went back.

As people I knew became infected, as the virus rampaged through the gay communities of America, the Caribbean, and the mining camps and villages of southern Africa, I struggled to keep AIDS and anything to do with it out of my mind. The ribbons, the walks, the quilts, the bike rides, the growing media fascination. I did what I always did when the word appeared in front of me: I turned the other way.

❁

My introduction to yoga had come in high school when I followed my girlfriend to a meeting on Transcendental Meditation. A week later with a couple of oranges, some grocery store carnations, and thirty-five dollars from my mother's purse, I had my own mantra. Ten years later, in the pursuit of mental stability, I found myself on the fringes of the University of Chicago campus purifying my soul with tantric poses. Yoga kept me inside my body, diminished my spells of depression, and curbed my addictions. Over the next ten years, I dabbled and experimented with one form of Eastern spiritual discipline after the other, coming back to yoga again and again for its pragmatic body-centered practice. After my diagnosis with HIV, I devoted more of my time to its study and practice. I went to classes two or three times a week; I went to retreats and workshops; I read the sutras of Patanjali, mouthed the verses of the Gita, and studied the commentaries of Iyengar, Feuerstein, and Eliade. Though I respected its ancient mystical traditions, I was never under the illusion that doing headstands and backbends had much more than a psychological effect on me. I had seen the numbers before and after the first few months on the antiretroviral cocktail, and I became a believer in the periodic table and the alchemic magic of the pharmaceutical industry.

I began to hang around these so-called yogis: people who'd given up jobs, divorced spouses, gone on pilgrimages to India and Nepal. It felt good to be around men and women who were unapologetic about their fascination with how their own smooth, sinewy bodies functioned. Even though, at times, they seemed ridiculous in their zeal and devotion to Indian gods and gurus and disinterested in the political world, I wanted what they had: a belief in the promises of the ancient Hindu sage Patanjali: "Whether old or young, man or woman, sick or healthy, all who practice can find freedom." When several of the yogis decided to make a trip to India to study under the guru of Astanga yoga, Sri K. Pattabhi Jois, I decided I had to go with them.

I'd heard the horror stories of travel in India: the bouts of dysentery, the days bedridden with typhus, the chills and fevers of malaria. But I persisted with my plans, ignoring all those who doubted my sanity. When I called my parents to tell them about India, I could hear my father sigh, and then after a long silence my mother's voice trickled out: "Honey, you do what you want; we gave up on telling you what to do a long time ago."

Hoping my yoga teacher would be supportive, I finally revealed my status and asked if that might be a problem. His eyes registered what I did not want to see: "Do you know what an Indian hospital is like? I've been sick over there, it's a nightmare."

But I was used to nightmares. Those nights before making my decision to go, I would lie in bed imagining Indian hospitals full of brown faces too afraid to touch me, or see my friends wheeling me through an airport with an IV bag dangling over my head. As I lay there in the dark, I thought about what it would be like if I didn't go. Was this going to be my future? A stripping away, one by one, of possibility and adventure? Where would be the next place I couldn't go? What would be the next thing that I couldn't do? Just the thought of traveling had given me hope. In my mind I heard the well-meaning words of my sisters and friends: "You know you can always stay with us if you get sick." "Don't worry, we can fix the basement up." Those nights alone in my room, the walls and the ceiling seemed to be closing around me, inch by inch, stealing my breath, boxing me in and away from the world.

The next day I drove to Devon Avenue, counted my money three times in the car, and hurried into the Indian travel agency to buy my ticket.

When I finally informed my doctor, he wheeled around in his chair and exclaimed, "India? Are you kidding?" When he heard yoga, he shrugged his shoulders. "Well, all I have to say is, you better have an open ticket back."

✤

Six weeks later, I was sitting on the cement floor of Mumbai's airport, frantically counting through bags of pills, making sure I'd packed enough to last six weeks. In total: 624 pills with three extra days of doses.

After another flight and a train ride from Bangalore, I got to Mysore, found a hotel, dropped my pack on my bed, walked to the window and looked down to see a corpse, covered in marigolds, being carried on the shoulders of bare-chested men through the narrow street. An ominous beginning, I thought, until I walked out into the evening air and felt the city and its swarm of children and shoppers absorb me into the kaleidoscopic dream that is India at night.

Early each morning, I rode on my rusty old bicycle through the empty streets to the yoga *shala*, passing women scrubbing the stone thresholds of their whitewashed homes and decorating them by sprinkling colored powder into the shapes of lotus flowers. Because I was not an advanced practitioner, Jois made me wait until his accomplished devotees had completed their practices. By then, the great guru was too tired to bother much with my tight hips and hamstrings, and left me to his grandson. But it didn't matter, the space itself had a power to untangle the body and mind. I would lie alone on the floor in the corpse pose listening to the jasmine vendors and the milkman calling until the housemaid came to sweep away our Western dirt. As the days passed, I began to realize that it wasn't the yoga that mattered. It was the faith in myself that allowed my body to open and stand as if I belonged again in this world.

On our first day off, I went with a couple of friends to take in the famous Hoysala temples near Mysore. I returned to my hotel exhausted and dizzy from the thousands of stone gods and maidens still dancing in my head. Hours later, I lay naked on the cement floor before the toilet, staring at a spider spinning a web in the corner. On a nearby rooftop I heard horns and chanting voices from a wedding party. Drink water, drink water, I kept telling myself. You must drink water. Somehow I pulled myself up and held onto the walls until I collapsed into my bed. I slept through practice and didn't wake up until I heard knocking on my door. It was the six-foot-two, red-haired, twenty-one-year-old Irish woman I'd met the week before on a rooftop, chanting devotional songs to Shiva. She opened the door, clapped her hands, and broke into laughter. I looked down at the sheet wrapped haphazardly around me and could see the stains of shit from the night before.

"Yoga fever!" she announced, as if offering both a prognosis and cure.

I took a shower and dressed, she waited in the hall.

She had warned me that I would get sick when we spent the day together a few days before, giving each other medicinal mud baths and making love: "Everybody gets yoga fever, the body must purge itself. Some recover and some go home." She shrugged when I told her of my HIV status, and scolded me for taking myself so seriously. "You Americans, you're always worried about something."

She ordered me to follow her to the market to buy flowers and fruit in celebration of my recovery and purification. Once there, she told me to meet her back at the hotel. Then she disappeared into the crowds along the street.

So I wandered through the market. I passed mounds of red roses. I watched men sewing marigolds into marriage wreaths. A man wanted to sell me hash. A silent little girl took my hand and led me to her grandfather's shop of scented oils. As I wandered among the narrow passages, sensual echoes of Senegal came back to me: in the smell of tomato paste, in the sounds of the muezzin calling the faithful to prayer, in the heat pressing against my skin.

I walked on, eating cashews and oranges, filling up sacks with flowers and fruit, trying to find my way out of the market, when I felt something grab onto to my leg. Looking down, a leper without hands held my shin with his stumps. Revolted, I yanked my leg away. But he refused to let go, clenching his teeth, pleading with his eyes for rupees. Searching my pockets, I only found large rupee notes, so I dropped some worthless half pence coins in his lap. As I wrestled free, he spat on my leg and cursed me, his stumps waving wildly in anger over his head.

I

Johannesburg, South Africa (July, 2000)

I arrive in rain. A chill pervades the airport. Immediately a swarm of outstretched, black hands pull, grab, plead with me for work. "Sir, sir! . . . Sir! This way. Just follow me, sir!" Exhausted and numb from a fourteen-hour flight, my mind is blank. After a decade of not smoking, I crave a cigarette, if for no reason other than to look like I know what I'm doing.

Nothing reveals fear like indecision.

Free from the pack of taxi drivers and their gofers, I dive into a guarded telecommunications office, take a seat before a phone, and open my notebook. I lift the receiver, but do not dial, staring at black men harassing businessmen from my New York flight.

I pick the man in the plaid sports coat: tall, lean, businesslike, handsome, or rather, he picks me, catching my eye and boldly walking by the armed guard to my desk behind the glass. I hang up on my imaginary caller, the plaid man takes my cart, and I follow him and my luggage to his car.

Like him, his taxi is worn but carefully cleaned and presented. We speed through the morning drizzle and drab industrial landscape outside of Johannesburg. This highway looks like it could be any highway outside of any large American city, until I see spirals of smoke coming from rows of small boxlike houses in the reddish brown hills in the distance. The townships.

The driver talks without prodding: petrol prices are up, business is down, he's broke, taxi wars and car-jackings make his work more dangerous. He fidgets, drives too fast, and keeps glancing over at me, making me think that I've made him nervous by not sitting in the back seat. Then out of nowhere, he launches into a monologue about fighting for the ANC rebels in Mozambique before Mandela's release.

"I come this close to death—dysentery." He pinches index finger and thumb and sticks it into my face. "This close."

He talks so fast that it's difficult to follow. "I was a soldier fighting for freedom and when I come back I got nothing. I lay in bed in a little dark room in back of my parents' house, wondering if I gonna live or die . . ."

I feel my lungs trying to breathe for both of us. His jaw juts out of his finely featured face, his knuckles turn pink as they grip the steering wheel. We finally come to a stoplight.

If this is his standard tale for the guilt-ridden white American, it's

19

working. He sighs, anxious, then takes off again nearly clipping a pedestrian. We pass clusters of weary-looking middle aged black workers in heavy, dull colored sweaters and coats waiting in the rain for buses to take them to work.

"Why have you come to my country?"

I know I don't have to tell him the truth. But what's the point in lying to people you will never see again? It's like knowingly going in the wrong direction. I recall the decision I made on the plane only hours before: *Someone asks? Come out with it. Make it easy.*

"I am here to attend the AIDS conference. You know, HIV?" He nods. "Well, . . . I have it. I'm positive."

"You?"

"Me." I point my thumb at my chest. "See the box in the back seat. Those are yoga mats. I'm going to teach yoga at the conference. In Durban."

"Are you married?"

"No."

"You are a teacher?"

"Well, I'm a journalist."

"Journalist?"

"Well, not really. I'm a teacher—English teacher at a college in Chicago."

"Chicago?" He gives me a sidelong glance, returns to driving, then asks: "Yoga, that's, like, for the body?"

"Right, you know, exercises, meditation." I explain, my hands miming karate chops. He is pensive. We weave through the elite suburb of Sandton, passing gated homes, offices with guard houses, dogs behind chain fences, windowless brick banks and businesses which look more like prisons.

"I've seen them," he says. "They're everywhere—the thin ones. Then one day you don't see them anymore." His voice changes, sounding less sure of itself. He tells me of a friend, a fellow taxi driver, who is sick.

"How does he know? Has he been tested?" I ask, trying out my new journalist's voice.

He smiles bitterly. "He knows he's just going to die." He shrugs. "People don't talk about it. Some woman give it to him. He doesn't care. He drinks and has sex just as before. He says if he has to die, so will others. But you?" He turns and pats me on my knee. "You look healthy. You got muscles."

I'm flattered but wonder why he has just touched my knee. He mentions a German journalist he took into Soweto a few weeks ago. "I can take you, I am a guide. If you want to go—go anywhere." He pats me on my leg again, laughing but not really laughing, as he describes the sexual overtures made by the German. "Can you believe it?" He asks, turning toward me with this forced grin on his face.

I feign nonchalance as the Hilton appears ahead. He pulls out a card and writes his name and number with a script thinner than an ant's leg. I take it. Just in case.

❄

A doorman in a maroon uniform with gold tassels and cap escorts me up to my room. His face is vacant. Scars mark his cheeks, sanctifying his manhood and tribal affinity. I wonder what he's thinking as he stands lifeless with my luggage. I tip him, and he bows and artificially smiles, reminding me of older black men of my Midwestern youth, who made livings as janitors, filling station attendants, and shoe shine men.

In my room, I rip off my clothes, take a shower, stare at my body in the mirror, open the liquor cabinet, and imagine two glasses filled with whiskey and ice: one for me and one for that taxi driver.

But the bruised, brown box by my bed reminds me that I'm here because I convinced a group of AIDS experts in Switzerland that I have transformed myself—body and soul—by doing headstands and sitting cross-legged with my eyes closed. They have invested in me as at least a role model. So I open the box of fifty used, purple yoga mats, pull one out, and unroll it on the carpet.

I do a sun salutation before the mirror, paying homage to myself for having made it back to Africa. After fifteen hours in a plane, my body works like an unoiled machine of cogs and cranks. As I raise my arms up over my head, they feel as if they might come out of their sockets. Bending over, my legs look like large ugly boots of dead skin. Coming up, I see myself in the mirror. My belly sags, torquing my pelvis; my shoulders droop, caving in my chest: gravity and age are taking their toll on my spine. My hips are like blocks of ice, my back like a winter branch. Cold sweat drips down my spine. Bored already, I go to the window and open the curtains to Africa from the fourth floor of a Hilton hotel in the posh suburb of Sandton. Tall cranes pierce the dusty gray sky. Workmen eat lunch sitting on two beams of steel. Below, women hawk food and sell fruit and cigarettes from off trays. Sleek new cars whiz about while black workers wheel barrels full of earth.

Looking at this new South Africa, I see another Africa in my mind: an older Africa, the one I left in 1983. My body remembers the heat of that last night in Dakar. The Wolof prostitutes in the hall. The single bulb dangling above our bed. The blue lights of the airport. The spongy tarmac. The darkness beyond the runway. Elizabeth's sad face and sick body sticking to her dress.

I'm hungry, so I head down to the dining room. The room is huge, chandeliers, wood paneling, displays of enough food for a banquet, fish the size of children, hams and sides of beef awaiting the long knives of the chefs. I'm alone except for a table of two men. Six people serve me: one takes my order; one brings water and bread; one brings wine; one serves the food; one takes it away; and one more hovers to make sure everyone is doing the right thing. My Midwestern upbringing demands that I not allow all that food to go to waste, and so I stuff pie and potatoes into my mouth as if I'm eating for an entire nation.

After sleeping for several hours, I've no idea what time or even what day it is. All I know is that I can't stay in this hotel any longer.

❁

I change hotels to one in downtown Johannesburg. There, at the Independence, a hotel from another era, I am the lone occupant on the twenty-second floor. My window opens out to this city of 2 million residents. In the distance, a brownish cloud hangs over a vast expanse of the other Johannesburg, named for nothing more than its location in relation to the city, Southwest Township, So-we-to. Nobody has any idea how many people live there. Perhaps 2 million, maybe 3 million. Collectively, the two cities and the surrounding townships have become a magnet for both legal and illegal immigration of peoples from all across Africa, making it the fastest growing city south of Lagos and an epicenter of the HIV/AIDS epidemic.[1]

Witwaterstrand University is only blocks away, so, fearful of venturing out, I spend all afternoon in the basement of the library, reading through boxes of South Africa's repressed sexual history. Old photos show dashing men in tails and top hats posing with other men, and beautiful women in evening dresses and boas in the famous Cape Town mixed-race neighborhood known as District Six. The same community that the apartheid regime bulldozed in the sixties, relocating nearly fifty thousand people to townships outside the city, virtually overnight.

Back on the streets, people hurry down the sidewalks, particularly whites. Doors slam, gates lock, grating rolls down over shop windows. The streets empty. A squat black woman sings as she shuffles along with her heavy bag, belting out a song as if she were in a church choir, and even though it's melodic, there's an eerie edge to it that makes me move quickly around her.

There's no heat in the room so I shower to get warm. When there is a knock at the door, I ignore it. But to my surprise, I hear a woman's voice: "Hello? Hello?" Annoyed, I fumble out of the shower and see a young, shapely black housekeeper with an arm full of towels in the middle of my room.

"Towels?" She asks, seemingly unfazed by my nakedness. "Where should I put them?"

"Don't you know to knock? Put them . . . put them anywhere." Embarrassed, I grab a towel from the bathroom to cover myself. She puts the towels down on my bed but doesn't leave the room. There's an awkward pause and then I realize I must ask her to leave. "Thank you, thank you, that's all." She smiles dutifully and leaves. I look at the stack of towels in the bathroom and wonder: What was she doing? I have towels.

❊

A friend of a friend puts me in contact with a lecturer in English and Media Studies at a local city university. His name is Buzo Mngadi. We arrange to meet for dinner and perhaps, if he wants, to listen to some music. Mngadi is from outside of Durban and working in his first year at his teaching post. As soon as we leave the hotel, he apologizes for everything—his car, the tape deck, the streets, the weather, Johannesburg.

At dinner, we chat about books and teaching and let the food and wine soak in. I like the guy; he laughs at almost everything I say. Reluctantly, I turn to the subject he knows that I'm here to discuss. Being the good academic, he gives a thoughtful sociological analysis, answering my queries kindly but with a noted weariness and discomfort at having to speak to a stranger about sexuality. Though he shows nothing but respect, he hints at resentment toward Western journalists, who sashay in and out of Africa and in weeks become experts on complex cultures and their social and political issues.

"AIDS is a sensitive subject," he tells me more than once. "Sexuality and morality are not easily understood." He reminds me of the role geography has played in shaping South Africa's history, and how the government had used its isolation to keep whites and blacks removed from the influences of not only the West but also the rest of Africa. "We are an exhausted people," Mngadi continues, loosening up from the wine. "We just went through our Truth and Reconciliation trials with testimony broadcast day after day on television and radio. A remarkable achievement for us. But AIDS? People don't want to talk about it. The government pretends to be concerned, but they don't know what to do."

Only six years had passed since Mandela's election and the sweeping changes that followed. What could I possibly understand about him or his country, except to see the heaviness in his body, the jittery way he took each bite of food, overly-anxious that I might not be enjoying myself or the food. What good would it serve to keep pressing him? I'd been waiting for the right moment to reveal my seropositive status. But looking at him, a man who admitted to me that he was too overworked and afraid to ever go out, I think, why burden him. The guy needs to get out and have a good time. And so do I.

After dinner, we amble across the street to the nightclub. We pass a cluster of street urchins in a parking lot, young black boys hovering by a fire of two-by-fours in a rusted out barrel. Behind their fire, cavernous brick warehouses parallel empty streets, billboards hawk luxuries and the fantasies that go with them. A black steel bridge arches upwards into the night. Kippies is a jazz club, named for South Africa's famed saxophonist, Kippy Morolong Moeketsi. The club recently reopened in Johannesburg as part of an arts complex trying to attract people back into the downtown area.

A saxophonist by the name of Khayam is playing; Mngadi tells me Khayam was once a part of Hugh Masekela's band. The clientele is primarily black. It reminds me of a blues club on the South Side of Chicago, which used to let in a few of us white souls from the divinity school. I flirt with the cigarette woman passing out Marlboros, making her light a cigarette I don't want but will smoke to keep her near us. She smiles with her sculpted shoulders and swaying hips, her long fingers flicking on her lighter, brightening my face with the flame. Buzo is enjoying himself, listening, as I am, to the dreamy reverberations of the sax, rooted in Khayam's legs, making our own bodies vibrate along with his.

Cape Town, South Africa (June, 2000)

I drop my naïve ambitions of finding my way about Johannesburg and Soweto and head to Cape Town. At the airport I pick up a newspaper and scan the headlines. Clinton and Blair, in a transatlantic joint press conference, applaud the completion of the DNA molecule map as the "greatest invention since the wheel." Locally, an oil spill has stranded hundreds of migrating penguins off shore and people are flying in from around the world to help in their recovery. Even the South African military is lending a hand, flying the birds up the coast where they were headed to nest. Then, in the far left corner a headline catches my eye: *UN Predicts 50 Percent of Male Teens Will Die of AIDS Before Age 30.*[2]

I check into my hotel and head across the street to a health club, barely noticing the magnificence of the mountains that tower over this coastal city. Craving adrenaline and the need for control, I swim, lift weights, and do a short yoga practice. Satiated, I take a long shower, noticing the array of mixed-race men who seem more comfortable in their bodies than the whites and the few blacks around. I see shades and facial types of all kinds, mixtures of Malay, European, Black African, Indian. *This is the future,* their bodies say as they walk through the dressing room with their dark hair and refined lips, their warm skin, glistening and moist.

❋

Restless and pumped, I search for Cape Town's famous nightlife. At a dance club, I'm invited home by a white tennis pro, a Malayan tailor, and a black teenager who wants to take me first to see the drag divas at another club. I'm exotic, I'm an American, I'm a new body in a tight-fitting blue t-shirt. No one has anything to say when I decline their offers and explain over the dance music why I've come to South Africa. Nobody wants to talk about the subject I want to talk about.[3] The tailor leans in close as if to kiss me, but asks instead, "Are you working for the police?"

I am deciding to head back to the hotel before the very handsome but very drunk tennis pro shoves another beer at me when I catch the eye of a man on the other side of the bar. He is thin, handsomely dressed in expensive, tight-fitting clothes, with a glistening, bald black head and unusually bright eyes. But something else attracts us and moves me past the tennis pro, who grabs at my arm as I cross the crowded dance floor. That something isn't necessarily sexual; it is some innate understanding of each other's bodies. Within minutes we've revealed the code visible only to others who share it. His name is Andre.

"I've been dead so many times people have quit coming to the hospital," he jokes. When I introduce myself and explain why I'm here, he assures me he can help. "I know everybody here." And when I tick off some of the names on my list of contacts, he knows almost all of them personally.

Andre grew up on the Cape Flats, the segregated city of mixed-race and black South Africans, a city built in the lowlands outside Cape Town near the sea. He, too, is of mixed heritage. Though his father was absent with another family in Germany, he provided support for Andre and his mother, which helped him escape a community that would have been brutal for a boy who fancied other boys. "I was good in school. I knew I had to get out of there. I was ruthless," he chuckles nervously. "They hated me there." He'd gone to university then worked his way up in one of the major department stores. He is now a marketing executive. He supports his mother and helps with his nieces and nephews, even though his brothers and sisters refuse to talk to him because of his lifestyle and his positive status.

Andre gives me sketchy details of his HIV history. He has stopped taking AZT, he tells me cavalierly, because he became too sick taking it. Now he uses an herbal treatment, which he swears is helping him, though he admits with a shrug, "What else can I do?" He is sick of being sick and knows unless he can stomach the side effects of antiretrovirals, he'll not make it. The last time he was in the hospital, he'd fallen into a coma and was surprised (as were his friends) that he came back.

Then Andre puts his hand on my chest; the brightness in his eyes turns off and something else turns on. I get the hint: the interview is over. "Let's go next door, the music's better."

Next door the crowd is youthful, dancing to a mix of European, Latin, and African music—soukous guitars, West African drums, Cuban rhythms—ethereal, earthy and unabashedly sexual. It is impossible to stand idly and talk, so we dance. Andre closes his eyes. I scan the room, envious of youth, realizing we are the oldest on the floor. I can't tell who is who or where I am or who is straight and who is not. Next to me, two women dance around each other, hips in sync, dark hair, their dark eyes smiling at each other, one Indian, one mixed-race. They seem to be in a world where bodies exist not to be questioned but to be expressed. My body finds those rhythms inside rhythms that take us into the beat of ritual time. But as these women dance and weave, their hips touching mine, I feel an aching sadness.

Others dance around us, drinking, laughing and talking, drunk on life. But I can't help thinking about the world that lies ahead of them in a country where it is expected that AIDS will not level off for another decade. How many in this room will make it? How many funerals will they attend? How many children will be born infected? But these young people are hardly the most at risk; they can afford to be in a nightclub in Cape Town. The vast majority of South Africa's youth live in poverty and powerlessness, particularly young black women, who are not only more vulnerable to HIV but increasingly to sexual assault.[4]

I kiss Andre outside in the cold. It's the heat that tastes good, the warmth of surprise and change. As his tongue rolls around mine, the Indian woman and her colored girlfriend dance in my head, reminding me of Sita, my last lover of months before, who for six weeks made me believe that fearlessness was the precursor to love. In every Indian woman, I still see the stabbing intensity of her black eyes, still hear her haunting voice, accusing me of not being able to take care of her: "Look at this hovel you call an apartment. You can't even take care of yourself, how could you ever take care of anyone else?"

I accept Andre as my guide. I'm tired. I'm sad. I'm alone. We speed away through the empty streets of Cape Town in his new BMW. He leads me onto a rooftop next to his apartment and points out the landmarks of Cape Town as though the city is his creation. Table Mountain looms ominous and dark behind us. Among the dark trees, he points out the old Parliament building, the historic first capital of the British Cape Colony. To the right is the Anglican Cathedral, where from his pulpit Archbishop Desmond Tutu called for Mandela's release and an end to apartheid. Beyond that stands the city hall where Mandela spoke to the world after South Africa's first free and democratic election only six years before.

Andre pours some orange juice for me and goes to the bathroom. I undress in his bedroom and wait. His fashionable clothes are strewn on chairs beside his glowing computer, fish tank and plants. Lying on his bed, I fold into a forward bend, more relaxed than I can remember in a long time, my face eventually touching my knees. I begin to wonder why he is taking so long in the bathroom. As I almost always do when I plunge into this other life, I begin to second-guess myself, thinking I should slip out now while I have the chance. The energy from the dancing and the dancers has worn off. Then the light is turned off in the bathroom, and out of the shadows Andre appears. I muzzle a gasp. His body is not only thinner than I'd imagined but covered in whitish scars like a leopard. It is Kaposi's sarcoma, a form of skin cancer associated with AIDS. Apparently, he has covered those on his head and neck with make-up.

I fold back into my forward bend to hide the shock on my face. Andre jumps into bed and covers himself quickly with blankets, shifting attention onto my body with flattery: "Look at you. So supple. Bending over like that." He rubs my back with his hands. "Those muscles in your back. I want to look like this." I flinch, unable to speak, unable to look at him. He turns out the light and explains: "The scars? You're wondering about the scars? They're from being stabbed and beaten."

"Oh?" I say, not sure if he is talking about his lesions or something else.

"I found them in my apartment, in Jo'burg. We lived there, did I tell you? Jahn and I, my lover. I'd just gotten home from Berlin, my last trip before Jahn's death. I caught them, going through our stuff."

"I'm . . . I'm sorry," I say, completely lost, forgetting he's told me, in the whirlwind of the evening's storytelling, about his lover's death from AIDS.

"They stabbed me with a broken bottle, see this right here, on my head and back." I try to find the scars, touching him for the first time on his smooth dark scalp. He points to the top of his head and neck, and then takes my hand so that I can feel them. But I'm fixated on what is so visible, the spots on his face and back, that I can't see the scars that mean so much to him.

"They nearly killed me," he says. I close my eyes to keep from having to look at him. "After that and after Jahn's death, I couldn't stay in that apartment. So I moved here."

His stylish clothes, his boots, his make-up, his silver BMW are all gone. I see now who lives behind the glowing eyes and charming manner. I see a frightened man's body that feels more and more like a boy's. Some other instinct arouses me. I caress his head where he told me that bottle was smashed. I pull him into my body and hold him, kissing the top of his head as his face is buried in my shoulder. Like an animal, I run my tongue to the creamy white splotch on the top of his head, and he moans.

❀

I am late and lost. I am to meet a woman by the name of Villas Tyeku, a community organizer who runs an association for women with HIV out of her home in the sprawling, dusty township of Cape Flats, where I'd driven through with an activists the night before. She told me she'd be at a bar on Long Street in one of the city's more fashionable areas. I can't find her. The bar is shabby and filled with pool tables. I'm angry with myself for being late. I called her five times to arrange the meeting. Someone calls out my name from behind. A black woman wearing a beret sits alone with two satchels at her side. "Are you Michael?"

"Villas?"

"You're late." She is suspicious, cell phone in hand and ready to go. "How did you get my name and number?"

I apologize and try to explain. She frowns, standing. "I've been waiting here almost an hour." Understandably, she sees me as another white journalist on assignment. So as quickly as I can move my mouth, out comes the HIV card and my story.

She sits back down, studying me, finally remembering the name of the man who gave me her name and number. "Oh, Michael Nixon, I know him, okay."

The waitress, whose eyes roll in suspicion that Villas is my pickup, angers Villas so much that we're forced to look elsewhere. "This is your town," I say, "where is a good place?"

She laughs, "I've never been to any of these places."

Across the street, we sit outside at a restaurant. Villas is built low to the ground with a round face and short-cropped Afro. She seems nervous and sad, and in her face I recognize the face of HIV loneliness. Reaching in my bag for my notebook, she stops me, "Are you married? Do you have children?"

I smile, "No wife, no kids."

She shakes her head, smiles, then begins her story without any prompting, her face drawing me in as she speaks. "I'm from Zambia. I'm a foreigner. That's where I met my husband. He came to my country to work. I didn't know he was infected. He didn't tell me because he didn't know. I went to the clinic when I was pregnant with my daughter and found out."

Villas's story is the story of how AIDS has devastated all of southern Africa; it's also the story of capitalism's appetite for migrant workers. Men must leave home for work, traveling far from family and community (in this case the mines of South Africa—gold, diamonds, platinum, and chromium). The labor is hard, tedious, and dangerous. The men spend half their day underground, live in dorms in worker compounds, and have little life outside of the mines. These miners do what all

28

exhausted, lonely men do—drink and have sex. The mining camps attract poor young women from neighboring towns and villages and migrant sex workers (female and male) who visit the camps. In the eighties, when AIDS was largely seen as a disease of gay men in America and Europe, it was spreading ferociously through the mining camps of southern Africa. Today in the gold mines of South Africa alone there are nearly 300,000 workers from across the region. They travel home to rural towns and urban townships and infect wives, girlfriends, sex workers. It's no surprise that the highest rates of infection are precisely in the rural areas where so many of the miners come from: the South African provinces of Gauteng and KwaZulu-Natal, and the neighboring countries of Zimbabwe, Botswana, Mozambique, Lesotho, and Zambia.[5]

As we eat, Villas tells me of her husband and how his family treated her when they found out. "They accused me of giving it to him because, you see, I'm a foreigner. Nobody trusts the foreigner." But Villas is not bitter. She sits up and her eyes show she wants all the world to know the truth about her husband. "My husband was sick, he was dying. I had to help him. I had to keep my family going. He died building our house. It's so big, so nice. It's got two stories with a balcony. He wanted to give us this. That's all he wanted in the end—to build this house for me and my daughter."

She fishes into a large satchel and hands me a grant proposal and a pamphlet with the ubiquitous red ribbon and the name of her organization, Wola Nani ("embrace" in Xhosa), printed on the cover. The grant asks for sewing machines, a computer, and some other materials to bring in money.

"You're a writer. Is it good?" Her face is so open, so hopeful. "You can help us, can't you?"

I bury myself in reading the grant to avoid her question. I want to return to the interview: "Where is this, this place, your organization, Wola Nani?"

"It's at my house in Cape Flats. My daughter and I now live on the second floor. The women come and stay, sometimes they bring their children. Many don't have any place to go. Their families are scared, they don't want them staying with them."

Encouraged by the possibility of my assistance, Villas explains how the monies would be used: "We want to work and make money to support ourselves, to feed our children." From her satchel she pulls out a catalog and some samples of the women's craftwork. Key chains and bracelets made of beadwork, tie-dye dresses and t-shirts, bowls made from intricate weaving of telephone wire, papier mâché toys, and bowls decorated with canned food labels. Villas pushes a key chain and a pen across the table. "Here, you take these."

The food comes, and I reach for my medications but pause and look at Villas. She carefully cuts her food with fork and knife, lifts it to her mouth and swallows. I feel the pills in my pocket—clumps of chemistry—that I have been living on for four years. I try to quietly pull them out of my pocket, but two spill onto the ground, and I pick them up and pop them in my mouth. When I reach for my water, she has stopped eating and folded her hands in her lap.

"You take the medications?"

I nod.

"I used to take some but they made me sick. And they didn't do much good."

She goes back to her food. I go back to mine.

"We got them in a special program at the hospital. You had to come and get them every week. Get on a bus, stay there until they decided to give them out, sometimes half a day, then get on the bus, and go home. I had to miss a half or more day of work. Sometimes I took my daughter. Sometimes someone looked after her. I got sick anyway. I decided they were not worth it. We don't even have much good water to drink out in Cape Flats. All the drugs, what good are they if we don't have the good water and the healthy food? This is what makes me so mad sometimes. I decided to just spend my money for good food for my daughter and me."[6] She goes back to carefully cutting up her food. And then, she looks back up, "But they work, don't they? Look at you, so healthy and strong."

I want to tell her that they made me sick, too. But the fact is without them I'd probably be dead. So what should I tell her? That they were the difference between life and death? That she, her daughter, the women of Wola Nani, and the other 99 percent of those like her in South Africa will all die, while I and others like me from wealthy countries will go on living? But Villas isn't interested in my emotions; she sees something else that has nothing to do with pharmaceutical know-how, she sees how I live in my body: she sees perhaps better than I can why I'm here. So I deliver the message I came to give: "The drugs, yes, they work, but it's yoga that has helped me the most." I lose myself and Villas in my rehearsed words about yoga's benefits, until she brings me back down to earth.

"Well, I want to learn this yoga. Can you come to our center in Cape Flats to teach the women?"

"Well, yes. I could, but I'm going to Durban for the conference, you know, and I'm going to do a workshop."

"I am going to the conference too, so I will come to your workshop. And when the conference is over why don't you come back to Cape Town and give the workshop?"

"Yes, yes, I'd like to do that," I say, nodding emphatically, wanting to believe that in the days ahead I will find the courage to fulfill her request and Andre's, who also asked me to return and offer a workshop.

❋

The convent for the Sisters of Nazareth sits high on the slopes of Table Mountain. Earlier that week, I'd tried to hike, or rather climb, to the top, getting lost, dodging thieves who'd jumped the couple in front of me, and bushwhacking up through vines and brambles until I found myself fingering holds on a ledge in the middle of a trickling creek bed, with arms and legs covered in bleeding scrapes. I admitted defeat when I turned and could see no further than a few yards below as clouds had blown in from the sea and swallowed the mountain.

I check in with two guards positioned in a brick guardhouse. They look at my ID and call to make sure I'm expected. The plant life of the Western Cape is like no place else on earth, and I can't help but stop and admire the vibrant yellow and red roses in a garden along the stone path. I wander up to the roses and smell them, and as I bend over, I see a name on the stone I'm stepping on. Looking around, I see others. Then it comes to me: I'm standing on a graveyard for children. I turn and walk back out of the garden. Just as I reach the gate, the guards who have been watching call from the gatehouse. "Sir! Up ahead! That is where you go!" I walk fast then break into a jog.

At the orphanage, a pleasant, old, white woman answers the bell and leads me to an antique chair in an anteroom. The place reminds me of my grandmother's: antique furniture, jars with striped mints, doilies; everything is drab and outdated, orderly and spotless. I fold my hands and wait in my chair like I am back in grammar school sitting outside the principal's office.

Sister Irene comes bustling in and I stand at attention. In a colorless tweed sweater, a practical, nondescript gray-green dress and black shoes, Sister Irene has that ageless look of Irish nuns: trim, milky complexion, sharp hazel eyes, narrow face. "Now Mr. McColly, tell me then, what can we do for you? You're interested in the orphanage, I take it?"

I hand her my university card. "Chicago. My sister lives in Chicago," she smiles warmly. When I tell her of my project, stressing the importance of trying to write about HIV from the perspective of someone with the virus, the acronym HIV brings the blink, the piercing look, and eventually that knowing nod. "A writer, then?"

She apologizes for her lack of time as I follow her down an echoing hall, passing elderly white nuns with canes and young black nurses and housekeepers; she greets all with equal energy. We stop at the Public Relations office so that I can be added to the long list of journalists who have come to do stories on the convent and South Africa's escalating population of AIDS orphans. The PR women tells me that there are over 500,000 orphans in the country and that figure is expected to rise to over 2 million by the year 2010, accounting for almost 2 percent of the population.[7] The convent has other missions—caring for elderly sisters and working with women's groups, children, and the poor.

Sister Irene then takes me to a site where they are building a wing for the ever-growing numbers of children they receive each month. "Here's the school area and here will be dorms for the children." Walking back to the main building, I can barely keep up with her. "My yoga is hiking up there," she says, pointing to Table Mountain. "I go as often as I can."

"Up to the top?" I ask, not wanting to hear that this older woman hikes up a mountain that nearly killed me.

"Certainly. Have you been?"

"I tried. But I kind of got lost."

"Happens all the time. You have to watch it when the clouds roll in. People have had to spend the night up there."

As we walk down a long hallway, I hear children. Entering a kitchen, I see a low table with abandoned bowls of cereal, half-eaten crusts of bread, little cups for juice. The sounds of the voices are bright, supplanting the image I fear of babies dying in cribs with eyes bulging out of disproportionate heads. Passing a small side room, Sister Irene stops. "Here is a boy who needs to be on a respirator." The boy sits in a miniature bed, hooked up to oxygen, rolling a red race car over his blanket, up the wall, and off into the air. His head lolls, his eyes regard us as if we are creatures from another world. "This little boy's name is Thomas."

"Hi Thomas," I say, hardly able to hear my own voice. He looks up and sticks out his little hand.

Sister Irene brushes back his hair: "The nurse says he is doing much better." I nod, trying to be the writer, noting the details of him and the room, but what I really want is to touch him again, feel his little hand in mine.

The main room is like any kindergarten: numbers and letters painted in bright, happy colors on warm wooden walls; toy boxes overflow with balls and stuffed animals; piles of red cardboard bricks; chairs and tables that come to my knees.

One by one they come out of a far room. A few run, heads bobbing, arms fluttering, legs in tights and dungarees, bending and bouncing, as they spill forth. Girls in groups of twos and threes, absorbed in talking, head toward the play kitchen and stacked boxes. Seeing Sister Irene, many of the boys run toward us, surround me, grab onto my legs and pull on my arms, like I'm a tree that needs to be climbed.

"This is Michael, and he comes from far away, in America," says Sister Irene trying to get their attention. "They just finished their lunch and now will have a resting time." I can see cribs in a far room. She sinks to her knees to talk with one of the boys.

A boy looks up at me with his head so far back I'm afraid he's going to fall over. He says something, but I can't understand his South African brogue. I lean down and he repeats his question, "What's *your* name?"

I kneel and put my hand around his back, placing my big palm on his bony shoulder. I look into his face, and a tremor moves up my spine. I stand, searching for something to steady me, something to do, some question to ask Sister Irene, but she has left me alone with these little boys. They take hold of my hands, playing with them as if they were toys. They call up to me, begging for me to come down and play, wondering what's wrong, wondering how I can be there but at the same time so far away. Fatherless three-year-old boys, their heads back, their mouths agape, hang from my knees. I tighten my jaw, smiling, clinging fiercely to myself.

Sister Irene, on her knees, her arms around two boys, talks with a swarm of other children. Entering the play room, she confessed that she had a room upstairs where she often sleeps at night to be near the children. She signals to me, pointing to two little girls, walking slowly, the last two to emerge from the nap room. One girl leads the other, holding her arm as if they were two old sisters. Step by tiny step, patiently they cross the playroom. "You see, they become like a family. They are always together, these girls. They even sleep together." Sister Irene explains that the little girl being led is blind and has been sick ever since arriving. I can see now too that the blind girl's face and body are deformed, making it difficult for her to walk. The little girls make their way through the chaos of playing children. I ask Sister Irene about how her work began with the orphans. "At first, we took children with incurable diseases. We were already set up for this, you see. Our mission is to care for children with incurable diseases. We began in 1991. Nobody would take them, so we began to take these children. We are just social workers. In most cases the parents have both died. We try to find homes with the relatives. But sometimes they can't always take them." I ask her about the plots out front among the roses. "Yes, we have a little ceremony for each of our children. Thirty nine have died so far, and many of them are buried out there."

Sister Irene needs to be on her way, so I thank her and prepare to leave. Some part of me turns back, half hoping a child will notice and come running to grab my pant leg, but they have returned to their world of play.

II

Durban, South Africa (July, 2000)

A screen four stories tall sits on a stage in the middle of a cricket stadium. On the bright green turf, hundreds of folding chairs face the screen, fanning out in long rows. The moon hangs in a chilly night sky over the city of Durban. Huddling for warmth at the corners of the field, clusters of boys without shirts are dressed as Zulu warriors in imitation leopard skin, drums dangling between their bare legs. People slowly file into the stadium and take their seats. Doctors, businessmen, government officials, and scientists get the best seats on the field near the stage. The rest of the conferees sit in the grandstands. In the far bleachers, without access to the field, hundreds of young people from around the country wave posters and banners from our march earlier that day through the streets of Durban. One poster stands out: it is nothing more than a white sheet with a five-foot-tall, bloody-red handprint with dripping letters that reads: DRUG COMPANIES—BLOODY HANDS.

The march fell short of the tens of thousands I was expecting, but the poor, the sick, and the young aren't easy to mobilize, especially if by showing up they might jeopardize their family's good name. But we looked good on TV. And what a picture we made for half a minute: a multi-racial throng representing nearly a hundred countries, wearing t-shirts that read HIV POSITIVE, shouting slogans, and holding posters and rainbow flags. At the head of the protest, arm in arm, were traditional elders, clerics from South Africa's diverse religious communities, and scores of activists from Africa and around the world, including Zackie Achmat from the Treatment Action Campaign and Winnie Mandela, who elbowed her way up to the front. I was somewhere toward the back tagging along, reluctantly wearing my t-shirt under a jacket.

Before the opening ceremony begins, men hired by the major drug companies toss day-glow necklaces and pens into the stands. I decide if one comes my way, I will throw it back, but when one flies up, the young man next to me eagerly catches the necklace and smiles holding it out for me to see. I have been watching this young man with the shaved head and sprouting goatee out of the corner of my eye, wondering what a young man (he can't be any older than eighteen) is doing by himself here at this event. He seems to be enjoying himself, talking with the three young women behind us and asking them to sign his commemorative t-shirt. Then he turns and asks, "Excuse me sir, would you sign my t-shirt?"

He watches my hand, reading out loud my name as I sign: "Mi-col, Mac-caw-lee, U-S-A."

He passes his t-shirt cheerfully up and down the rows. Then he gets up and walks it down several rows to what looks like a group of traditional elders in magnificent robes of canary, forest green, and striped indigo. I'd seen them make their grand entrance. It was impossible not to notice: women wearing cowrie shells in their long beaded hair to match their brightly colorful gowns and head wraps; men erect as posts sitting like royalty with elaborately carved canes and fedora caps. One man without shoes wears a tunic with a sash made of animal skin, and around his triceps are copper amulets in the shape of snakes swallowing their tails. All the elders sign this young man's t-shirt as if it were a document of the greatest import.

He introduces himself as Miamiza Norman from a small town north of Durban in the state of KwaZulu-Natal. "I'm HIV positive," he says in a voice that startles me in its directness and pride. "I'm here to help my church group learn how to help people so they don't have to live like I do." All in one breath it comes out, as if composed and practiced. "I'm so glad to be here. I feel so good. I'm so proud of my country."

"SHOW THE WORLD! BREAK THE SILENCE!" an enthusiastic voice barks over the sound system. People in the stands pick up signs at their feet, stand and wave them, including Miamiza.

"BREAK THE SILENCE! DURBAN SHOWS THE WORLD!" comes the voice again, stirring up the crowd as if we're here for a soccer match.

We are on the screen, waving our signs, waving to the world, waving back to ourselves in the stands.

In the middle of hubbub, Miamiza turns to me and blurts out, "Michael, my family and a few friends, and my girlfriend are the only ones who know." I nod and consider telling him about myself, but I sense he wants to talk. He tells me he had to drop out of school because the books and fees cost too much for his family. He tried to look for work but hasn't found anything yet, with South Africa's unemployment rate at nearly 40 percent, and the black male youth rate much higher.

Miamiza has no access to medication. But when I ask if he takes any other treatments, he describes a medicinal powder that his mother procures from a traditional healer, which he boils and inhales. "I put a towel over my head and breathe it in like this." He demonstrates, inhaling and lifting up his chest and letting it out. "It makes me feel strong, good." And to prove it, he makes a fist and flexes his biceps.

"BREAK THE SILENCE! HOLD UP YOUR SIGN, PLEASE! SHOW THE WORLD WE'LL BEAT THIS VIRUS!"

Mostly young people stand but also some adults. I look around at those standing, the young women Miamiza was flirting with and wonder, them too? And those behind them? How many of us here?

Hundreds? Thousands?

Miamiza proudly introduces me to the young women behind us, who like him are thrilled to be a part of this historic event. They are from Johannesburg, but why they are here I don't know, because Miamiza stops in the middle of my introduction, realizing that he doesn't know much more about me other than I am from America, and asks, "So, why are you here?" I look at them, youthful, energized by the crowd and each other but refuse to tell them. "I am a journalist."

The choir is now set, the little drummer boys are lined up, the dignitaries are seated, the crowd waits in anticipation. But I, the "journalist," am feeling little of the excitement and consider heading back early to my hotel.

Thabo Mbeki, the president of South Africa, climbs the podium, and his fuzzy gray face fills the big screen behind him. He reminds us of how far South Africa has come in such a short time, how historic the changes have been since Mandela was released from prison. Yet, as he faces his own people, like Miamiza, who can't hope to survive without the government providing HIV medications, he sticks to his claims that AIDS is caused by poverty and not necessarily by the virus HIV. Miamiza is too respectful to show his displeasure, but the AIDS activists and international intelligentsia are infuriated, and many boldly walk out in protest.

The journalist gets out his notebook and begins to scribble.

A film begins with an image of an African boy kicking a ball through the streets of Soweto. A series of talking heads with ties and white coats follows. Now we see the world of AIDS montage: African mothers with their babies, children in an orphanage in Ukraine, Thai woman, Chinese farmers, Indian doctors, and of course the forlorn dying young white man in a hospital. It always comes back to that image of a homosexual in a hospital.

Agitated by this sentimentality, I take out my own camera. And when Miamiza asks to see what the stage looks like through the lens, I hand it over to him: "Take any you want, go anywhere." He looks back at his friends, decides to take their picture, and then heads off into the crowd. I think, as I watch him, that now would be a good time to pop the pills and get something to eat with it. But as I get up, he reappears. When I ask if he wants anything, he says no and insists on going to the concession area for me.

"Sure. Okay," I say, digging in my pocket full of rands, and as I pull them out, out come the pills. I stuff them back quickly before he notices.

While he is gone, I listen to a South African doctor tell us: "Knowledge will bring us a solution." An ice cream man catches my eye and I buy some ice cream to go with my pocketful of solutions.

Miamiza returns with my Coke. Cells are on the screen now. I eat my ice cream and listen to the science talk that's supposed to give us hope for the future. Looking over at Miamiza, I try to think of how to tell him, knowing that if I don't I will feel even worse than I already do. He is so serious as he listens, wanting to get it all right, so that when he returns home he can explain everything to his church group.

"Miamiza. You know something, you know, really, why I'm here?"

"You're a journalist writing about AIDS."

"Yes, I'm a writer but I'm also like you. I'm—I'm HIV positive, too."

He turns to look at me. "You?" He reaches over and grabs my biceps. "But you are a strong man?"

"I exercise. I do this thing called yoga, it's like exercise. I'm going to teach a class at the conference to show people how good it is for us. You should come to it."

Though I don't intend it as a challenge, his body language changes, he looks scared, sits up straight and explains. "I play soccer sometimes. I like to, when I have time. That's good isn't?"

"Yes, that's good."

His face is no longer relaxed, his confidence gone. He seems confused by my sudden intensity. He looks at me and then away, then quickly back again. Selfishly, I think he's going to ask me about medications, or worse, how I contracted it. But I am wrong. "My girlfriend, can she get it? Just kissing, I mean, can she get it? You have a girlfriend?"

"Uh, I did." Searching for what advice to give, my tongue thickens, I hear the voice of Sita seething through the static on her cell phone: "I can't believe how stupid I was to let you jeopardize my life!"

"You have to be honest," I say weakly, trying my best to find my own voice in the clutter of anger and emotion. "Kissing is okay, but be careful," I remind him, offering the party line about sores in the mouth and cuts.

"I want to show you something." I put down my can of Coke, reach into my pocket and pull out my medications. "See these? Do you know what these are?"

He shakes his head and looks up at me, "No?"

"These are the drugs, you know, for HIV?"

"They help you? Don't they?" he says looking younger each time I look at him. He picks one out of my cupped hand, a tablet in the shape of diamond, and holds it up to get a good look, as if it were a precious stone.

He nods, returns it carefully to the palm of my hand, and then turns to the screen without saying a word. I tip back my head and swallow them down, chasing them with a sweet, syrupy gulp. Together we listen to a scientist from the International AIDS Society talk about all the advances since they first convened an AIDS conference.

Finally, Nkosi Johnson, South Africa's AIDS poster child, walks onto the stage and into the beam sent out to the world. Nkosi is a boy of twelve, who has lived with the virus since coming out of the womb of his now dead mother. He became a hero for those with the virus, as he and his adoptive parents demanded that he be able to attend his local school. He is so small he can barely be seen on stage, but his voice sounds like a herd of animals stampeding in the distance, shaking the ground and everyone out of their chairs as they give him a standing ovation.[1]

❀

Outside the conference, Durban goes about its work. Cargo ships that look like incoming cities dominate the harbor, while a few miles up the coast a surfing championship highlights its beach front of hotels and parks. Durban's architecture reflects the layers of its history and its disparate populations, from its 19th century Victorian municipal buildings and churches, to its stolid, muscular, Dutch buildings of commerce and trade, to baroque, Hindu temples, to the informal markets that exist everywhere between. This is the center of Zululand. And it's the Zulu, not the British or Dutch, who first claimed this part of South Africa, pushing out or killing off smaller nomadic peoples who had been living relatively peacefully on the land.

The conference itself is enormous, filling up Durban's new convention hall and spilling out into municipal buildings, hotels, and a nearby university campus. It is clear, upon entering, what this conference is about and who it is designed to attract: doctors, scientists, academics, government functionaries, officials of various international health and development agencies, and, of course, those footing most of the bill—the multinational pharmaceutical industry. Over twelve thousand people are in attendance, making it the largest international conference ever held on the continent of Africa. And Durban is primed to cash in.

I have never been to one of these conferences, nor have I ever bothered to follow what happens at them. I am stunned to see the hundreds of suits and ties walking around with cell phones and papers under their arms. Huge halls are devoted to the business of AIDS with most of the floor space taken up by high-tech, multi-media displays advertising the major players in the business: Roche, Abbott Labs, Pfizer, Bristol Myers Squibb, GlaxoSmithKline.

The first day I attend as many sessions as I can, from the role of the media to strategies for working with MSMs[2] in Latin America, but the majority of the presentations have to do with the hard sciences related to treatment and the development of vaccines. Notebook in hand, I try to follow their Power Point presentations. Their lectures seem smart and measured and understandable up to a point, but when "projectiles attack the protein's outer armor" and "drugs are designed to carry loads to destroy enemy cells," I become lost in a barrage of militaristic metaphor and abstract jargon. The only signal that the lecture is finally over is that the lights are turned on.

Between sessions, I meet a woman at the bar at the Hilton and strike up a conversation. She is a research scientist from North Carolina who has been working in Thailand on vaccines with several other virologists. I ask what brought her here, and she laments, "Not much, unfortunately." What she means, I learn, is that Thailand's infection rate has dropped so quickly that they can't test the vaccine because they don't have a high enough percentage of infected to test it. "We don't know what we're going to do now," she sighs, aware of the irony, but obviously let down.

❊

Eunice Odongo sits next to me drinking tea outside the conference hall. Her skin is gray, her body fragile. She reminds me of a broken dish that has been carefully put back together. She is from Nairobi, where she works as a community organizer for a group of women who are HIV positive. It is called WOFAK, Women Organized to Fight AIDS in Kenya. Her story is one I've now heard several times: once she discovered that she was HIV positive, she was fired from her government job without reason, and then her husband, who'd infected her, left her and her two children.

She's anxious, checking her watch again and again. Looking around, inviting people with her eyes to interrupt us. My first real interview at the conference and it's going nowhere. She lectured the day before on WOFAK's work in Kenya trying to provide traditional medicines to its members: a subject I'd like to write about. But I'm no doubt the tenth writer to approach her today for an interview. She's an AIDS feel-good story that everyone wants to hear: educated African woman, betrayed by her husband and society, who survives nonetheless by working with other women like herself. She responds to my first question by staring right through me; her words are as stiff and lifeless as her body. Her weary, wise eyes belie her age. They silence me and my greedy desire to get her story into my notebook.

She's exhausted and I apologize to her, wondering why I thought I could hunt people down and bother them. I collect my things, and as I prepare to get up, I remind her of the yoga class and that, if she can't come, I'll show her some of the poses sometime that week. She turns to me, "Oh, so you're the one who is the yoga teacher? I saw that someone is doing this. What is it? Do you have anything I can read?"

Even though her face stills me with its ghostly aura, I tell her the phrase I repeat to myself: "Yoga can't cure me, but it helps me learn how to live with this disease." As I say this, I hear how hollow my words sound to a woman whose body has been tortured by this disease. She looks at my body, especially my bare legs, as I've worn shorts to distinguish myself from the suit and tie crowd. "Your eyes are very blue, and as you talk they get bluer."

"Really?" I laugh nervously. "Nobody's ever said that to me." Now it's me who is looking around hoping to find a way out of this conversation.

"How did you contract the virus, Michael?" she asks.

"I don't know exactly. I'm bisexual." Her gaze holds me on that thought. "It was most likely a man." Most likely?

"Yes," she says, nodding in satisfaction, making her seem less ghostly.

We drink our tea in silence. She nods and smiles. "I'd like to learn about this yoga. Maybe you can come and help the women in Nairobi. We do some exercise sometimes. And it always makes us feel so good. I will do more when I am healthier. I am better but I was very sick. I know I don't look as good as I used to. But, once I had sores all over my face," and she slowly reaches up and runs her bony fingers down over the right side of her face. "I hid my face with my hair and with scarves. I had my hair cut to hide my face. I looked down all the time. I was so embarrassed. People knew. I had only my children when my husband left. Without them," she pauses, looking up as if seeing them in her mind. "Without them, I wouldn't have stayed alive. They took care of me. They made me live."

I take out my notebook.

"Then one day I got sick and was taken to the hospital. I was very sick and I didn't know if I would live or not. But every day the women from WOFAK came to see me and pray for me and my children. I told myself that if I got better I'd commit myself to those women, and then, like that, I got better. The women did it. And my children."

"One day last year, I walked on a bus and someone said to me, 'This is you? This is you here in the paper, isn't? You are this woman.' I looked and there I was in the Nairobi newspaper in a story about WOFAK—my picture, my face, not covered with my hair or a scarf. I'd become a celebrity." Her thin face opens into a smile, and so does mine.

"You should come to our seminar on traditional healers tomorrow. We are organizing a demonstration. Talk about yoga, tell people what you are doing. Michael. It's important."

❋

Eighty-five percent of those infected in Africa will use some form of traditional medicines to treat the spiritual and physical suffering which accompanies HIV and AIDS.[3] Yet, if you type the word "traditional medicine" or "healer" on the diskette that holds over five-thousand titles of abstracts sent to the conference for display or discussion in seminars, only five titles show up. So it's no surprise that the seminar on the role of traditional healers is held some distance from the conference center. At the door, I listen for the right moment to slip in, scanning the list of panelists: Eunice Odongo, from Kenya; Dr. Gbodossou of Senegal; Merci Mancy from South Africa; but there's no Indian name to match the voice I hear inside.

Creeping in, I see Dr. Rebello, the ayurvedic doctor from Mumbai, his chair askew on the outside of the speaker's table. It appears he has invited himself onto the panel. He is delivering the same harangue I had to listen to the night before over dinner. I had been curious to meet a doctor who was treating HIV with the tools of ayurvedic medicine: diet, herbal treatments, breathing exercises, and yoga. He is a strong opponent of the antiretroviral drugs, believing them to be poison. "Only the body can heal the body. You must know that being a yogi. These AIDS drugs are not natural; they are killing people. They need immune stimulants, good food, and purification, am I right?" All through dinner, I had listened to him with the drugs in my front pocket, wondering if I should take them, revealing my status and my blasphemy, but I had chickened out.

I head for an empty chair in the back, but before I reach it, Dr. Rebello announces to the room: "Here is Michael. He is the one teaching yoga from Chicago. Ask him about the benefits of yoga." Exposed, I'm not sure what to do. Then he asks: "Why are you late? I told you about this meeting."

Saving me, another panelist jumps up to cut off the feisty doctor: "You are Michael? The yoga teacher? You called me. I'm Merci. I want to talk to you, afterwards, okay?"

Gratefully, I find a chair and agree to talk afterwards.

The room is full of Africans, believers or practitioners of traditional medicine, including the royal elders I saw at the opening ceremony. They are discussing ways to make the conference more responsive to them.

"We need a march with all the healers!" one man calls out.

"We need a press conference," a large man from Cameroon demands.

Dr. Rebello continues to interrupt: "AIDS is world problem, pandemic means world disease. We must have people representing all the different regions where it is a problem. We have Africa, Latin America, Asia, but we need someone from Western world, from America. We have to have someone from America: white person. I will speak, I'm from Asia; and you Doctor Ghodossou are West Africa; and you are from Cuba, you speak for Latin America; and Merci, you speak for South Africa, and we need an American. Michael, you be the one to speak from America, okay?" He turns back to the panel, "He'll speak. He's from Chicago."

I can't believe this guy. "No," I say, standing, waving my hands. "I'm no healer, just teach yoga."

"Yes!" Dr. Rebello insists, pointing his finger at me. "You are healer, Michael."

Disappointed, he shakes his head, and the panel settles on an anthropologist from Switzerland. The meeting breaks up and I want to avoid the Indian doctor, but I must speak with Merci Mancy, who opens her arms and hugs me. "So it's you who has been calling? The yoga man? You will be at the march won't you? Then we can talk more, okay?"

"Yes, of course." I say, seeing Dr. Rebello waiting for me at the door.

"How's your cold? Did you take the pills I gave you?" (He'd insisted on giving me an ayurvedic treatment when he saw me coughing at dinner.)

"Yes, feeling much better, but I have to get going."

"I must tell you that when you are given the power to be a healer, you should never back away from it. I will come to your room tomorrow morning at eight for the march."

❋

The next morning, I'm out before Dr. Rebello comes for me. A mile from my hotel, I hear them before I see them, whistles blowing, drums beating, rattles and shakers keeping the beat, the voices of women chanting and singing, maybe fifty, seventy-five tops, mostly women recruited by Merci Mancy. The women wear scarves and skirts of the same cloth pattern, black with traditional Zulu shields in red and white. Several of the men wear clothes and caps of a green and white tie-dye print. PROMETRA it reads on their caps and on a large banner, which stands for the international organization to promote and protect traditional medicines and practitioners.

They march to the steps of the conference hall. As planned, Dr. Rebello speaks first, rather convincingly to my surprise. Next, Merci Mancy lifts a sprig of leaves over her head calling on the ancestors to protect the "sick and the poor." The traditional women respond to her prayer with an eerie ululating of their voices. She then passes on the branch to Dr. Gbodossou, the stately Senegalese doctor, trained both traditionally and in the West, who needs no microphone. "We know they are using our medicines at night. Please give us a chance to speak and participate in solutions."

The press invades the crowd with cameramen pushing people aside. A rowdy handful from the Paris ACT UP chapter see the crowd and the cameras and chime in with their conference chant condemning the drug companies: "Abbott Kills. Abbott Kills." To my left, CNN's Charlene Hunter-Gault, microphone and notepad in hand, has cornered Merci, who slumps in shyness, yet boldly responds, "Please listen to what they are saying, don't ask me anything."

An elderly man with a cane, wearing a sky blue cape and thick, broken glasses hobbles to a chair and sits while Dr. Gbodossou holds his microphone. The press jams more microphones in his face. In a gravelly voice, he condemns the conference for coming to their land and ignoring their traditions. He reminds them that African healers had been treating their people without Western medicines just fine until they came with their diseases and drugs. The crowd of conferees is suddenly quiet.

After the speeches, I follow the traditional healers back to the university and finally get my chance to talk with Merci. Her work is to go from region to region and give workshops for traditional healers, helping them to recognize and better treat HIV. And if that wasn't enough, she also has the impossible task of setting up councils of traditional doctors in each region to weed out the charlatans who are increasingly undermining the credibility of traditional practices. "Why not come to one of our trainings and meet some of the healers? We are going out in a couple of weeks. You can come, right?"

Merci races ahead and leaves me pondering her invitation.

When we get to the university, instead of heading indoors, the marchers huddle under a few shade trees and sit in the grass. After handing out sandwiches and drinks, Merci leads me by the hand to Credo Mutwa, who sits in a plastic chair next to his wife.[4] I sit cross-legged at his feet, as Merci introduces me, exaggerating my credentials. At the base of his necklace of stones and teeth is a monkey's skull. He leans on an old wooden staff, which is crooked and carved with a bronze eagle's head for a handle. He barely looks at me, staring up into the branches of a tree, his old, thick glasses taped together at one corner, resting low on his large nose.

He needs no prompting. Shaking with emotion, his mouth opens like a lion's, and he asks me questions instead. "Please sir, tell me why. Why are our people being destroyed? Why? Why is this old, man-made disease taking more of our people than slavery and all the wars combined in the past century? Why?"

He looks up into the tree above us and poses another of his koans: "Do you see this tree, sir? It has the power to heal some and to kill others." He pauses to give me time to look at the tree not as a tree but as a source of life and death. "You have to know the person to heal them," he explains. "We need our own medicines and our own food. We have to listen to our grandmothers. It's the only way to stop this monster that behaves like an intelligent creature."

"AIDS has come to destroy Africa," he asserts with cold certainty. "It is a plot to keep Africa down and to destroy our nations." For him, a storyteller of African legends, AIDS is a weapon in a cosmic war of good

and evil, where white men come from across the seas to steal "his people," "take the riches from their land," and "poison its young people
with disease and ideas."

His face squints as if he can see the virus in his mind not as some par-
asite visible only to scientists behind a microscope but as a beast
unleashed upon the world by evil forces. Unable to keep my mouth shut,
I ask if what he means by "old disease" might have something to do with
the theory that the virus came from monkeys in Central Africa. But
quickly and angrily he silences me: "Sir, you've been told a lot of shit!"

"AIDS has come back to haunt the world," he claims, explaining that
it is a curse that comes from the tomb of King Tutankhamen.

When I bring up the fact that many women in South Africa have the
disease because they do not have the power to refuse sex, he fumes:
"You, sir, do not know our women. Crossing a Zulu woman, you can
have a war on your hands." I look at his wife sitting stoically beside him
with hands folded in her lap.

He seems disgusted with me and I can see my time is up.

A healer from Cameroon opens a bottle of Orange Fanta and pours
it out at the base of the small tree, and Credo Mutwa addresses the
group, calling on the ancestors for their protection and guidance.
"Medicine is like a broom cleaning out illness," he tells them in a tone
noticeably different from the one he used with me. "We need nourish-
ment. We need our own food—our own medicine."

Though the traditional healers have been essentially ignored in their
own homeland, what is important to them is not so much how others see
them, but how they honor their traditions and ancestors. They define
themselves outside the frame of a CNN camera and the dispiriting AIDS
statistics that Westerners associate with their countries. They see themselves in ways that few on the outside can understand as we have buried
the notion that our futures depend on how we honor the past.

❇

On my forty-third birthday I climb up the steps of Durban's old City
Hall, my arms full of yoga mats and blankets. They are the same steps
where, only days before, activists and religious leaders raised their fists
and voices in support of the thousands of young people wearing t-shirts
proclaiming their status: HIV POSITIVE.

The first person I meet upon entering is Villas Tyeko and her daughter reading on a bench.

"Villas!" We hug, and they help set up. People file in timidly.
Eventually all thirty mats are taken. I begin as always: with a meditation,
instructing them to close their eyes, relax their faces and listen to the
rhythm of their breath.

Shafts of afternoon sunlight pour through the windows, giving the room a golden glow. I study their faces: their eyes tightly closed, straining, trying to follow the rules. Unlike the workshop I taught the day before, most are African women. While they meditate, slowly and unconsciously, they let go of the muscles in their faces, dropping their jaws, their mouths opening like children. How vulnerable we are without the mask of thought.

I am supposed to be meditating too, but my mind is anything but calm. Worries weave themselves into the sounds of traffic and the street vendors below: What should I do if Dr. Rebello comes to my class? Will people understand what I have to say? Will they notice that I'm coughing and sick? A sick yoga teacher? What message will that send?

I glance around to check on the students and see that the courtroom next to us is named for Nelson Mandela. I can see the bench and a chair where the judge sits. Is it here, I wonder? In this room or somewhere in this building, where, ninety years ago, a young Indian lawyer by the name of Mohandas Gandhi first practiced law, and discovered that the rules—so beautifully written, so rationally argued in the law books in London—didn't apply to his people or to anyone who didn't have white skin?

I walk around the room as they meditate. I adjust chins and lower backs, my fingers inviting them to sit up and feel their spines lifting and rooting them to the Earth. Some jerk their bodies into their idea of a correct posture, others moan—audible only to me inches away. When I touch the backs of their necks and shoulders, some of them cringe and cower. Many of them have a sheath of skin, cold and leathery, in which they shield themselves from the world. When I feel them, I feel my own spine and the muscles around it tighten and tingle, reminding me of those days when my teachers put their hands on me and felt the same hardened shell.

In the few classes I've taught from Cape Town to Durban, the men, particularly those with HIV, seem fragile, a bundle of bones held together by defiance and a determination to survive, galvanized from growing up under the cruelty of apartheid. The women have adapted differently. Some are as fragile, but many have endured the ravages of AIDS, it seems, by wrapping a thick blanket of flesh around their bones and nerves, making them appear somehow larger than life.

I come up to Villas and knead her neck. Behind Villas are a couple of South African high school girls. One proudly wears her status on her t-shirt. I check for her name on the nametag and can't believe what I read. I lean down to make sure. Her name is PRECIOUS. Earlier, before class, it is Precious who came up to me and asked: "Will you be teaching us how to meditate? I want to know how to do that. I read in a book once that it might help me. Do you think it could?" She'd smiled like any other curious eighteen year old, yet behind her smile, I could see in her eyes a hint of the panic that comes from dreaming too hard. What epidemic is worse, I wonder, the one that has infected over 40 million people around the world, or the one that paralyzes the other 5 billion into such fear that it can mangle the spirit of an innocent young woman?

While they are meditating, a man enters the room. He is an Indian in the traditional, conservative dress of a Brahmin, long loose-fitting pants with a folded tunic of the same crème color draped over his shoulder. Three lines of white ash mark his forehead, signs of his devotion to Shiva. His face is bright, his eyes glow. He's an older man, maybe sixty-five, seventy. He smiles so kindly that I can't help but to put my hands together, bow and invite him in.

He stares in amazement at the people sitting on their mats and folded blankets, and then he looks back at me. We walk toward each other, and he hands me his card, whispering, "I noticed on program board downstairs class on yoga. This class is yoga?"

I ask him to hold his questions, as I need to arouse the students from meditation. I look at the card. He is a doctor, a psychologist, from Mumbai. I offer him some handouts. He smiles gratefully. The participants open their eyes and before them is this man in white. "I want to say something to them, please." I nod and give him the floor, fearing a long discourse on yoga. Dazed from meditation, the students hardly know what's going on, some, no doubt, think this was just all part of the workshop.

The man offers his apologies, but just wants to thank them: "This makes my heart so happy to come here from my country and see you here at this conference doing yoga, learning about my traditions. I'm very happy."

"Do you want to say anything about yoga?" I ask.

He smiles, "No, you are the guru." Then he bows and exits.

We begin by doing simple forward bends, using chairs and walls to help them feel stable so that they can stretch their spines. We do the poses I've been taught by all the teachers who have come through my life. We do various poses to develop flexibility and stimulate the immune system: *Suryanamaskar* (the sun salutations), *Trikonasana* (the triangle), *Virabhadrasana* (the warrior), *Marichyasana* (the sitting torso twist), and *Salamba Sarvangasana* (shoulder stand).

I keep watch on the teenagers in the back of the room and hover near a man from Zambia, who came in with a suit and tie, bony and fragile but so determined to do every pose that he nearly crashes into the woman next to him. I let him lean on me in tree pose, and he laughs hysterically, bordering on tears, until I slowly, finger-by-finger, release him and let him stand on his own.

Not all of the participants in the workshop are Africans or HIV positive. There is a social worker from Chennai in a flowing red sari-like exercise outfit who is named after the Indian goddess of good fortune, Lakshmi; a nurse from Indianapolis; activists from Britain, Brazil, and Peru; a Russian activist and sex worker with a pack of cigarettes beside her mat; a gymnastics coach and activist from Hong Kong by the name of Charles Chan, who went about helping others around him, knowing exactly what to say, having taught children for years. I ask him if he has a pose we could try, and he leaps up and we all follow him. Then the social worker from Chennai has a pose, and we do that.

Toward the end, I ask Villas to come up to the front of the class to help me demonstrate a back bend. She squints, "Me?" With Chan at her feet and me at her shoulders and with encouragement from the rest of the participants, we talk her through a back bend, supporting and working with her to raise her solid body and push her pelvis up into the air, her back bending with more suppleness than she or I expect.

"I feel so light," she says looking up at me, her back arched and face beaming.

"That's because you are," I say. And as we slowly lower her back down on the mat, the class breaks into a burst of applause.

Then it is time for the class to end. As they lie in the corpse pose, their chests supported by rolled up blankets, I walk around the room adjusting shoulders, propping heads, opening fists and spreading fingers. "Let yourself be here, be in your breath, be in your body."

Finally I sit down before them, cross my legs, close my eyes, and take a few deep breaths of my own. I listen to the sounds of the street below, the traffic, the market, the people of Durban going about their lives, and I feel content if not a bit exhausted. Despite my worries, it has all gone quite well.

After the class, several stay, some help me clean up, some hover around looking at the handouts. They do not want to go. Some ask me how they can keep practicing if there isn't anyone to teach them. "Are there some video tapes?" someone asks. They've grabbed the photocopied stick-figure diagrams of the poses and my essay explaining yoga's benefits for people with HIV. But they want more. A young woman representing a church in Soweto comes up to me and shyly asks if I might consider coming there to teach a workshop for at-risk teenagers. Then the teenagers from Zambia ask the same. The activist from Brazil wonders: "I don't suppose you ever come to South America, do you?"

I don't know what to say to them. I'm flattered, but I have a flight in three days back to Chicago and an adjunct teaching position that begins in a few weeks, a job which I can't afford to leave for fear of losing health insurance. I take down their names, knowing there is no way I can possibly fulfill their requests. But I'm afraid of telling them this. My feeling of self-satisfaction is gone, and I begin to wonder if what I've done is only introduce yet another means of giving hope that they cannot have or afford.

❋

Eunice Odongo and a Cuban-American Santeria healer and AIDS activist from New York City have asked me to offer one more yoga class. This time we practice outside. Several teenagers join us, along with Chan, the Chinese gymnastics coach. We do some partner poses, some standing poses, and headstands—using two chairs and blankets as props, while Chan and I hold up their legs. Even Odongo gives it a try. By the end there is a crowd watching, including Miamiza, the eighteen-year-old from the opening ceremony. I ask him to join us: "No, no. I see on a sign that you are having the yoga class, so I wanted to stop by and say goodbye to you."

After the class, a grayish-blond haired woman approaches. Romy is an activist from Switzerland and also seropositive. "I tried to get here, but we just finished with the press conferences and then later we have to take Danny Glover out to see the grave of Gugu Dlamini."[5] Romy came to work with a dance company in Soweto and then decided to stay and help with Durban's chapter of NAPWA, an organization for HIV-positive people, co-founded and headed by one of South Africa's leading activists, Mercy Makhalemele. Mercy, from a well-known family, revealed her HIV status on a popular television talk show in 1993, one of the first South African women to do so. "Mercy wants to meet you. I told her about you and your yoga. Where are you staying?"

"Well, nowhere now that the conference is over."

"Come to our apartment. We have an extra room. You can show us some yoga. Mercy will be there tonight."

They live in a large, second story apartment in a working-class neighborhood near Durban's port. Romy tells me how she'd met Mercy at a conference, and was so moved by her work that she decided to come to South Africa to help her. As if she were reading my mind, she asks: "Why don't you stay with us? You can teach yoga. Write. There's so much you can do to help."

Makahalemele arrives with her son. She plops down in a chair, too tired to say much to me, her eyes appear permanently pasted open in an otherwise warm and finely-featured face. Yet she exudes strength in her compact body, like a fist, calling people to battle. Her twelve-year-old son, as weary as his mother, bolts to his room and shuts the door.

We go out to a porch. Romy rolls a fat spliff of dagga (South African marijuana) and lights it. She uses it almost every day to ease the nausea that accompanies the combination cocktail treatment. My muscles relax at the scent. The women pass it back and forth, assuming I don't smoke, so I must help myself. "Oh, sorry," Mercy apologizes, "I just thought your yoga and all."

I suck in far too much smoke, burning my throat, already raw from a lingering cold. Romy serves tea and biscuits. And for a while we are silent, smoking that single joint, drinking our tea, settling into the evening as the last light of day fades. They look ready to collapse, spent after an intense week. But I want to talk to Mercy; I want to hear her response to Mandela's historic speech that afternoon at the end of the conference.

His presence had sent a message not only to those of us sitting in the packed conference hall, but to the South African government and the world. I'd never witnessed anything like the response Mandela received as he entered the hall. Drums shook the hall, a chorus of singers chanted his praise, dancers whirled and stomped, the audience—particularly the Africans—exploded with thunderous outbreaks of emotional cheers. For ten minutes people stood and clapped.

The warmth in Mandela's voice made everyone sit back down. He told a story about a group of crippled children who'd come to his home, and the faces of those around me were like children themselves, holding their hands up to their mouths. "We must not ignore these people, they are our friends, our teachers, our family, we must love the people with HIV and AIDS." He is not talking only to Africans, he's talking to everybody, he is talking to me. I fumble for my pen, trying to hold myself together by scribbling down his words, but choke on the emotions that have been welling up inside me for the past month. How hungry we were to be spoken to about the courage to love. Mandela ended the speech with a line from Julius Caesar that rings through my body as these women and I recall it together: "A coward dies a thousand deaths, a hero but one."[6]

From Romy, I'd heard how painful it was for Mercy to speak out at the beginning. At that time in South Africa, no one was admitting their status for fear of reprisals, including death. In fact, Mercy's husband went berserk when she returned from the prenatal clinic and told him, throwing her and her baby out of the house. The next year, both he and her baby daughter died of AIDS. It was difficult for her family, as her father, Mike Makhalemele, was a respected jazz saxophonist who'd recorded with Paul Simon on his Graceland album. To have Mandela embrace this struggle and those who were fighting it, calling those like Mercy who worked at the grassroots the "real heroes in the fight against HIV and AIDS," affirmed her suffering and her work.

Sitting with these women, I feel an affiliation I'd not allowed myself to feel before coming to Africa. It had begun in Cape Town three weeks ago with Michael Nixon, the musician and AIDS activist who worked with young people developing scripts for community radio. Nothing was said, but he drove me one night up into the mountains outside of Cape Town. We pulled off the highway and looked out at the lights of Cape Town and down at the surf rolling on the beaches at the foot of the mountains. In that silence with Michael, I felt as I did with Andre and Eunice and Villas and Charles and now Mercy and the others; I felt understood, not just as someone with HIV but as someone whose life has been transformed by HIV. There is a difference. These women sitting on the porch next to me knew that helping others realize this distinction was what gave them hope and ultimately their health.

They ask me about yoga, curious as to my story and what my classes were like. "I'd wanted to go, but I had so much to do," Mercy confesses shaking her head, "I want to do something like this with my body."

I nod, recalling the same sentiment in the participants in my yoga workshops. I wonder, out loud, why so much of the conference was geared toward the intellectual. A British friend of Mercy's describes the responses she received from her painting workshop with those with HIV and families who've lost members to AIDS. Romy, who has been working with a theater company of teenagers from Soweto, concurs, remarking how their passion and energy have helped her more than all the drugs she's been taking. I'd seen this company perform and I was struck by how rooted they were, their voices and gestures shaking with emotion.

"I worked with people's bodies," I tell them, reminding myself. "I can't get over how hard they felt, it's like they are living in shells. People are in such pain. Couldn't you feel it?"

Mercy has come from six days of little sleep in front of the international media, answering questions, giving interviews, sitting on panels, listening, and strategizing. She begins to break, her hand trembles as she brings it to her eyes to cover them. "I know, I know, I know, there is so much pain here, so many people—and you, and people coming here from outside and seeing it and feeling it—it reminds us." She tries to compose herself, blinking away the tears. But she can't hold back, and tears roll down her round, black face as she crumbles before us. My body tells me to go to her, but I sit there with the other two women, dumbstruck, too afraid perhaps that by touching, I will fall apart too.

Mercy's cell rings. It is a journalist from the *New York Times* who called earlier. She closes her eyes and stiffens, wiping her nose, trying to compose herself.

"Hello? . . . Can I talk to you later? Please? I'll call you later, thank you."

She puts down the phone, wiping away more tears. "This man keeps calling. I've told him everything. I've got so many things I need to do and . . ." She looks at me. "I'm sorry, but they want too much. They don't understand." She bows her head, embarrassed, the tears freely falling again.

A full moon rises over the warehouses along the port, filling up the porch and bringing with it the reminder that we live to rhythms beyond our control.

Later that evening, after dinner with some Canadian doctors, I drive Mercy and her son to the bus station. On the way, Mercy asks me if I would consider staying, the fifth time someone has asked in the last forty-eight hours. "After I finish this TV show in Cape Town, I will be traveling. The apartment will be free. It's sort of our base. People are always staying there. Stay as long as you want. It would be good to have you here. It's not much, but you can have the back room. Think about it."

I get lost trying to find the bus station. Then it begins to downpour. Miraculously, we find the bus station just before the bus departs. We don't have time to say goodbye. They run to the bus through the rain, hand in hand.

I leave their apartment the next day, cold and sick. I find an expensive Holiday Inn on the beach and spend my last two days getting sicker, eating crackers, and drinking lukewarm tea while from my twelfth-story window I watch surfers balance in the rolling surf. On my last day I take the blankets and yoga mats from the conference center and drop them off at Mercy's and Romy's apartment. I put the key on the table and lock the door behind me.

❧

Somewhere over Africa I lock myself in the toilet of a 747 bound for New York and spit into a steel sink. There is nothing more than a few vermilion strings of blood, magnified slightly in the spittle, shiny and dark against the clear mucus and stainless steel. But it is enough to sustain the anxiety I have been living on like an addict since well before traveling to South Africa.

My face has shrunk, exposing hollow jowls and cheekbones, extending my Pinocchio nose. If I were to take off my pants, every vein in my leg would surface, blue and red through translucent skin. But it is the eyes that startle me. They have retreated deep into their sockets, reminding me of my grandfather, who left this world by his own hand long before my arrival. The ghost of my father's father stands before me now with his protruding forehead and deep eye sockets, stands as he always stood in the few photos grandmother did not purposely lose, shoulders slumped, arms folded, alone even when surrounded by family, in a garden behind a gray farm house in that black and white world of rural America in the thirties. And so he has come, my namesake with his sad, sunken eyes, to ride with me high over the savannahs of central Africa where, as traditional Africans believe, the dead wait for their final release from the memory of the living.

I wash my face and retreat to my seat. I wrap myself in thin airplane blankets. I'm not sick, I tell myself. Other people get sick. Indeed thanks to the genes of that same man who stepped off the stepladder into his homemade noose sixty-five years ago, I live a suspiciously healthy life for someone with a compromised immune system. I rarely get a cold or the flu. But I'm always waiting for the other shoe to drop.

New Hampshire, USA (August, 2000)

After spending the night at the home of an old Peace Corps colleague's, I am back on the road in leafy Massachusetts heading toward New Hampshire where I have a residence fellowship at an artist colony. The road weaves its way through American perfection. Engineered bands of asphalt bank and curve, carry me along it seems on nothing more than intention. Gone is the wintry, rainy gloom of urban South Africa. I pass lakes, imagining myself in some other body, a boy's or some animal's, lying on a rock baking in the sun and then slithering in through the mud. I have gone the last five weeks without feeling warmth. The brilliant white reflection of light on the water makes my body ache for the sun's penetrating heat. I take off my shirt, not even bothering to stop the car. As the sun heats the oil on my skin, it awakens the memory of other bodies touching mine: the insides of Andre's mouth, the hard shoulders of Villas in down dog, the little hands of the motherless boys pulling on my leg at the orphanage.

Long before HIV came into my body, swimming had become a cure for the ills of the heart. I swam to escape, to dream, to heal, to love—if not someone else, then water. For that reason, I have stolen into private ponds and pools or traveled far out of my way to find a lonely lake I've spotted on a map while driving. Perhaps it isn't the lakes, themselves, that sustain me, but the effect they leave in memory: that the freedom of water is always within reach.

As a boy, my grandparents had a cottage on a small lake in Northern Indiana, so small you could hear the echo of screen doors slamming in the evenings across the lake. My mother's parents had saved all their lives to retire in their little brown cottage along with the other working class folk from the industrial belt of Indiana. Formed in the Ice Age, the lakes of Northern Indiana are all that are left of the lands of the Miami and the Potowotomi, the black bear and bobcat; the rest had been clear-cut, drained, plowed under and put to productive use. The lake was a kind of island of magic in my childhood. It was here that I learned to swim, wading off into the weeds, sinking into the silt and muck to my knees, dog paddling with my sister out to the anchored raft off shore, made of oil drums and plywood. It was here too that I first tasted sex, putting my fingers inside a red-haired girl in the suffocating heat of an empty trailer that was for sale on the side of the road.

When my grandfather developed emphysema, my grandparents abandoned that cottage, and then died on the edge of town in a trailer court. But that lake stayed in my body, as memories do of the landscapes of our youth, like the instinct of birds that carry them back to where they first learned to fly.

As I get closer to the colony, I imagine myself entering a room full of intense and accomplished artists. My self-confidence will soon be under assault. I fear them thinking I am a fraud, or worse, a charity case, invited to make them feel good about themselves. I shudder to think it is only my HIV that has allowed me the honor. I twist a joint and turn on the tape I made of Mandela's speech. I roll down the highway hearing a very bad recording of a voice that doesn't need to be understood to have its effect.

❋

My fears, as usual, are exaggerated. My fellow colonists are full of questions and concern and I do something I've never done before: walk into a room of people from whom I desperately want respect and admit my status. These artists live in their own private tortures and admire boldness, irony, and self-revelation of all kinds. I pass the test, at least for the first day.

Later, sitting at a table next to mine at dinner is a writer I'd met at another colony, when I was living from month to month thinking that my time was running out along with my dreams of writing. From South Africa, Rob Nixon was instrumental in helping me find contacts. When I enter, Rob rises from his table to grab me in a hug that braces me with his emotion. After dinner, he leads me outside with glasses of scotch. We sit on a stone wall and look out at the rugged pines across an open field, facing the fire of an August sun reluctant to set. I try to summarize my experiences in his country. But it doesn't really matter what insights I have gathered, what tales I can narrate, or what cruel fact of Africa I have witnessed, because Rob's haunted by that world I only barely tasted. It lives there in his tight jaw and careful syntax. There is nothing I can say that surprises him. He nods and sighs as if reading a newspaper, as I speak of the traditional healers and the work of his old friend Zackie Achmat. It isn't until I describe the beaches of the Western Cape that he brightens and reminisces about swimming in the ocean with his brother as a boy.

❀

The green water reflects the thick-leafed hardwoods and shadowy pines that circle the lake and roll gently up the slopes of the surrounding New Hampshire foothills. I stand on a boulder of granite and survey the dreamy sheen before me, as Rob and another colonist, Alex, a filmmaker from New York, dress on opposite sides of a boulder behind me in the privacy of the empty lake. Finally, I have found my lake—and what a lake it is, free of cottages, fishermen, or echoing children. It's pure silence save for a pair of loons nesting on the opposite shore where we are headed. Rob tells me he has been coming here almost every afternoon for the last couple weeks. I'm still coughing and finding blood staring back at me in wads of Kleenex, but I assure my swimming mates I am feeling fine.

The water is cold, but I've swum in Lake Michigan for years. My body knows that the chill won't last long, once the muscles heat up. It's Rob and Alex I'm concerned about. Perhaps they won't want to swim all the way across. But they quickly take off and are well out into the lake ahead of me.

It feels good to be surrounded by the lake's emerald glow. Swimming in fresh-water lakes is as close to paradise as swimmers get. There is something almost sexual about pulling the body through passive water, the rhythmic oars of the arms beating and slapping in motion against the wetness, the legs thrashing, the chest engorged by the effort of halving the surface. Framed by elbow and eyebrow, the land blurs in the corners of the eyes, and from water level the mountains and trees tower in mythic stature. Then comes a moment when the body, under the influence of internal chemistry, blends the boundaries of the self, and the brain becomes drunk with adrenaline, allowing the skin to become the sole intermediary between the world and the world within.

But the long-sought release will not come; my muscles remain cramped from what seems like days flying over the world. The water feels heavy, dragging me down, making every other stroke laborious, and I find myself doing what I rarely do while swimming, checking ahead to see how far I have to go.

I make it to the other side well behind Rob and Alex, who are picking and eating blueberries along the shore. I want to join them, but when I drag myself from the water, the air is cold and my teeth begin to chatter. I sink back in up to my neck to keep warm. It begins to gently rain. A lone canoe glides off to our right looking for loons. We wave. The canoeists lift their oars. I look across the lake and know it is going to be a long slog back in the cold rain.

"Maybe we ought to get back since it's raining?" Alex suggests looking at me with concern. "You look like you're cold."

I don't need to reply and take off ahead of them, hoping with a head start I can at least keep up with them. I don't even know this woman, Alex, but I can feel the withering of my pride, as she has that unapologetic strength that some women reveal when in the company of men. In no time, they pass me, which only makes me feel that much more exhausted and pissed off. Sure, I rationalize, I am still tired from the flight and I'm not feeling well. Still, I put my head down and push on like the coach's son that I am.

But after barely ten yards, I'm spent. My lungs can't take in much oxygen. It's like someone has grabbed me in a bear hug. I slow down but still can't catch my breath. I stop and tread water, hoping to give my lungs a break. It helps, but as soon as I begin my stroke, they tire again and I'm hyperventilating.

Panic seizes me, making me jerk and splash, as if I've never learned to swim. My mind scans the lake for options. I see Alex and Rob ahead but dismiss the idea of calling for help: Too dramatic. Don't embarrass yourself. I look back to the blueberry bushes, thinking: Then what? Stand on the other side of the lake and call for help? But it doesn't matter what my mind thinks, my body is running out of air. I'm sucking so hard, my lungs hurt. Stunned, my mind demands logic to prevail: I can't be drowning! I'm a swimmer. I can't die! God damn it! I'm already dying!

My body awakens with fury. Blinded by rage is not a metaphor.

My vision blurs into chaotic swirls of green and gray. In this whirlwind of emotion and blindness I recognize the stark and brutal reality of biology: my body is sick, it's losing heat, my lungs are collapsing, panic is shutting down my rational mind, if I don't find a way out of this water, I will sink to the bottom of the lake. Why am I so surprised? Didn't I learn anything from the land I've just returned from?—where teenagers bloom only to die, a million children have no parents, women are stoned to death in the streets, and men rape children in hopes of being cured? This is your life! Wake up!

I try to focus and find the shore again; my lungs heave involuntarily, each intake more painful than the next. Fatigue is winning out over will. My feet churn in weary loyalty, gleaming in the jade-colored shadows, and then, as I feel the coldness climbing up my legs, instead of terror and anger, I feel relief. The searching, the striving, the saving face, the work—could it be no longer necessary? I imagine my body sinking without fear into watery annihilation, and coming to rest in the soft mud at the bottom of the lake. Parts of me fall and sink away, the coward and the hero, the addict and the teacher, the man, the boy: all take their bow. As my mind floats off toward this blissful death, a memory pulls me back: I am lying on my back next to my sister in the warm shallows at my grandparent's lake, my mother standing between us, her head just above water, her fingers barely touching our spines, as she teaches us to float.

Instantly, I flip onto my back, pulling myself up onto that image of my sister floating next to me, the memory of my mother's fingers tingling my spine, her simple rules whispering in my mind: "Relax your body. And when you feel yourself beginning to sink, move your hands and feet very slowly, and you will float."

I look up at the colorless sky as sprinkles of rain drop on my face. Now I hear my own voice, speaking to me as if I were one of the students in my yoga workshop, lying on that wooden floor in Durban: "Listen to your breath, inhale completely, exhale until you are empty." My mind, however, still fights, intensifying the panic. But I keep to my mantra: breathe, breathe, just breathe! Finally my body lightens and energy returns.

Thinking I'm out of danger, I turn back over and make a beeline back to the other side of the lake, but my lungs quickly collapse. I return to my back, and intermittently ease my way onto my stomach until I reach a boulder off shore.

Too tired to pull myself out of the water, I hang on the granite rock, my cheek holding as tightly as my fingers. Shaking violently from shock and lack of heat, I try to catch my breath and will myself upon the rock. On the third time, in tears, I drag myself out. My muscles are locked, my jaw aches, my teeth rattle. I crouch, shaking uncontrollably. Across the lake, Rob and Alex pace on shore, stopping to look out. I call to them but nothing in my body projects sound. Speechless, I try to wave but can barely lift my arms. Numbed by the cold and what has happened, I can do nothing but shiver and stare across the lake, hoping that they see me.

Soon, however, a canoe cuts through the gray green water heading toward the rock. It is the man and woman who have been watching the loons. Embarrassed, I apologize but only to myself as my voice is inaudible.

"I'm a doctor," he says as he stabilizes the canoe against the rock. "It's a bit cold to be out for a swim today, eh?" he offers in a laconic New England lilt; "Your friends are right there waiting with the car heating up."

They paddle me in a hurry to the beach where Rob and Alex help me dress, then pull me into Rob's heated car. Without a word, Alex begins to massage my arms and shoulders and then Rob goes for my legs, transferring their heat, rubbing my body like I've been lost from the pack, cleansing me of the fear they can smell clinging to my cold flesh.

Back at the colony, I struggle through dinner, relishing the normalcy of each simple act of eating. I stay after dinner, pretending as if nothing has happened, wanting to watch a screening of a film by one of the artists. When the lights go out I feel such an intense claustrophobia and panic, I nearly knock people over while scrambling to get outside.

Walking back to my cabin, I feel better. But even thinking of the panic in the screening room makes it difficult for me to breathe.

My cabin is a little house on the edge of the woods, slept in by hundreds of writers over the years; their names on wooden tombstone-looking tablets hang on the wall by the fireplace. I take a long hot bath, staring up at the ceiling, afraid to close my eyes for fear of the panic returning. When the water cools, I climb into the old-fashioned brass bed and cover myself with four layers of blankets. By my bed I have stacked a pile of books from the colony's library. One after the other, I lift them into bed, feeling their spines and weight, opening them at random and reading, then lying them face down next to me.

My mind, normally full of chatter and ideas, particularly after sitting around such interesting people, is still and quiet, feeling almost a sense of mourning. Propped up by pillows, I stare into the corners of my room, absorbed by the sensations of that afternoon that continue to reverberate through my body. If I close my eyes, my mind returns to the lake. The memories are so vivid, my legs churn like obedient dogs, so I place my hands on my thighs to calm them.

III

Ko Chang Island, Southern Thailand (May, 2001)

Under a milk-white moon, the surf turns silver, and the shadows of tilting palms shudder in the breeze. Down the beach, the lovers in the cabanas have extinguished their passion, and now the night and the ocean are mine. With my arms wrapped around my naked legs, I watch the waves like surfers do, reading the rhythms and falling under their spell.

I have come to this island off the southern coast of Thailand to pace the beach and try to convince myself that it wasn't a mistake to sell my furniture, give up my apartment, and leave my job to travel through Asia to chronicle the surging AIDS pandemic. After three days in Bangkok, I pulled up my shallow stakes, hoping that my failure to make it no further than a few blocks from my hotel was only jet lag and Bangkok's heat and smog. But as I sit before the wide, forgiving emptiness of the sea, I'm not thinking about Bangkok or my ambitious plans. I'm thinking of a fantasy that haunts me when I'm alone near bodies of water. Like a recurring dream, this fantasy had returned while I was swimming in the surf earlier in the day. It was nothing more than the force of the undertow, testing my will, pulling me out when my body wanted in. But it triggered the drama that has replayed itself in my mind many times since that night in Africa twenty years ago when, after announcing my love for Elizabeth in front of our parents, I took off my clothes and swam as fast as I could into the darkness of the sea.

Since the incident in the New Hampshire lake and the troubling memories of South Africa, these seductive suicide fantasies have become more frequent. For the rest of last summer and into the fall, I swam alone in the cold waters of Lake Michigan, trying to reproduce that sudden twitch of panic and momentary loss of control I'd felt in New Hampshire. This had become a ritual. I would swim out just beyond the buoys where the boats were free to speed, take off my swimming trunks and place them around my neck. I waited for the panic to return, relishing the terror and the near ecstatic relief that eventually followed, as I swam in a frenzy back to shallow water. To me, it was like sex, perhaps even better. After these episodes, as I scrambled to get my swimming suit back on, I began to laugh nervously at my little stunt, performed in front of the towering apartment buildings along the shore.

My swimming fetish, however, was not always so apt to end in self-amusement. There was a time when I sought to use it for its ultimate purpose—to push myself so far to the edge that to fall off might look like an accident rather than what it was, suicide. In the years before I was infected with HIV, when I used my struggling writing career as an excuse to isolate myself and churn out solipsistic tracts I thought were short stories, I cultivated this particular fantasy. It had to do with Lake Michigan and the water intake cribs two miles off of Chicago's lakefront. Like I'm doing now, I would sit and stare out into the water at these feats of engineering, round like temples with a single spiral, built of bricks a hundred years before to provide water to the people of Chicago. In my fantasy, I walk to the lake in the middle of an autumn night when the water is calm and cold. I take off my clothes and bury them, shoes and all, in the sand. I point myself in the direction of the lights on top of the crib off Belmont Harbor and plunge in. I know it's a risk. I know if my blood temperature cools, my body might shut down, my muscles tighten, my lungs collapse in hypothermia. I know it's possible that I might panic in the darkness and fight myself to the death with the lights of the city laughing as I sink into the lake's frigid depths. Even if I make it to the crib, I know I must climb onto a platform, my body trembling, and stumble to a door and present my shrunken naked self to a shocked, pale-faced engineer. But my fantasy is a test, a test of the body and will. I want Nature, you see, to answer the question that has plagued me since that day in my youth when I knelt before the naked legs of another horny thirteen-year-old boy: Am I worthy of living in this body? If not, then I want Nature to mercifully take me, and hide me forever from that world of work and dreams, of children and real estate, of love and loss. I want to be released from the cycle of sadness.

If, however, I prove myself to be strong and able to take even the ignominy of my triumph, which would surely make the papers—*Botched Suicide: Naked Man Saves Self by Swimming to Water Intake Crib*—then I would accept this as a sign of grace and devote myself to the pursuit of good works and become like the bodhisattvas of the East.

At first, I imagined this fantasy for the narrator of a novel I tried to write. At the time, I was living in Seattle and I had other suicide fantasies: hiking into the Olympic mountains and accidentally slipping off a cliff, diving from the top of Snoqualmie Falls, or jumping off the back of the last ferry to Bremerton. When I began to spend too much time hiking alone and taking ferries, I boxed up my things and sent them back to Chicago. Actually, I wasn't so much afraid of the mountains and the waterfalls as I was of telling a woman I'd begun to admire that I was having sex with men in the parks and staying up all night on ecstasy, catching my hair on fire while fucking another woman who was as fucked up as me.

If you are in love with the idea of being a writer as I was at the time, the difference between fantasy and fiction is dangerously slight. As my life unraveled, those water intake cribs became an obsession for both me and the "I" that lived inside my head. I moved back to Chicago to an apartment near the lake. From my apartment, I would look out at the blue green dreamscape as I tried to write, lost in thought, wondering in the back of my mind if tonight was the night. I pretended to myself that experiencing the ice-cold water and the fear of getting caught naked on the beach by the police might give me insight into the troubled mind of my main character. But the fall passed and the lake froze over. I found other more immediate means of putting my will to the test.

My sexual addiction—for that is really what it is when you wake up weekend after weekend in a stranger's bed and don't know where you are or how you got there—was already putting me at risk. I didn't need to take off my clothes, bury them in sand, and swim in fifty-five degree water. I could float into any bar on Halsted Street and find death in the eyes of too many men. And by January on the coldest night of the year, with the wind blowing stiffly off the lake, icing the windows so that we could not see out, I found him.

Perhaps this fetish for panic has something to do with why nine months after returning from South Africa I boarded another plane, this time for Bangkok, with this vague idea of writing about AIDS activists and activism. Others might argue the trip has to do with my well developed talent for using some unquestionably idealistic project to mask another escape from having to face the realities of my life: as a lonely, stubborn, bisexual man with HIV but without a career and or financial security. For them, for friends and family—who have watched me nearly self-destruct several times—for the way they live, they are right. But I don't live in their world. I tried to. I spent a good twenty years thinking that all I needed was to just make the right move, get the right job, meet the right person at the right time, and I would be right back in there with the wife and kids and the two-car garage. When I got rid of my belongings, it wasn't the things themselves I released, it was me.

I admit, I am happier to be moving than standing still, happier to be lost in lands where I can't speak the language than in places where I can predict the content of every landscape and conversation before I enter them. Though I'm not sure where this trip will lead me, I do know that I want to be back among people, among activists, who, when they meet me see someone who is not a victim but a man as innocent and passionate for life as he was when he was thirteen.

I stand, look up and down the beach, and run like a boy into the surf. The water is warm. The salt stings my eyes. My muscles swell with blood, making me believe I can swim all night if I have to.

Chennai, India (May, 2001)

All I have is the name and phone number of a man who runs a community organization for poor, young men who are sex workers on the streets of Chennai. I'd gotten his name from an activist I'd met in Cape Town. At the airport, when I call the number in my notebook, Sunil Menon answers, informs me that he has already booked a room for me, and asks me to hand the phone to the taxi driver so he can explain where to take me. Things are already out of my hands.

Chennai, formerly known as Madras, is a city of 7 million residents that spreads out from the coast, where it began as a tiny fishing village on the Bay of Bengal, into the rural farmlands of Tamil Nadu. A manufacturing center and one of India's major ports, Chennai has become one of the main incubators for the spread of HIV, tuberculosis and malaria.[1]

As I'm driven through the haze and clamor of the city, the streets are a blur of moving vehicles: three-wheel rickshaws, oxen carts, antique taxis, buses, bicycles, and thousands of motorbikes. My body recoils. My eyes squint from the smog and the dusty brightness. The chaos and cacophony remind me that India can feel like a cosmic war: too many souls trapped with nowhere to flee.[2]

The taxi pulls to a curb on a tree-lined street. A man with a cherubic face appears, waving a heavily ringed hand and calling out my name. He is my contact, the director of Sahodaran, Sunil Menon. I climb out of the taxi and Sunil grabs my hand and counts the bills. "What? One hundred rupees?" Behind my back a diminutive young man with coal-black hair takes my heavy duffle bag, lifts it onto his head, and disappears up a flight of stairs. When Sunil finishes lecturing the stunned taxi driver on his poor manners, he takes my arm and, in a flourish, escorts me up the stairs to his three-room office.

Inside, young men play a board game at a table, two more man phones at desks; others mill about looking at tattered movie magazines. Upon my entry, hands quickly go through thick waves of shimmering black hair, shirts are straightened, pants dusted. One by one they dutifully approach me, offering shy handshakes but piercing gazes, as if I am some kind of celebrity.

Sunil calls out for someone to serve tea. "You must excuse me, we are having a meeting in a few minutes."

Tired from my six-hour flight from Bangkok and not sure what's going on, I think it best to go to my hotel first and then come back after the meeting, but when I suggest this plan, I'm quickly corrected, if not almost scolded, by Sunil.

"Oh, no! Why would you do that? The meeting will be interesting for you. Besides you'll meet the boys." He disappears into a side room. *The boys?* I catch the men staring at me until they break into playful, curious smiles, laughing among themselves. They invite me to play the board game, but since I can't understand Tamil and they can't speak English very well, I am at a loss as to the rules. The door opens and more young men enter; there's more giggling and staring. Finally it dawns on me. These young men are *the boys*—the male sex workers.

The office door opens and out steps Sunil with another man, dressed in black down to his cowboy boots. I'm introduced to Shivananda Khan, the field director from London for the Naz Project, the group that has created this community organization as well as others throughout south Asia. A computer printout in hand, Khan is all business, with a fierce look that matches his leonine face. He sizes me up, tilts his head and listens as I blurt out why I am here, beginning with my calling card: "I'm a writer with HIV and I'd like to—"

Khan interrupts: "Yes, Sunil, told me. How are you doing? Are you taking the cocktail?"

Taken off guard by his directness, my mouth doesn't quite work: "Yes, taking the pills. I'm taking the cocktail. I'm fine, thank you."

Khan nods, staring intensely at me. "We're having a meeting here. You can listen; it'll help you see what we do." He heads out for a cigarette but then turns back at the door, "D'you mind if I reveal your status to the boys? They need to meet people like you." Then he turns to Sunil: "You should have him talk to them while he's here."

I swallow the tea that one of the boys has handed me and agree. "Sure, I can talk."

Khan returns after his cigarette. The boys assemble on the floor in front of him and a flip chart. Sunil hands me a worn copy of a homemade pamphlet, which explains the center's mission. Sahodaran, which means "friends" in the south Indian language of Tamil, hopes to establish a community among these generally uneducated and poor young men. It offers them a safe haven, basic health care, and training as peer educators. This means handing out condoms in public spaces where MSMs or male sex workers frequent and inviting these men to join them at the center. As I glance through this pamphlet, Khan begins a training session in English, while Sunil translates into Tamil.

Khan breaks down the types of men and the particular sexual behavior that the peer educators will encounter in their fieldwork: *kothis,* with a feminine construction of gender identity who usually take a passive or receptive role in sexual interactions; *panthis,* usually heterosexual males, who take an active role in recreational sex with men for various reasons; a third they call *double-deckers,* who, although they don't see themselves as *kothis,* will either take a passive or active role in sex depending upon the partner.

Khan wants to focus on the *kothis,* because sex workers are often *kothis* and the ones most at risk for contracting HIV. Khan leaves off the sociological talk and puts down his pen. "Look," he says, "we're all at risk in here, we all like cock, right? Maybe not all of us, I can't speak for Michael over here," and then he turns to me and brings with him the eyes of the whole room. I hesitate, but the corners of my mouth slowly form a smile. "I thought so," Khan nods. And with a quick translation by Sunil, the "boys" are beside themselves with laughter. My initiation has begun.

Khan perceives my embarrassment and makes a point of telling them why I'm here. "Michael is here to write about you, and he *knows* how serious this is. We all do don't we?" Then he asks how many people know someone who has died of AIDS—everyone raises a hand. Khan pauses in silence for effect, looking slowly around the room at each of us.

Khan's no-holds-barred discussion goes on for a good hour. His message is that they must work together to protect themselves and those they counsel as peer educators. Khan is passionate, reminding them of what their sex work can be like: "It's brutal, fast." He slaps his fist into his palm a few times, the slapping louder on each hit. "Anal sex is dangerous. *Panthis* just want to discharge; they want relief. They don't care if it hurts you. That's why you must protect yourself and teach others to do the same." For these young men, who may have several sexual encounters a day, some lasting little more than a few minutes, it doesn't take much medical knowledge to figure out how at risk they are.

As Khan speaks, the boys fiddle with each other's shirt collars; they take notes in worn, coverless notebooks, shifting uncomfortably from side to side with their faces drooped and serious. Khan is trying to teach them to take responsibility for their own sexual health. Sure, he wants them to pass out condoms, to record the numbers of those they meet on the street, to encourage their friends and clients to come in to see the doctor and get tested. But it's these boys sitting here whom Khan and Sunil have dedicated themselves to saving. Khan knows that AIDS is a disease of the young. He knows that well over half of those infected in the world are between the ages of fifteen and twenty-nine. So he doesn't mince words. He doesn't have the time. Neither does India. It's either act now or face an epidemic that may well prove worse than in southern Africa.[3]

After the meeting, Sunil arranges for me to be escorted to my hotel by one of the peer educators, a serious-looking young man who speaks not only English but also several other languages. Neat in appearance, with a stylish flowered shirt, Anto tells me he lives with his mother. He wants to open his own business someday to provide for her. He is on his way to work at Chennai's train station. I ask him what he does there, forgetting why he was there at the meeting.

"We ride the trains and give the condoms, talk to the men around the station."

"How much do you make?" Sunil had told me that they are paid a small salary for their peer counseling.

But Anto thinks I'm talking about the men he meets as he works—his clients. "Not that much," he tells me. "They sometimes give us clothes, the businessmen do, or they buy us things we need, take us to eat." But he wants to make sure I understand that he doesn't consider himself a sex worker. "A lot of the times we meet guys for the fun, but the older men, they know they must give us something."

At my hotel Anto helps me with my bags. I give him money to pay our fare and to make sure he has more than enough to get to the train station. Anto looks down at the money in his hand and then sadly back to me. Something is wrong. *Have I given him too little? Too much?*

"I will see you again at the office?"

"Oh yes, I will be back." But he doesn't leave. He stares, holding me there in the hot sun, his eyes opening wider and wider until he folds his money, puts it into his pocket, and climbs into his rickshaw to head for work.

❋

I barely have time to take a cold shower, rummage through my bags for a wrinkled pair of pants before I'm back at the front desk asking how to get to another address. Earlier, after the meeting at Sohadaran, I called a woman I'd met in South Africa at the AIDS conference, a social worker at a rehabilitation hospital for drug and alcohol abuse in Chennai. Instead of a polite hello, she insisted I come to a farewell party for her cousin, who was moving to America to join her husband.

After two hours circling neighborhoods in the dark with a taxi driver who couldn't speak English, I arrive at a large, multi-level cement and wood home. The interior is furnished with exquisite taste: Victorian furniture, intricately designed tapestries from Rajastan, Hindu iconographic statuary and other ancient artworks and heirlooms. Lakshmi appears, beaming with excitement, casually dressed in jeans and a white cotton shirt. At once, she grabs my arm and leads me into an enormous sitting room. "You must meet my family. I have so many ideas for people you can interview." Her warmth intoxicates, just as it did the first time I met her when she entered my yoga workshop at the AIDS conference, her billowing red-and-yellow-striped silk pants and shirt lighting up the room.

Her relatives are among the Indian elite: doctors, lawyers, businessmen, even a filmmaker. Her husband, a jovial, bear-like man, who works in the booming South Indian software industry, brings me into the cluster of men who have gathered around an extravagantly stocked bar. Soon I'm floating on some of the best scotch I've ever tasted.

The family chef brings bowl after bowl to fill a long table with Indian specialties and desserts. Politely, the men slip away from me one by one when I mention my work. Lakshmi rescues me, pulling me into the circle of women, who are giving the departing cousin advice on what to expect in America. When the conversation turns to my work, the women show much more interest. They are angry about the Hindu Nationalist ruling party and their policies toward women and the poor. I am not sure what to say, having arrived only that day and still overwhelmed by my afternoon with "the boys." I want to say something about the young men I met at Sahodaran, seeing them now in my mind on the streets and train stations doing their work, their peer counseling between blow jobs, but I realize maybe I'm too drunk and just smile.

❈

The next morning Lakshmi phones and tells me she has already set up appointments for me to see another social worker, a government health official, several doctors, and her yoga instructor and the director of the renowned Krishnamarcharya Yoga Centre. I brave the toxic air of midday traffic in a rickshaw, getting lost several times before I reach my destination an hour late. Covered in a fine layer of dust and soot, my shirt plastered to my back, I walk down a shady street next to a girl's school where I spot a bronze statue surrounded by a short brick wall and shielded from the sun with a white canvas cloth. As I enter, I see the name of Patanjali etched in the marble pedestal.[4] Patanjali sits in meditation with his hands in prayer; a cobra, poised to strike, shields his back with his hood. Red rose petals litter his lap, trickling down onto the marble floor while marigolds rest on his folded arms. Before him, I close my eyes and open up my lungs for what seems like the first time since I got off the plane.

Krishnamarcharya is actually the father of two of the most influential styles of yoga now practiced in America—Iyengar, as taught by the B.K.S. Iyengar, and Astanga or Vinyasa yoga, introduced by Sri Pattabhi Jois, with whom I briefly studied. Both teachers were taught by Krishnamarcharya, here in Madras well over fifty years ago. So I have come to a kind of yoga Mecca, as directly or indirectly every teacher I have ever studied under has been influenced by Krishnamarcharya.

Here, all students are first given an assessment or diagnosis; then a series of poses (asana) and breathing techniques (pranayama) are prescribed to correct imbalances and retrain the body and mind. For centuries, Indians have used these traditional methods of treatment along with diet and ayurvedic medicines to treat both minor and major physical and psychological maladies. Even with doctors and private hospitals comparable to those in Europe and America, Indians, particularly the lower classes, still rely heavily on traditional practitioners and their ancient methods and medicines.

The Centre is a simple, one-story building with a series of thatch buildings surrounding it, where teachers work privately with students or patients. I sit outside on a porch and wait for my chance to meet with the director. Next to me, a man clothed in folds of traditional white muslin trousers and a sleeveless tunic sits reading a book. I don't want to bother him but it's impossible to keep my eyes off his glowing, erect body. From his perfect pearl-like toenails to his symmetrical face, the young man projects that rare equipoise that comes with devoted study. He possesses what is known in yoga as shakti, the animating, feminine energy of the divine. It's a term often bandied about in yoga classes in America but rarely understood or embodied. My body rises sympathetically with his, my spine welcoming his corrective influence. I take one of the books in the rack between us, a book called The *Healing Power of Yoga*, but I can barely comprehend a sentence. I want to say something, engage him in conversation, ask him who I should study with, but before I can summon the nerve, he rises and gracefully crosses the sandy road, appearing almost to not touch ground.

As this princely Brahmin body floats away, I'm left with the question that has haunted me since those days living among the Wolof and Mandinka of West Africa, when I would watch the men crowd into the mud-brick mosque each evening and listen to the their chanting voices echoing across the village. Then as now, this kind of devotion eludes me, terrifies me even, and I don't know why.

From inside, a woman calls my name and leads me into the director's office of the Krishnamarcharya Centre. The office contains two basic, wooden chairs, a desk and examining table. The director bows and offers his hand. He wears no flowing shirt, beads, or priestly Brahmin's outfit, just a simple white shirt, black pants, black-framed glasses and hard-soled shoes. He gets a sharp pencil from his desk and takes notes as I answer his questions. I offer that I'm a yoga teacher and have studied for several years, mentioning Pattabhi Jois, but my resume has no effect on him.

"So you've come here from America to study yoga?"

"Well, yes, but I'm really here to write about AIDS."

"AIDS?"

"That's right." For a moment I consider telling him that I am HIV positive, but don't want to chance that they'll think I can't handle the more advanced poses, or worse, that they'll refuse to work with me altogether.

He nods, asking me to hold out both hands so he can take my pulse. "You've a very slow pulse. Have you had any illnesses or serious medical conditions?"

I really don't want to tell him. But I know I must. "Well, yes, as a matter of fact, I do have a condition."

When I tell him my status and explain why I've come to India, he slowly puts down his pencil. "I see," he says, relaxing his body. "I have worked with some of the patients at the government hospital, but I must be honest, it was not a good experience and I had to drop our program as they could never be counted on to come to our class." Then he pauses and takes a deep breath. "Mr. McColly, I have a question. Forgive me, but why would you want to put so much stress on yourself in this condition. India is not an easy place to travel; with this disease you must be careful, no?"

"I was here before in Mysore and nothing happened. On the contrary, I've found that traveling makes me stronger."

He nods again. "Just asking." He smiles and continues with his examination, seemingly unaffected. "Stand up, please, and touch toes." I try to do the best forward bend, pushing my palms flat to the floor, my hamstrings pulling with pain.

"More flexible on your right side," he observes matter of factly. Then he leads me to the examining table and asks me to sit in lotus. My thick khaki pants make the pose difficult. I mumble excuses under my breath as I try to bring my left foot over my right thigh. Finally, he asks me to lie down and breathe, counting how long I can comfortably extend my inhale and exhale. I'm sure I can easily extend my breath to at least a count of ten, probably more. But he stops me at five. "That's fine."

"But I can go further."

"No, you were straining at four."

Back at his desk, he writes some notes and prepares his diagnosis. I try to sit up straight now, worried that maybe I've failed this test and will be misplaced in a beginner's class.

"You are strong, but you have a shallow breath. You are very tense."

Tense? Of course, I'm tense! I nearly blurt out, suddenly annoyed with him and his ridiculous examination. He wants me to come three days for the time I'm here. "We will work with you on this tension."

While we wait for my teacher, he offers his view on the AIDS epidemic in India: that it has spread along lorry routes by drivers who traverse the country. I agree, but when I make the comparison to the same trend in southern and western Africa, he flinches, unable to accept the similarity between India's poor and Africa's. "I know this doesn't sound fair," he says, "but it's mostly the fault of the women." He pauses, seemingly unable to even say the word, prostitutes. "If *they* weren't there, or if *they* didn't do this, the men wouldn't catch the disease." He frowns. "We have many poor, uneducated people in our country, Mr. McColly, and it is their ignorance that causes many problems." Among traditional Hindus and middle-class Indians, his opinions on sex workers are accepted as common truths. Impurities in the body affect the mind, creating impure thoughts and actions, which in turn affect the family, leaving a karmic residue for all to absorb and overcome. I take my piece of paper with the drawings of stick figure bodies bending and twisting to show me the path toward purity, pay my fee for my diagnosis, and set up my next visit.

❀

For several days I have been bothering Khan for an interview. He agrees to meet me, but first I must meet with the peer educators of Sahodaran. Khan wants them to hear my story, not just for my perspective on living with HIV, but so they can meet a professional man who is not straight.

Sunil and Anto serve as translators and I sit on the floor after lunch in a packed room of young men. "Just tell them about yourself, Michael, and how you take care of yourself, the yoga and all that," Sunil tells me before I speak. I'd figured I'd admit I had some problems with drugs and dealing with my bisexuality and then reinforce how yoga had helped me embrace my body again after the diagnosis. But when I look out at their faces, so eager and real, I know I must tell them things I've never publicly admitted. I try to recall for them the days before I became infected, but I fall into embarrassing blank silences, unable to control my emotions, as I confess how often I took drugs or got drunk to silence the shame I felt about my desires for men and that I was so fucked up that I couldn't remember where I was or who I was sleeping with. I tell them how depressed I was when I learned of my diagnosis, how I'd wanted to kill myself. Their eyes are so penetrating, I can barely look at them. I rush to the happy ending, give my spiel about yoga's benefits, eager to get it over with.

"Do you want to ask Michael some questions now?" Sunil suggests. Immediately several hands go up. One bold question follows the next: "Why do you look so strong if you have AIDS?" One young man asks, while another crawls over to me and pinches my biceps, swooning dramatically as the room explodes in laughter. I laugh, too, but it's not funny. It's only a reprieve as the questions become more personal: "Why did you have to take drugs so that you could have sex? Why did you keep it a secret from your friends that you were having sex with men?" My body shrinks with each question; I hunch and stare at the floor. There's no letting up: "Do you like Indian men? Who do you want to sleep with here?" (Followed by roars and nervous pushing and shoving among them.) "In America, I've heard you can live like you are married to your boyfriend, walk around and kiss on the street, is that true?" "Do you have a boyfriend? Why not?" The questions probe deeper and deeper, each questioner trying to out-do the next in audacity. One young man cuts to the quick: "You said you thought of killing yourself, why would you think that?"

It isn't the question that silences the room; it's the way the young man asks it. Even before I hear the translation from Anto, I know what he has asked. The sadness and surprise in his voice constricts my own throat. *Why, sir? Why take your own life?* My head sinks to my chest, my eyes fix on my bare feet. I can't bear to look at their faces, young men who struggle daily to survive, who have been beaten and robbed, who are ridiculed and humiliated, but go on with their lives. How fitting, that it is these boys who serve as my confessors. No answer comes to describe the blackness that was my life then; language itself was what I wanted to annihilate. Words, my own words, betrayed me day after day. Only silence kept me alive, and I reach for it here out of habit.

Khan hovers in the back, coming in and out from doing work in the other room. For someone like him, a gay man from London who has lived through the onslaught of AIDS, watching friends and lovers die, and now works to prevent the plague from spreading across South Asia's MSM communities, mine is an old, old story. My silence must have pulled him away from his computer, or perhaps he anticipated my response: "I wanted to die because I was ashamed."

My answer lingers in the air. Then Khan interrupts the silence: "But see, he does yoga. He takes care of himself. See, he's strong." Khan underscores one more time what he wants the boys to hear, that HIV can strike anyone, even the blond man from America with the strong arms. "Do you have anything else that you want to tell them Michael?" he asks, looking at me with his warrior's face. "Yes. It's your body," I tell them lifting my head and pointing to my chest. "Take control of it, take care of it. Don't let anyone make you feel bad about it."

I meet Khan at a tea stall around the corner from Sahodaran later that day. The late afternoon sun pours into the shop, steam rises from vats of chai, biscuits bake in ovens in the back, and the walls drip with condensation. Sweat smears the words in my notebook. Khan is oblivious to the heat: "This is nothing compared to Delhi."

Chain-smoking, in a voice that alternates between bitterness and compassion, he shares his personal story, with asides on Foucault and Marxist theory, and a cold analysis of India and South Asia's impending AIDS explosion. He seems pressed for time, but I get the impression that he is always in a hurry, flying from Lucknow to London then back to Delhi, giving trainings, meeting government officials, setting up new programs like Sahodaran. He is working against a ticking time bomb: "It makes me pessimistic when I think about it. India is going to explode. 500 million males, 300 million sexually active men and a huge number under 30." He shrugs and lifts his eyes. The math is clear. The Indian government has no idea of the gravity of the problem, he says. They're getting the message but they don't know how to respond. "It's too difficult to talk about, because it deals with sex. So, publicly, they don't know how to speak about it." It's politically expedient, he believes, to see the rise in AIDS cases as a sign of Western decadence infiltrating Indian society, further illustrating the need to maintain Hindu traditional culture. "We have a serious problem here with the gap between what politicians say and what they do," he spits out in anger.

India's public health system is already stretched beyond its means. He reminds me that India already has an STD and Hepatitis B epidemic. With rising rates of malaria and TB, persistent malnutrition, and a severe and growing shortage in potable drinking water, AIDS is just one more crisis for India.[5] Khan shakes his head and drinks his tea.

As passionate as he is about politics and public health, it's India's cultural attitudes toward sexuality that disturb him most. He blows smoke through his nostrils but it might as easily be fire. "MSMs and commercial sex workers are social outcasts here," says Khan, and so the epidemic continues unabated as these people are seen as impure and, like the Dalits (the untouchables), unworthy of much concern. To help them would appear to condone their practices. "There are many doctors who refuse to treat people with HIV," he says, frowning, "they even ostracize those physicians who do."

To understand Indian attitudes about sexuality, he tells me, you have to understand, first and foremost, the preeminence of the family. Identity is shaped by the family, not necessarily by what one does for oneself outside it. What successes individuals have in business or in school are a direct reflection on the family that supports them. To remain single is unthinkable for most Indians. Consequently, according to Khan, men who are sexually attracted to other men would never consider not marrying, but rather act discreetly on their desire while still maintaining their duties to their family. Khan reminds me that many of the young men I've met at Sahodaran are married and that most of those who are single will eventually marry. Without a wife or family, life can be very difficult for a man in Indian society.[6]

Khan believes a profound revolution is occurring as Western commercial culture seeps into traditional social systems and beliefs. "The middle class is trying to learn how to be behaviorally heterosexual," he explains. He uses as an example that teenagers now date and go to movies without chaperones, whereas before, and still in rural and traditional culture, men never met their wives until the wedding night. Even in the middle class, sex is still seen as something for procreation alone, particularly among women. One has *duties* to fulfill, as I have heard Indian men and women describe it. "All of this is in flux now," says Khan, "and it is complicating how to address STDs and AIDS, as people want to believe in the older ways while wanting to liberalize society and look to the West for how to live and advance economically and technologically."

I am puzzled by the dramatic difference between the ancient religious symbols of Hindu beliefs and practices, which still permeate Indian culture, and the conservative attitudes toward sexuality that he describes. How does one explain, I ask him, Shiva devotees placing flowers and fruit and prostrating before a stone phallus? Or the many depictions of the Kama Sutra's arts of love chiseled beautifully on sacred temples? What happened?

"The British, of course," he wryly retorts. "Indians have re-imposed a Victorian, neo-colonial morality denying their own past." Those lively forms of sexual expression in Indian mythology and history found in dance, theatre, literature, iconography and daily life, Khan believes, have been manipulated to suit a patriarchal ideology in rural India. Here, he explains, in rural India, where women were once repositories of tradition, they can now only be interpreters of it, following the rules of men. He also cites the changes in the gender separation of labor and the way in which boy children became rural capital for families. According to Khan, these changes in Indian society are a direct result of the British occupation. Now they are believed to be authentic Indian aspects of tradition, particularly by those living in urban India who want to romanticize rural traditions for political and economic gain. Consequently, India's complex and multiple cultural histories are being silenced.

Ironically, Khan points out, India is responding to HIV and other STDs in much the same way the British did when thousands of their soldiers contracted syphilis during Britain's rule of the subcontinent. The solution then was to blame prostitutes, close down brothels, and condemn those men who lowered themselves to the level of the uncivil behavior of Indians. Similarly, India's government believes the solution to its AIDS outbreak is enforcing stricter laws on immoral behavior, that is, by penalizing sex workers and drug users. Khan shakes his head at how little people have learned in a hundred years, still refusing to open their eyes to the social, sexual, and cultural context that underlies and spreads sexually transmitted diseases.

He also doesn't have a lot of praise for the so-called AIDS experts in positions to make policy. "Doctors, politicians, and international donors don't have enough understanding of the problems, because they themselves really can't see from the mind and the bodies of those who are living in these worlds." What India has, he believes, is mostly a donor driven policy, well-meaning people who really don't understand those they are trying to serve. "Oh, they know all the right buzz words and can speak the language," he sighs. "And they have been reinforced by those who admire them for what they are doing. But this is charity work, which is different than community development."

He points to the boys working in the tea stall: "the boys at Sahodaran service them," he tells me. In the back of the shop, these shirtless, thin boys slave away, running back and forth between the ovens to take trays of tea out into the streets to the shop owners. In India, as elsewhere in the developing world, those who live at the bottom must survive by exchanging goods and services in the underground economy. It's in this invisible economy that at least half the world's people must eke out a living.

Khan sees the work of the Naz Foundation as radical but essentially pragmatic. "We are trying to make the young men at Sahodaran into a cohesive, self-sustaining community. It's the only way they are going to survive not only this disease but this life."

Khan's activism is about demanding that the world pay attention to the forces at the root of this disease: declining resources, poverty, powerlessness, cultural beliefs that mock human dignity and preserve only the rights and security of the powerful. Fittingly, the HIV virus is itself a model for Khan's brand of activism. Like the virus, the work of activists and their organizations replicates themselves, latching on to new sources of strength in order to distribute its message ever more broadly. This organic social movement spreads resistance not only to the indifferent biological machinery of HIV, but also to the more deadly indifference of human beings to the suffering that surrounds them.

❊

Y. R. Gaitonde AIDS research clinic sits off by itself behind an aging colonial-era government hospital. Once a tuberculosis and leprosy clinic, this clinic serves all of South India.[7] On the grounds outside this pink, two-story building, women are doing laundry and spreading green bedding on weeds. Men sit under shade trees. Inside, patients cluster in corners. They are mostly men, but there are families and couples, too. I talk with the clinic's office manager, a calm young woman named Rochelle. She tells me that many of the patients have traveled sometimes as far as three hundred kilometers to get here.

Though there are twelve beds, YRG mostly serves outpatients. Those who are too sick either die at home or are brought to the government TB hospital, a facility that Sunil warned me away from: "Don't go there, Michael. The patients are dying on the floors and hallways. You don't want to see this."

The doctors at YRG Clinic are harried and worn down, not only by the ever-increasing patient load, but also by a stream of international benefactors and doctors interested in their research. The woman behind YRG, Dr. Sunita Solomon, has become a kind of AIDS superstar, and is constantly in demand to speak at the proliferating number of international commissions and medical conferences. While I wait to see the other doctors, I recognize in the faces of the patients that blank stare, that feeling of trying to shrink oneself into invisibility.

A hand pulls open a curtain: behind it appears a doctor who looks more Chinese or Tibetan than Indian. He wears khakis and a blue shirt with black-rimmed glasses; he is standing beside a man who sits in a chair, his body stiff and unable to move as if stunned or drugged. Doctor Yepthorani keeps talking to him, patting him on the shoulder, then looks at me, "One more person, please and then I will have some time, sorry to keep you waiting."

Dr. Tukugha Yepthorani (or Tuku as he suggests I call him) is not easy to understand; he speaks in quick rushes of words, as if his mind is somewhere else. He begins, before I even ask, with a sarcastic summing up of the AIDS business: "It's really a way for a lot of people to make money, get better jobs, and gives them a chance to travel and see the world." He points to the patients outside the curtain of his cubicle: "There is a long line, you see it, right? There will be more tomorrow, and the day after more still. It is much bigger than anyone believes. We only see those who are coming in because they are sick. We are just now beginning to see how bad it really is," he says, frowning. Dr. Yepthorani provides another stark example of the magnitude of the epidemic. A community health project sponsored by the U.S., he tells me, allows doctors like him to go into poor neighborhoods each month to offer basic care and evaluations for any number of health problems. "Each time we go on these health camps we find four or five out of about seventy people who test positive for HIV," he says, raising his eyebrows. "Who knows how many people are infected—eight, nine, ten million?"

Dr. Yepthorani seems bitter and tired of talking to journalists. When I talk about how activists have inspired my writing about the epidemic, he scoffs, saying they are always arguing among themselves and can't do much for those who need medications. Suddenly, he looks at me and asks: "Why do you want to do this? What kind of story do you want to write? Are you from some newspaper? Perhaps I can help you, but today I just don't have time." His attitude provokes me. I can see that if I'm going to get anywhere, I'd better reveal my status and purpose myself. "I represent nobody, no paper, no magazine, I am HIV positive and I want to write . . ."

"When were you infected?" he interrupts, eyes narrowing.

"1996."

He moves closer. "What are your counts?"

"Uh, I don't know. I'm off the drugs right now."

"Oh yes, but before."

"Three hundred or so T cells last time they checked. My viral load is pretty low."

"Have you heard of me? Do you know of the Indian Supreme Court case banning the marriage of people with HIV?"

"No, I haven't."

"That is me, the case. It was in response to a suit I filed." For the first time, his tone changes: "We were diagnosed in the same year."

I am confused: What court case? Banning his marriage? Did he just tell me he was positive?

"It's a sad story," he begins as I pull out my notebook. "I was an ophthalmologist in my home city in Manipur, (a state in the northeastern part of India near the border of China and Myanmar). I was to be married; bought the wedding dress, everything. I donated blood for my cousin who needed an operation. Then I went to Kolkata to get the wedding things and the dress. When I came back, everything was ruined. You see, the hospital had told them, told them before I got there. Everyone knew. Everyone except me."

"I became an activist. You know, INP?" I nod. I'd interviewed a Muslim man, the secretary of India Network Positive, the day before. "I was the first president. We started it. I took the hospital to court. Big case. You want me to tell you about that? . . ." He looks at his watch. "Where are you staying? Are you hungry? Go eat something and come back later and I can talk to you between patients."

I agree, rushing out to find some place to write out my notes from the interview, but before I can sit down, I am told that the other doctor can now see me. I am ushered into another room to find Dr. Madhivavan sitting behind her desk writing. She smiles politely, rises, offers me a chair, and orders tea. Thin, with hair pulled back in a bun and piercing, intelligent eyes, she is far more relaxed than Dr. Tuku. I like her immediately and surprise myself by telling her my status at once.

She sits up and leans out of her chair, inviting me to tell her more. "Have you spoken with Dr. Toku—the other doctor?"

"I just spoke with him. He's—he's exactly who I want to write about."

She nods, gravely, "Yes, yes. He inspires us all here."

"My story is not that interesting," she begins. "I was drawn here by Dr. Solomon. I volunteered one day a week, then two, and after three days Solomon asked me to come on board full time. They had no one who really understood or had the time to work with women and reproductive health; I thought I could help." Like Dr. Yepthorani, she has a ring of exhaustion and bitterness in her voice. This is a research center, she says, and she herself has contributed an important study for the use of the effective drug nevirapine to reduce mother-to-child transmission. She is very proud of this work. But she tells of spending far too much time on meetings, entertaining American doctors and health officials who are constantly streaming through the clinic. "We spend all of this money and time on them; it really is upsetting at times. We have all these people to see and there we are with these nice people who—; sorry, you don't want to hear this. I'm a little tired, today."

She *is* tired. I am not sure if I ought to tell an Indian physician about yoga, but I do, wanting to know what she thinks about it. When I tell her how important it has been for me, she agrees. "I know, I know, I do some pranayama and some poses. I wish I could do more. I swim, that's what relaxes me . . . when I can get some time. I have a son, and my husband is always traveling. It's hard."

Recognizing her fatigue and worried that I've taken up too much of her time, I tell her, by way of a farewell, how impressed I am with the work of the clinic. She smiles, but wearily. "My parents asked me when I came here, 'when are you going to get a real job?' People don't think very much of what we are doing. Doctors in India don't want to deal with this at all. They refuse to treat people, find excuses, or simply ignore what they see. They don't want to be seen as someone who treats people with AIDS."

I ask her what she considers the most difficult problems India faces in responding to HIV. She pauses to think for a moment. "These women are so ashamed when they come in here. They won't even look down [at their own bodies] when I ask them to point or show me where they have pain or have been experiencing sores. They say things like: 'He does things to me down there.' I've seen at least 1000 women over the last year and one, only one," she says, raising her finger, "has told me that she believed sex was something that gave her pleasure."

Her anecdote typifies the problems that lie ahead in confronting this epidemic for India. If it continues to deny women their rights to avoid conceiving children, protect themselves or even experience pleasure, how can they ever expect women to learn how to prevent themselves from being infected?

She shakes her head. "I'm burned out. I'm going to America to get a post doc in public health, so that I can be with my son and take a break from this. Then when I come back, I'll try to open another clinic somewhere else. We need so many more of these." Then she pauses and changes her tone: "Have you eaten?"

I've had nothing but cups of tea since breakfast, but of course I beg off. "No that's okay, I'm going back to my hotel." She makes a face, returning to her role as doctor. But before I have a chance to thank her and make my exit, in comes Dr. Yepthorani with several plastic bags of food. The two doctors relax in each other's company. Dr. Yepthorani is glad to see me. "You eat with us? Here, you like curry chicken? We don't have a fork, but you can eat with the bread, you know how, right?"

Doctor Madhivavan apologizes, "I know it's not exactly the best place to eat, but I can clean off my desk, sit here." So I sit and eat, as they talk shop and dollop more food onto a piece of plastic I use as a plate. "Here, eat," they command, pointing to the food before me.

✻

Two days later, after another afternoon sitting in another clinic wait-ing to see a doctor who didn't have time to see me, I'm back in another rickshaw looking for a community organization called Positive Women Network. Traversing the city reveals the multiple worlds within India: mosques next to Hindu temples, international hotels next to tea stalls, open markets next to shopping complexes, small motor fix-it shops next to internet cafés. School children, in uniform, parade down the streets alongside an old man and a little girl with straggly hair who leads an emaciated monkey on a string. Maybe it's the afternoon I'd spent at this clinic, where female sex workers sat slumped in chairs with their chil-dren crawling on the floor, but Chennai is starting to take its toll on me.

I find the street and begin to look for the address. Walking along a narrow road barely wider than an alley, I cover my head as forty-year-old buses leave billowing clouds of dust and diesel smoke as they pass. Walking feels like wading through water. It's so hot that it burns to touch my hair.

I have to call for the third time from a phone shop. As soon as I hang up, a woman crosses the street and waves to me. "Madame Kousalya has been waiting for you. We thought you might not come." She is shy, refusing to look me in the eye. "I am a social work student; I volunteer for the women here, translate and write things for them." She takes me through two hallways into the back of an old cement block building, up a narrow, dark stairway to the two-room office of PWN+ (Positive Women Network Plus).

Dwarfed behind her desk, Ms. P. Kousalya, the president of PWN, has the stature of a teenage girl. She is well under five feet. Her dress hangs too loosely from her small frame. The dress is made of tradition-al khati cloth, the cloth Gandhi had instructed Indians to spin and wear to boycott the cloth from Britain during the independence movement. Her face is thin, her skin unhealthy; yet when she smiles and begins to speak, her eyes flash an intense, but calming, green that belies her meek-ness and sickly body.

Kousalya comes from Namakkal, one of the areas in Tamil Nadu hardest hit by the epidemic. Her story is another tale of the struggles of Indian women to stand up to the age-old injustices meted out on them. These stories begin to sound like folktales, with the same plot and char-acters. Mother dies. Father marries evil step mother. Step mother works her and siblings to the bone. Greedy father forces her to marry against her will to secure property. She hides from her villainous husband, cry-ing in her room every night, until he catches and rapes her. When hus-band becomes sick, she learns he is HIV positive. She leaves him, becomes sick, and discovers she too is HIV positive. Ex-husband tries to marry another wife, but she attempts to file a lawsuit to prevent him from infecting another woman. Husband dies. But here the story changes dramatically. Broke and ostracized, and against all odds, Kousalya begins a second life as an activist, creating India's first support group solely for women living with HIV.

PWN serves over eighty women, she tells me. It is an offshoot of India Positive Network, the support group started by Dr. Yepthorani. "We felt we needed to have our own group to address our own problems," she explains. The group provides support for women and their families; they also pass out information on women's health and medicine. She shows me a little bear and some other stuffed toys and trinkets that they make; "soft toys," she calls them. Toys are part of an income-generating project. The organization has begun to branch out around the country, especially in south India, offering workshops for women and helping them to create their own support groups.

I try to keep up with her intensity and the earnest translation of the volunteer, but I am so tired from the heat I can barely form legible words in my notebook. I float in and out, my mind in a haze, and at times it seems as if her voice is coming from inside my own head. They order tea, but it doesn't help. I give in to the fatigue and realize that the important thing is to listen to her words and look into her eyes.

She sees beyond her life now; her energy and will seem to come from her motivation to help other women, and no longer from her anger at what she has had to suffer. And it's this voice, this power that I selfishly find myself sucking into my heart. "We are not treated good at the hospitals, not given respect. They tell us we will die and that there are no drugs. We go home crying, but we don't let anybody bring us down," she says with a matter-of-fact tone. "Sometimes we have to go to two or three hospitals before they see us. Some doctors say they won't treat us because we deserve our illness, blaming us for the disease. They think we are the sex worker." With this kind of treatment and advice, it's no wonder that, along with opportunistic infections, depression poses a serious threat to the health of HIV-positive women. She gets depressed, she says, worrying about money and food for her children. But her work drives away the depression: "When I come to work, I forget all the sad things. We have picnics, we shop together, we help each other with childcare."

I inquire about what treatment she uses. She tells me that she and other woman at PWN are offered free samples from doctors who get them from drug reps,[8] but she knows that can't go on forever. The government is beginning to provide drugs, but they are still too expensive for most people.

Mercifully, the sun is finally going down. More tea is served, and Kousalya repeats a now familiar refrain about her fears that the government is spending too much time and money penalizing those they think are spreading the virus, rather than on protecting and educating those most vulnerable—young people and women.

When I ask her about traditional treatments, such as ayurveda and siddha, which use herbal medicines, massage, and special diets to heal and purify the body, she has mixed feelings: "Many women get their hopes up for these promises that they see on television and in the news-papers." She, too, has tried some of the traditional treatments, which she says are a mix of steroids and other mysterious medicines. "You feel good for a while and gain weight, but they give you side effects and you must stop taking them." Yet, she adds, "at least they touch us, the tra-ditional doctors. The hospital doctors don't."

❖

I return to the YRG clinic a few days later and spend an afternoon with Dr. Yepthorani, as he sees patients. Most are poor lorry drivers in soiled pants, who somewhere along the routes of their migratory lives, have contracted the virus. His patients are so anxious about what the doctor will tell them, they barely notice that I am there. He asks how they are feeling, takes a household flashlight from off his desk and looks inside their mouths. Then he feels under chins for swelling in lymph nodes and checks their lungs with a stethoscope. With a warm demeanor, he coun-sels, gives prescriptions, and answers questions. One man wants to know if he should get the CD4 and viral load tests to determine the progression of the disease. Dr. Yepthorani tells him it's a good idea, but the drugs cost a lot of money—1,200 rupees ($30) for CD4 and 6,000 rupees ($120) for viral load—and that once they begin to take the medications, they must take them for the rest of their lives. The men look confused and saddened, knowing they can't afford it.[9] At one point, trying to cheer him up, Dr. Yepthorani points to me, "See, he's from America, he is still alive and has it many years." He says nothing about the fact that I have been taking drugs for four years, nor does he tell them about himself. "I only tell peo-ple," he tells me later, "if I think it will really help them."

After hearing the costs of tests and medicine, one man asks about a cure offered by a siddha doctor in the state of Kerala. With a stern face, Yepthorani lectures against going: "Don't go there! Waste of your money." The man is disappointed; clearly he's looking for some good news.

I envy doctors like him in the middle of this epidemic. Not because of what they must face every day, but because they have a tangible skill for alleviating suffering—a talent for conveying hope, a touch to allay fear. Writing about this is my only act of healing, and a debatable one at that. How much more good could I offer if I wore a white coat?

Watching patient and doctor interact, I see how intimate we become with our doctors, and how doctors become intimate with us. We are their work, mirrors reflecting who they are, if, that is, they take the time to see themselves in us. We need the hope that medicine represents, the possibility of a cure, but more than that, we need the firm grip of the physician to lead us into the redemptive cure that comes from accepting our bodies and facing ourselves. The men look at me, and I try to exude something from my eyes that might give them strength, or at least the sense that I know what they are feeling. But *I* don't know; how could I possibly know what they must face? People with little chance of ever being able to afford or receive the same treatment I have. People who fear for their family's survival if they die. People who are terrified of neighbors discovering their status, knowing their families will be shunned.

"They want to know when the cure is coming," Dr. Yepthorani says, looking at rashes on a man's back. "They ask every time."

"What do you tell them?"

He shrugs. "We tell them it is coming, it is coming."

Dr. Yepthorani steps to a window and lights a cigarette, embarrassed that he smokes, but it only makes him that much more human. I ask him to elaborate on the story he told me of his return from Kolkata with the wedding dress for his fiancée. He tells me that after he found out, there was nothing he could do but leave his family, his hometown and his medical practice. He muses: "We all have our problems: poor people, rich people, people with HIV." Then he pauses, trying to hold on to his role as doctor. "I was shattered. Everything I had was gone." He exhales smoke out the second story window. "I went back to that hospital in Kolkata, and I asked them: 'Why didn't you tell me? I am a doctor.' Total breach of confidentiality." He returns to me in the room, his anger still there. "Why did they have to embarrass my family, and my fiancée's family? I was thinking of suicide then. I was heartbroken. I came here to Madras because of the clinic. Dr. Solomon, she saved me, she knew it would be best for me to work, so she mentioned that they could use me to help patients and counsel them. And now, here I am."

"What about your court case?" I ask.

He chuckles, shaking his head. "The case was eventually taken to the Supreme Court. But they threw the case out for some made up technicality."

The story doesn't end there. The morning after the Supreme Court threw out his case, he woke up to find camera crews and reporters outside of his apartment. Incredibly, overnight the court decided to rule against him and in favor of the hospital. In so doing, the court created a new law, barring all people with HIV from marrying. Today, because of this case, it is illegal for any person in India who is HIV positive to marry.

At the time of his court's decision, he was engaged again to be married, this time to a woman who works at YRG clinic. "My picture was in the papers," he laughs, sarcastically. "I got married anyway," he says. "Now I ask everyone who is positive to get married. They call me the matchmaker. I want to help everyone get married to defy this ridiculous law. What about you? Are you married?"

I shake my head. We laugh together, but awkwardness dampens the humor. There it is, that word, *marriage*, like a plate shattering in a restaurant. He senses my sadness and apologizes for not being able to invite me to stay with him and his wife, lamenting that they don't have the room.

As I'm getting ready to go, he calls his wife, dialing the phone in front of me. I get the sense that talking about her made him want to call. I try not to listen, pretending to fuss around in my pack, but I can't avoid overhearing him. He has nothing more to say than that he's coming home soon and he will pick up something to eat. We say goodbye in that abrupt way men have, avoiding the eyes, avoiding that last touch of the hands.

On my way out of the clinic, I glance into the ward one more time. I see a woman lying in a bed in the corner with her arm over her face. Outside, a few patients sit under a tree, others on the steps of the clinic. Away from the rest, a man sits in a chair with a bloodstained bandage on his wrist. Glassy-eyed, he looks away into the evening as a woman, perhaps his wife, gently rubs his neck. Dust turns the setting sun orange, as the heat releases the city from its grip. It is a bittersweet image: the pink hospital, the patients leaning against what is left of their lives, the long warm shadows of the clinic on the red earth, the black birds in the dirty trees; death blending into life as day fades into night.

❋

Almost every day Lakshmi leaves messages at the hotel wanting to know how I'm doing. She feels remiss that I must stay at a hotel and worries that I'm not eating well and that the stress and pollution of the city are unhealthy for me. More than once she has invited me to her home, but it is too impractical as she lives outside of the city. But when she asks me to address a training session for social workers at the hospital where she works, she insists I come for dinner and spend the night. "It's by the sea, so much cooler, you will like it."

At the hospital, she parades me around floor by floor, introducing me to everyone. She also takes me to see her patients, men lying around in pajamas rehabilitating in dimly lit wards.

Lakshmi's students are young, earnest, and naïve. As I speak candidly about contracting HIV and my own problems with addiction, introducing the idea that sex, too, can be an addiction, they sit bolt upright in their chairs. In back of the room Lakshmi and her female colleagues nod politely, faces frozen, hands tightly clasped in laps. When I ask the trainees to try some yoga, many nervously look around wondering if they should follow this wild man from America. A few stiffly refuse, including a young nun in her habit with a crucifix staring back at me. I try to convince her that many practicing Catholics do yoga, but she is defiant.

Most of the trainees reluctantly stand and follow my instructions. I ask them to reach their hands over their head and other simple poses that they can do sitting in a chair. After doing a few breathing exercises and a short meditation, I ask them to write about the differences they feel in their body. When they are done, Lakshmi asks for questions. Nobody lifts a hand. So she asks me about yoga's benefits for people living with HIV. After telling them it helps me care for my body, more students find the courage to speak.

When the class is over, a few students come up and shyly shake my hand, including the nun, who seems afraid to touch me, but I extend my hand, forcing her to take it or reject it. "I agree with you. Prayer and meditation can heal people. I will pray for you." With her tiny hands together at her heart, as is the Indian custom when addressing a teacher, she bows and exits.

Weaving through afternoon traffic on her motorbike, Lakshmi drives us to the outskirts of Chennai. On our way, rising out of the poverty and dust, we pass a gleaming, cobalt-blue, glass multistory building. Quietly Chennai has become an attractive home along with neighboring Bangalore for many software corporations and their subsidiaries, although no signs identify them. The incongruity of thatch shanties clinging to the tall security fence and women carrying bricks on their heads building the road leading into this modern corporate center detracts from the promise these corporations might hold for India's poor.

Lakshmi's neighborhood is indeed much quieter. We bump along streets of sand flanked by palms and tall eucalyptus trees, passing single-family dwellings of stucco with potted plants on tile porches. Then we arrive at a low-rise, breezy condominium, with men hovering about watering flowers and guarding cars. I immediately head out to the beach, breaking into a barefoot run along the surf. Energized, I think of pulling off my shirt and diving in when I realize that nobody is swimming and no man has his shirt off. In the evening breeze, women stroll along the beach with saris flapping behind them, children run in the surf, and young men play cricket on the beach head. This place is a welcome relief from the smog and claustrophobia of Chennai.

Lakshmi's home is a modest, two-bedroom condo with a small porch on the ground floor. In the kitchen is a two-burner gas stove and mini refrigerator. Krishna, their six-year-old daughter, introduces herself and then goes off to a neighbor's for the night. Lakshmi's husband comes in from jogging; we exchange awkward greetings, realizing we passed each other on the beach without speaking. He grabs two beers and gives one to me, turns on the TV, and goes into a long explanation about cricket and the hopes of India's national team. He watches the game with me a while and then retreats to the porch to make phone calls in the dark and smoke. Disapprovingly, Lakshmi comes in and turns off the TV, frowning, asking me to carry some snacks onto the porch. My attention is on what is smoldering in the ashtray, and I can't seem to think of much to say, until I make my move, "Do you mind if I have some of your smoke?"

"Oh! I'm sorry, sure. Take all you want."

The awkwardness quickly melts away under the pungent smoke. We sit in the candlelight talking until their friends arrive for dinner. They are old college friends, activists and lawyers who work part-time on legal aid for various community organizations. The lawyers reinforce what others have said about the fears of the middle class concerning AIDS. They mention the archaic infrastructure of laws and customs that hamper India's evolution from a disparate collection of cultures and states into a more prosperous and egalitarian society. "The problem," one of them sarcastically observes, "is the government just wishes half a billion poor people would go away so that we can modernize and not have to be burdened by them." The friends take apart the government, ask questions about my work, eat and smoke, and drift naturally onto subjects I can't follow. But I don't much mind. The smoke has me drifting away, too.

How narrow my life is, I think, as I listen to these couples, content in their simple apartment with motorbikes and two-burner gas stoves, eating with friends, articulating their nuanced views of politics while laughing and reminiscing about some hiking trip they've taken together into the Himalayas. When the guests go home, I retire to the daughter's room and lie in the dark with her stuffed toys, listening to the surf, feeling the loneliness that accompanies the intimacy of travel.

The next day Lakshmi gets me up early so that we can attend her yoga class down the street. The yoga center is on the top of what appears to be someone's home, a rooftop covered by thatch to shield students from the sun. The rooftop fills with a mixture of men and women of all ages. It's a basic class, taught by a doctor, who receives no pay for his teaching. The usual self-consciousness and competition one usually finds in American yoga classes are noticeably absent. People's bodies are softer. They are in less of a hurry. Each pose is followed by a moment of rest before beginning the next. Normally, this slowed-down style would annoy me. But this is the same style I am learning from my teacher at the Krishnamacharya Centre, and I like the mellifluous voice of the doctor/teacher as he counts out the breath. He watches me carefully, asking me to slow down several times, slapping the tops of my feet as I do what I think is a pretty good shoulder stand. "Too tight, too tight; too much effort." Afterward we all sit together, students and teacher, and calmly drink tea before heading out into the day.

❋

I am back on the beach a few days later, albeit Chennai's beach, where thousands of the city's poor come each night to escape the heat, amble among the makeshift food and trinket stalls, and mingle in the darkness. The beach is where Sahodaran's peer counselors hand out condoms as well as meet some of their clients. On the way, Sunil wants to show me another area where the counselors work. We stop along a polluted, stagnant river. Behind us are the backs of two- and three-story commercial buildings. The wooded strip along the river might have been a park at one time, but now looks more like a dump than a park as piles of rubbish and mounds of old bricks and debris line the road. Hidden from the life of the city, rickshaw drivers sleep and men meet to have sex behind the trees. Sunil points out a man moving among the shadowy branches. I nod as if astonished, but I've frequented places like this in almost every city I've ever lived.

The rickshaw driver drops us off in a wooded park next to the beach. Sunil, Ravi, one of his trusted field workers, and I walk under a canopy of trees until we hit sand. It's growing dark, and I can't see where I'm going. But I follow closely behind them until I see rats hopping out of the weeds and scurrying ahead. I pull up, concerned. "I thought we were going to a beach?"

Sunil laughs, "It's up here. Watch your step; it's like a toilet here."

We hike up and down mounds of sand, through dry weeds and trash, and around small leafless trees; then out pops a man from behind a clump of bushes by a miasmic pool of stagnant water. Ravi greets the man and they walk back into the shadows. Sunil and I follow at a distance. I have gotten to know Ravi in my visits to Sahodaran. I watch him disappear into the darkness, a young man who might be in his late twenties but looks much younger, as do most of the other boys, being shorter and more feminine in appearance. I feel nervous for him, seeing, now, the world in which he works. But there he is opening his satchel to hand the man some condoms, who then is gone again, back into the bushes. Returning, Ravi explains that the man in the bushes has a client.

Though dark, it is still steamy even by the beach. Lanterns glow and an invisible mass of people murmur in the distance. We slog through the sand. Finally, I hear the surf and children playing and begin to see clusters of people sitting on their haunches eating. We meet other sex workers or they have been following us, I can't tell. Ravi and Sunil greet them.

I'm oblivious, under the spell of the ocean, wanting to sit beside it and be mesmerized by the silver luminescence of its waves, which, like these boys, seem to emerge out of darkness.

Stepping into the warmth of the people and the bazaar, I can see the sex workers who have followed us out of the darkness. They have thin, bony bodies with handsome noses. Their oily black hair catches the light from the lanterns, their unbuttoned shirts flap in the breeze from the sea. They study me, too: the blond man from America with the smiling teeth and the anxious body. We amble up to a long line of vendors that have set up shop on the beach. We pass wooden tables with vats of sauce and rice, women frying chapati, piles of samosas on platters, pastel colored candies in glass boxes, tea in tin urns, sweaty bottles of Coca Cola, biscuits stacked in plastic jars. It's a playground, picnic ground, and a place where men can float off into the darkness and meet other men. As we walk down a row of vendors of shells, bangles, toys, and t-shirts, I see that we have drawn some attention. At first I think it's me, but no, it's me with them, the *kothis*, who are as much a part of this nighttime beach bazaar as the vendors. "They all know what these boys do," Sunil whispers, pointing to a couple of guys selling sodas who smile knowingly at us.

I buy everyone sodas and offer to take pictures. Combs come out and they tuck in shirts and primp, using each other as mirrors. Another peer counselor spots us. I remember him from the center, always wearing a baseball cap and flowered shirt. He's the artist who paints signs for storeowners and sews clothes. He shows me his mini portfolio tucked in his satchel along with his condoms. I study them, abstract human figures drawn in pastel chalk without faces or feet, sexually indistinguishable, languid and willowy.

We walk back toward the dimly lit street where couples and groups of teenage boys stroll under the large banyan trees. Three women scurry toward us, waving, bangles jangling, sari scarves flowing off their necks. Their gaudy, made-up faces, nose rings, and diamond bindis don't quite camouflage their masculine chins and cheeks, nor do their saris and dainty shoes so gracefully fit. Sunil and Ravi and the other peer counselors greet them with hugs. I offer my hand and they nervously giggle, not sure who I am. They are the hijras, transgender men, hermaphrodites, or neutered men.

From ancient times, hijras have served in various ceremonial purposes at certain temples, particularly those devoted to the worship of Kali, the dark goddess, who represents the terrifying destructive element in the cosmos. Today, except in the southern region of Kerala, hijras are generally harshly ostracized by society. They are believed to be a sign of bad luck if crossed in the streets. Thus custom has it that you must give them money if they ask for it, or else suffer their evil will. They run off back into the darkness of the park, fearful of being seen by the police, who frequently beat and rob them as they do the peer counselors and other sex workers.

In the merciful dimness, on a beach strewn with litter and shit, one still finds the brightest saris, the mirrors framed in seashells, the sugary sweets, and the photo galleries, where the poor can pose next to a cardboard Bollywood star.

One can look at these young men crawling about under the bushes and think how pathetic to be reduced to performing these acts, but in their work, as in their lives, they have learned a very basic lesson: to trust the human need for affection. And like the tantric teachers from ancient times, these boys see that the body can both trap the soul or free it.

❋

I've been told about an AIDS activist who travels alone into the rural villages and towns devastated by AIDS in southern Tamil Nadu. Anto, the peer counselor, accompanies me as we head through densely packed neighborhoods, in search of Mr. B. Sekar and his community organization for MSMs.

Sekar is thin, with that ghostly, gaunt face characteristic of those with HIV, yet his energy and spirit belie his physical form. He takes us into the offices of SWAM (Social Welfare Association for Men), which is also the house where he lives. We sit in a whitewashed, cave-like room overlooking a shady courtyard of mango and eucalyptus trees. Sekar's English is understandable, but he talks so fast Anto has to translate. He recounts his story as if on remote control, and I try to ask questions to slow and break him out of his rote responses.

He begins with a frank history of his sexual coming of age: "I was confused. I felt like God had punished me because I can't be excited about women and sex with them. At first, I didn't know anything about AIDS. I'd heard about it, yes, but I really didn't have any idea about it. I thought condoms were something for child planning. My father kept insisting I prepare to get married. But I said no, not yet."

Then, he tells me, his father asked him to go with him to buy clothes for his marriage. At about the same time he got tested. "I had a rash and I had some doubts. You see, I had been with many different men."

When he got his results, he collapsed on the floor of the clinic. "I came home crying and my family knows something is wrong. I went into my room and my father came in and I told him." He pauses for effect, then mimics his father wailing, startling me and Anto, and making me wonder if Sunil's warning about him beginning to lose his mind might be true. "My father cries out to the deities, cursing them: 'Why has this happened to my son? He has done nothing wrong.' Then my mother begins to wail too. And then all the neighbors hear, and they come over." With an eerie laughter, he shrugs, "This is India. Soon everybody knows."

"All in one day?"

He nods. I shudder, glancing out the window at two neighbors who are staring at us over the fence. Sekar waves. "They are always looking at us; we wave, we give them food, things for their children."

I can't help but recall my own parents and how they took the news. My mother the compassionate social worker, who'd taught special education in high school, who'd gone to the city jail and tutored prisoners, could only say that she couldn't understand how people could let something like this happen to them. *People? It's me, mom!* I wanted to shout, sitting as far away from her as I possibly could. I can still see her shattered face, her body sunk in my father's chair in the family room, unable to move even when I came over and tried to hug her.

Sekar continues his story, telling me he left his parents and stayed with his grandmother, who slid food through a window in his room where he stayed afraid to come out for weeks. "Nobody would touch me, not even my mother," he tells me finally beginning to slow down. "My father was dark and sad and didn't do anything, very sad all day long, always looking down. Once his old friends found out I had AIDS, they no longer came to visit. He was shunned like me."

"My friends told me not to think about suicide, but I do," he confesses. "They told me to get involved: 'You are going to die, why advance it? Help people. Educate them about HIV.' So I became a counselor." Now Sekar speaks at schools and community groups. Some people are critical of his openness; homosexuals are angry that he is too open about his sexuality, fearing the connections people are already making between AIDS and homosexuality. He is determined, though, to tell all and leave no misconceptions. "I tell people that I'm positive and gay.[10] I'm the first one in India to do this," he says proudly, showing me an article in a national magazine. Because of his outspokenness, he was condemned and beaten up by a man he'd slept with. Tenants in his apartment moved out. His brother and sister have left Chennai, embarrassed by his publicity and the effect it would have on their marriage prospects. Like a drug, the telling of the story overwhelms him emotionally and his arms fly about dramatically. It's almost a performance. I give up taking notes at one point, put down my pen and just watch.

It's the people around him, he says, that mean everything to him. Sekar points to the staff standing around listening, one leaning against the door jamb, the other two sitting on the edge of the window sill— three men and one woman—young, street-wise, warm and confident. They work with him for SWAM: providing health services, offering basic job skills, and training MSMs to serve as peer counselors and hand out condoms in streets and parks.

When I ask him about his health, he shrugs. He takes a form of the cocktail, showing me pills I know quite well. One pill is AZT, for which he pays 1,500 rupees (about $30) per month, but that is only one of them.

I want to hear more about his work in the rural villages of Tamil Nadu. He tells me he goes out to see them twice a month, traveling by bus, if he is not sick and has the energy. "I go to be with them, help them however I can. I bring them things." He explains that there are ten or more new cases each month. "They don't have enough firewood to burn the bodies [referring to the Hindu tradition of cremating the dead], so they have to buy the tires, the old tires to burn the dead."

His staff has been kindly preparing lunch for us almost since my arrival. But before we sit down to eat, I ask him about the future and what will happen in India if the epidemic continues to spread. As if back on stage, he pantomimes putting a sari over himself, symbolizing India's conservative culture. It will have to change, he says, nodding seriously. "I protest, but not many join me, some of the gay, but not so many." He shrugs. But with a flash in his eye, he adds: "When I stop my heart, I will stop my life."

❋

Sunil and three of his peer counselors decide to take me to a play performed by a troupe of musicians and actors that do educational theatre involving issues with HIV and AIDS. The play is in a fishing village on the edge of the city. Sunil asks a lover of his to drive us, a police officer who has the use of a jeep. He is, no doubt, married, but he acts nonchalant about his escapades into the world of khotis. Sunil tells me with a wink that they are going to have a little "quickie" after he drops us off. Sunil is frank about his sexual life. And why not? His work is dedicated to helping young men confront the realities and responsibilities of sexuality. Yet the ease at which he and the peer counselors talk about their sexual lives makes me at times a little uncomfortable. Repeatedly, Sunil and the boys ask me if I have met anyone or *had* anyone since arriving. I'm evasive, because if I say no, I suspect, they will feel somehow responsible and the overtures from the boys will become more overt. I'm trying to walk the line between befriending them and keeping my own privacy, but it's not easy.

Our police escort drives us down a winding, sandy path to a cluster of old, whitewashed homes and thatch huts surrounding a small temple to Ganesh with a blue roof and a cement fence circumscribing it. I walk along the beach watching the men pull up their long dug-out fishing boats, which look much the same as the boats the fisherman used in Senegal. Children crouch and shit in the surf as the sun begins to set. I look down the beach, and recognize where I am; it's Lakshmi's beach-side neighborhood. And then, just as I'm thinking about them, Lakshmi and her daughter walk up the beach.

"We are going to watch a play," Lakshmi's daughter announces surprised to see me.

"Me too," I say, then turn to Lakshmi: "I'm here with Sunil and Sahodaran."

I get the feeling my association with Sahodaran makes her uncomfortable. We had a long talk that morning after the yoga class, discussing not only the AIDS situation in India but also my own complicated sexuality and how I'd contracted the virus. I told her, too, about Sita, my former Indian girlfriend. In spite of Lakshmi's professional experience and frustration with the moralism that dominates India's response to AIDS, when it turned to the reality of homosexuality and then to me, she became quiet. The more open I have become about my own bisexuality, I've noticed that people can intellectually accept the sexual expression of those outside their normative heterosexual world in the abstract, particularly if they are of another class or race. But when that bisexuality involves someone close to them, a family member or friend, attitudes often shift and shame compounds their true fears.

We listen to the music for a while. The Sahodaran boys watch me, and the young men and boys of the village watch them. But I gather the Sahodaran boys are used to the role that they play in Indian society; in fact, I've noticed that they find pleasure in eliciting responses from men, even if it may result in ridicule. What, really, is the difference between those acting on stage in costumes and make-up, who flamboyantly strut and sing to please an audience, and the Sahodaran boys who like to excite and entertain on a less public stage?

Lakshmi asks if I've eaten, suggesting I come to her home after the play. But I decline. I drift toward Sunil and the boys, stopping midway between them and Lakshmi. There, I assume my most comfortable role—that of the observer—and I watch the performance and the amusement on the faces of the villagers.

Eventually, Sunil comes to my side. We watch together. From time to time he whispers translations of dialogue. Then in the middle of the play, a tanker truck rolls into the village halting the play. "What's this truck doing?" I complain to Sunil. I have noticed many of the villagers watching the play are holding basins and plastic jugs, but I assume they are taking a break from some work. "Why doesn't he park somewhere else? There's a play going on here?" The actor in me is vexed.

"It's water, Michael. See the buckets? These people have no water." Sunil looks at me like the privileged American that I am. India's water problems are critical and getting worse every year. Embarrassed, I watch as people politely form their nightly queue to get their ration.

The truck leaves and the play resumes. The plot revolves around a couple that is going to get married. When the woman goes to the doctor for her blood test, she discovers she is HIV positive. The boyfriend is furious and ashamed, as are both sets of parents. The young woman is condemned, accused of having had sex outside of marriage—the sin of all sins in Indian society. She is barely given a chance to defend herself. Alone and sad, knowing she is HIV positive and having lost everyone's respect, she thinks of suicide to spare her family the ignominy. The audience is enraptured, and as I look at their faces in sympathy with this actress, I recall a story Sita told me during our brief affair. Because she was writing a novel set in India, we often talked about India and the work she'd done there with a legal organization that advocated changing India's archaic and terribly unjust dowry laws. She was haunted by the cases and the stories she'd heard of young Indian women who would be found burned to death in kitchens supposedly by accidental stove explosions. In reality, they either set themselves on fire out of despair at their enslavement, or mother-in-laws torched them in order to get out of paying the remainder of the dowry price. But the scene I recall now is of a young wife, barely sixteen, who was thrown out of her husband's compound on suspicion of having had a flirtatious episode with her husband's brother. Left on the streets of Mumbai, this terrified teenager found her way back to her parent's home. But when she pounded on their door to be let back in, she heard her mother's voice warning her sisters and brothers not to open the door. All night she cried, pounding on the door, but was never let back in.

But here, in the world of educational theatre, we get a happy ending. The good doctor in the white coat comes back on stage and reveals that they had unfairly accused this innocent woman. She was infected by a needle at the hospital and therefore is blameless. The couple is married. The families are united and all is forgotten. The safe ending disappoints Sunil and me. The number of people being infected by tainted blood or by accidents is minuscule compared to those being infected by drug injection and sex. A question and answer session follows, and the actors pass out condoms. Then the music blares over the speakers, and the show is over. The villagers retreat into the darkness of their village by the sea, and we amble back to the main road to find a taxi to the city.[11]

❋

After three weeks in Chennai, crisscrossing the city in rickshaws to meet with doctors and activists and returning to my hotel room too tired to eat or type notes, my body and mind are beginning to revolt. My throat is sore and I'm losing weight. I take several showers a day to get the dust and diesel soot off my skin. The heat is unbearable, climbing to well over one hundred degrees every day. But it's my psychological state that worries me. I argue with rickshaw drivers over fifty-cent fares. I drop my yoga lessons, unable to get to them and frankly annoyed with my instructor: "You're not following directions, sir. Your breathing is still too shallow . . ." Even Sunil and the boys are starting to get on my nerves: these young men, I keep thinking, need more skills, schooling, and English, not just condoms to pass around. But of course, when Sunil wonders if I might consider staying to help them with their English, since I'm the English teacher, I make excuses. I know if I don't get out of here, I'm going to get sick.

So on Lakshmi's advice, I travel south along the coast to the old French colonial city of Pondicherry, where she tells me I can find a bungalow on the beach and relax for a few days. Mistakenly, I board a local bus without air conditioning, and it takes half the day to go eighty kilometers. By the time I arrive, I feel like someone has hit me with a hammer. I have a splitting headache from hearing sacred music blaring between intermittent horn-blowing. The beach bungalows are all taken. I sulk and go for a swim, slapping my arms as hard as I can against the salty water until I collapse on the rocky beach. Here, I listen to the rocks roll in and out until sunset.

I head inland to find a bed on solid ground in Auroville, a spiritual community just outside of Pondicherry. Auroville, "the city of dawn," was founded by Sri Aurobindo, the revolutionary turned mystic poet and philosopher, and "the Mother," a French woman and follower who helped run his ashram and carry out his vision of transforming the world through the practice of karmayoga.[12] Those who follow Aurobindo's teachings, a pragmatic synthesis of both Tantric and Vedantic yoga called Integral Yoga, believe that Auroville is the manifestation of the "New Age." And so I have come to the cosmological center and birthplace of the New Age Movement.

I find a guesthouse that looks like it belongs in Tuscany, with charming gardens and stone cottages with tile roofs surrounding a gargantuan banyan tree. Indeed, throughout the two-square-mile community, which has been collectively purchased (some say unfairly), from the local Tamil farmers, are architectural showcases made of experimental materials environmentally appropriate to South India. There are schools, art studios, a visitor center, a performing arts center, and clusters of homes, or abstractly designed villas like nothing I'd ever seen in India. A Dutch resident at my guesthouse calls the whole experiment "basically a retirement community for Europe's aging hippies." The centerpiece of this visionary city of the "divine life on earth" is the matrimandir (the soul of Auroville), which is an eight-story geodesic dome that rises out of the rural Indian savannah like a golden spaceship. In fact, when I first see it, I nearly run off the road on my rented scooter and hit a tree. It's not sur-

91

prising to learn that Christo, the famous French installation artist, is a community member and is assisting with this monumental ongoing project that began in 1971.

The next day, I find myself standing barefoot in a long line to climb eight flights of precariously built cement stairs to see inside the matri-mandir and meditate in the only part that is finished, the "inner room," which is at the top of the dome. In this circular room with white carpet and white walls, we sit on white cushions and face a giant crystal. Sunlight hits the crystal as it falls through a skylight at the dome's azimuth, which gives the room the look of a disco club rather than an aura of spiritual calm.

For two days, I ride around on my motorbike like a teenager on the sandy roads of Auroville, take trips into Pondicherry to see the Shiva temples, buy things to make myself happy, stroll along the boardwalk with Indian families eating ice cream, and pay homage to the original ashram of Sri Aurobindo.

On my last night, it's too hot to sleep, and I lie on the floor naked and listen to the frogs and the Indian forest and the laughing couple next to my room. Images come before me of the white lotus and dark red chrysanthemums floating in the pools of Sri Aurobindo's ashram and of the children patiently waiting in line to bow and give their offerings to his spirit.

On the way back to Chennai, I stop at the ancient sea temples of Mahabalipuram. On giant granite boulders, carvers have depicted the scene of the Ganges River descending to Earth. I study the figures, the monkeys, the humans lifting their arms in awe, the nagas, serpent demigods with human bodies and snakelike torsos, swimming up into the heavens. And to the right, an elephant observes this mythological scene, monumental but fashioned with such reverence and realism that it seems as though its granite skin is gently breathing. I am drawn by their mysterious supernatural shapes and the emotional life created by the nameless carvers who carved them over a millennia ago. Looking at this mythical story etched in stone, I again feel a ghostliness, where everything I believe seems to no longer matter. I think about the carvers and what they must have believed as they released these iconic dreams, chip by chip, from the rock where they had been waiting from the beginning to emerge.

❋

"Why haven't you called? The boys keep asking me: 'When is Michael coming back to teach yoga?'" Sunil's voice is a mixture of disappointment and relief when I return to Chennai and call him.

I have not forgotten my offer to give a basic yoga class at Sahodaran for the boys. But frankly, if Sunil had not reminded me, I wouldn't have brought it up. The thought of returning to Sahodaran and trying to teach yoga to twenty young men staring at me is too much; besides, my sojourn south has convinced me that it is time to leave India and head to Thailand. But when I arrive at the Sahodaran office, my anxieties vanish into the vibrating atmosphere of a room full of young men who are eager to know where I've been. They circle around, greeting me, asking where the pictures are that I took of them. After giving them the pictures, we crowd into a small back room. On the walls are posters promoting safe sex: handsome and stylish European men embrace with the outlines of condoms in the back pockets of their tight-fitting jeans. We can barely close the door, and Sunil has to exclude more than half of the boys, literally pushing them back and closing the door, promising that he will show them the poses later. We have no mats. They aren't wearing appropriate clothes. Most can only understand a fragment of my English. "Take off your socks and lie down." I tell them through my trusted translator Anto, who volunteers while Sunil takes the class himself. "Close your eyes and listen to your breath," I say wondering whether this will work at all. They fidget and whisper with one another. I take a deep breath myself.

As I count and they breathe, the room quiets, the whirr of the air-conditioner meshes with the street sounds below, and I begin to take note of their bodies. Sympathetically, the rhythm of their breathing brings us together.

After a few minutes of silence, I ask them to open their eyes and come to a sitting position. I see individual faces, softened eyes, and looks of disorientation. We do a few poses on the floor. I'm winging it, watching them and thinking of what to do next. I show them a simple salutation to the sun. Kneeling, I raise my arms over my head on my inhale and lower my forehead to the floor on the exhale in prostration. We do it together. I tell them to move with their breath, recalling the slowed-down version I'd learned working with my teacher at the Krishnamarcharya yoga center.

We do camel pose: they lean back, some grabbing ankles, chests lifting; then I tell them to fold down into a child's pose, stretching their torsos and arms out in front of them on the floor. Going around the room, stepping over bodies, I gently press down on their backs to lengthen their spines, knowing that touching them is the most important thing I can do.

They stand. We try full sun salutations, but confusion reigns. I stop them. "Let me demonstrate." I point to myself, "Me. Watch me." Sunil and Anto bark out my orders in Tamil.

I do a simple sun salutation, right leg back, arms up, left leg back, stick, cobra, down dog, and so on. The look on their faces almost makes me laugh. "Just follow me, *Suryanamaskar*," I say, suddenly remembering where I am and thinking that maybe saying the Sanskrit might help them.

"Suryanamaskar, Suryanamaskar," I hear them whispering, smiling openly to me, as if I'd finally figured something out: the name itself is the pose and the movement only something you do if you don't know the word. As I watch them, smiling uncontrollably myself, it dawns on me, that it *is* the name, the word itself—Suryanamaskar, the first pose we all learn—that has brought us together in this room. The pose I recall learning in an acting class in college in the seventies. The pose Indian children learn from their grandfathers. I have to stop the boys, as they are becoming like wind-up dolls set in motion and unable to stop.

We do more standing poses and I use all the Sanskrit I can effectively pronounce. "*Virabandrasana*!" I stick out my arm and bend my knees. They follow, relishing our new relationship forged through my bad command of Sanskrit. I hold them in Warrior pose, wanting them to feel it, adjusting arms and legs. They strain, eager to please me. I am moved by their sincerity, their yearning, desperate to embody this image of the warrior-hero.

Yoga, the discipline of the Brahmins and priests, has now become ironically the new trend among the Westernized elite and educated class in Mumbai and Delhi. How absurd, I think, teaching yoga in India to Indians? Or is this part of the absurdity of modern India itself? A nation that exports grain while its people starve; a nation that honors the ethical wisdom of its founder, Gandhi, while maintaining beliefs that deny basic human rights to women and people of lower castes; a nation that educates hundreds of thousands of its best engineers and scientists so as to create a technological and economic boom primarily for those in the West to exploit.

As we continue the more challenging poses, I see some of the young men wither from lack of stamina and no doubt from lack of food as well, but for most, I see that shimmer in the eyes, that brightness in the face, that quickening of the body, that is yoga.

I want to end with some partner poses. I know Sunil and Khan have told me that one of their goals is to get these young men to realize that they have to learn to depend on each other, if they are to going to survive. So back-to-back they sit, folding forward to the floor then backward to open their chests, exchanging energy, the spirited feeding the sluggish, the calm the anxious.

I try to help them feel the pose, pulling back shoulders, planting feet, and massaging necks. At first, they feel fragile—tending to tighten or recoil when I touch them, but now as we reach the end and the corpse pose, they sigh and seem to spill out onto the hard tile floor. As they let me press and pull and sooth, they expel their own tenderness.

Before I awake them from the corpse pose, I pause to look at them once more. One by one I take note, a belly slipping out, a skinny leg, a scarred arm, an open mouth. If you really look at people, study them not as people but as bodies, a feeling of terror suddenly comes upon you. You see the defects, the marks that reveal how they are made, the places where, if they were cut or injured, their life would surely end. But the terror comes not because you see their bodies as fragile, but because you see their bodies as if they were your own.

Afterward they line up to offer me their gratitude, shaking hands, bowing, the bold hugging and kissing me on the cheek. Then, one young man comes up, eyes a blur and full of emotion, grabbing my hand: "Oh, sir. Thank you. Thank you! I never do this before." And before I can respond, he's wrestling with the door and his emotions as he bursts out of the room, pushing through the throng of the other young men, and vanishing into the street.

※

In the darkness, my plane flies over the Indian Ocean carrying me back to Bangkok. My eyes are cold from looking into the night. My fingers, though, are warm, my checks almost burn, my lips still taste the hot air and skin of their faces, my feet cling to the sensation of warm water and their touch.

I want to sleep because sleep will transform these sensations into ideas so that I can understand them and record them in my notebook. For now, I am too full, too afraid, too awake. Thailand will soon eclipse what India was. I sift through my readings in my catalog of articles on Thailand in my shoulder bag. I try to attach myself to the new facts, study the names of the cities on the map, look at pictures of gold Buddhas in the guidebook. But how can you file away touch, a sensation that does not end when someone's hand lets go?

Before I left for Bangkok, one of the young men of Sahodaran insists on giving me a massage. "He wants to give this to you as a gift before you leave," Sunil tells me while we wait at his apartment to depart for the airport. It is Ravi, the young man we followed as he worked along the beach that night. He takes off my socks, puts my feet in warm water, and baths them, toe by toe, heel to arch, arch to heel. Like Jesus, he lets his hands remember me.

At the airport, I abandon my role as distant observer and grab Sunil and the other two peer counselors to me, holding them with a force I didn't know I had. Sunil and the men of Sahodaran had been there for me from the first day to the last, like I was part of their family. When I told Sunil it wouldn't be necessary for him to accompany me to the airport, he laughed like it was just another absurd thing that came from my mouth.

How do we arrive at these distances, traveling without knowing names or languages, ignorant of manners and custom, drunk on childish fantasies and meaningless bits of facts from books? Perhaps we are like migratory birds, born with a terrestrial truth that directs our passage. We seek that particular smell of the sea, we feel for that angle of the sun, we see in the stars a map that tells us where we are.

IV

"O, Sariputra, all dharmas are marked by emptiness . . ."
—The Heart Sutra

Bangkok, Thailand (June, 2001)

From my hotel, I gaze at Bangkok's mountainous terrain of steel and glass, its buildings half empty from the Asian economic crash of four years before. The sky turns purple and gold with the help of the monsoon and carbon monoxide. The Chao Phraya River snakes along markets, hotels, and the stupendous triangular temples of The Grand Palace, holding the city in place, connecting the past to the future. The futuristic Skytrain figure eights and disappears behind a flank of commercial and banking centers. A metropolis of over 10 million people, Bangkok stretches from horizon to horizon covering over 1,600 square kilometers. Another sprawling monstrous mass of people, another set of contacts to make, another culture to comprehend, another set of stories to record. I'm weary as I contemplate the weeks ahead, knowing I'd left India just when I began to hear the real stories and not what people wanted me to hear. Now I must start over in a culture that seems to have learned how to feign openness as a means to protect itself from marauding foreigners.

I want to pick up where I've left off in Chennai and explore Thailand's vast commercial sex industry. I want to understand, too, how Buddhist monks figured into Thailand's remarkable turn-around from having nearly 140,000 HIV infections a year to only around 20,000. I have a couple of names in my notebook: a coordinator of the UNAIDS program, some activists who work with sex workers in Bangkok and several Buddhist monasteries I cannot pronounce.

My plan is to stay a month before moving on to Vietnam, maybe go to Cambodia, then back to Thailand as my return flight leaves from Bangkok. It will all depend on my health, of course, and on whom I might meet, and how far I can afford to go into debt. If India was any sign, it isn't going to be far.

After a day and half catching up on sleep and writing about India, I wait until evening to let the city finally suck me into its steamy cauldron of flesh and capital. I'm apprehensive, recalling those few days I'd spent here the month before in transit. I had recoiled from the commercialism and the way in which I was commodified as a Western man carrying cash and a cock in his deep pockets. I hope that was just a first impression.

At nine o'clock, the streets are still thick with people. I pass table after table, stall after stall, shop after shop. Every square inch of the city seems devoted to selling something. Stacked and sorted, packaged and picked over, organized and displayed: underwear and undershirts, jeans and wallets, cell phones and CDs, sunglasses and shoes, and millions of watches. The industrious Thai can turn an eight-by-four square foot of space of concrete into a mini-mini mart or noodle shop or bastardized Calvin Klein outlet.

Before long I'm hit by the pimps and three-wheel tuk-tuk drivers trolling for men: "Hey mister! You want fuck girl?" A frenzied man pulls out a stack of nude photos, showing his wares: "You like her, huh? She nice, no?" I'm polite at first, nodding, trying to race on by, but they nag and pull on my shoulder, thrust photo after photo of young Thai women with their legs and arms akimbo. I'm more interested in the ubiquitous spirit houses that the Thai set out in front of their shops to honor deities and spirits who bring them good fortune. Each morning in these minia-ture wooden temples, shop owners and home owners place enamel plates of food and drink: balls of sticky rice, oranges, incense, flowers and cans of Coca-Cola. One temple, festooned with strings of yellow marigolds, catches my eye. I peer inside the intricate woodworking and see a plump rat enjoying a plate of rice. Passing massage parlor after massage parlor, my body aches to stop. But each time I linger to look in a window at the row of bored-looking young women waiting to work on my back or feet, I'm accosted by more desperate pimps.

❉

The next day, since I can't find the energy or nerve to make cold calls to my contacts, I decide to plunge into the world of the commercial sex industry and hit a go-go club. I ask the tuk-tuk driver to stop at a group of Thai women hanging over the railing of an outdoor bar. I tell myself it won't be difficult to meet and talk with some of these women because I'm not a customer. But I no more than cross the street and two women shout: "Hey you! Nice looking guy!" Startled, I hurry past. With no idea where I'm going, I march swiftly down a dark street. A tuk-tuk passes, then another, more interested in whether I want a woman than a ride. This is not going to be easy.

Rock music blares out of a bar with flashing, pink lights framing a marquee advertising: GIRLS! GIRLS! GIRLS! Inside, identically dressed women in baby blue swimsuits prance around on a wooden bar. I speed by, thinking maybe tonight isn't the right night. It begins to rain. Heading back to the main road to find a taxi, I'm back in front of the first bar I tried to enter. Before I can cross the street to avoid notice, I'm caught: "Here! here!" several girls wave from the bar, "Come for visit us!" So I stiffen and push myself through the door.

The bar is nearly empty except for a few men sitting in a corner drinking, uninterested in the bar girls who outnumber patrons three to one. A woman in a short skirt and blouse, the uniform for most of these young women, comes up and puts her arm around mine and guides me to a stool looking out on to the street. "You look no happy. What you want to drink?"

I order a beer, not wanting the drink but knowing the poor woman, who up close doesn't look quite as young as she looked from the street, must sell her quota of drinks or have her pay docked. The bar is decorated in palm trees and tinkling lights, fish netting, buoys and driftwood. Many of these go-go bars have been around since the late sixties and seventies, when GIs turned Bangkok's rather benign sexual entertainment business (catering mostly to Thai men and Asian businessmen) into a major part of its economy.[1] GIs from Vietnam came to Bangkok for R and R or what they more appropriately called "I and I" (intercourse and intoxication).

She tries to make small talk. But my tongue feels too heavy to move. I mumble a few breathless questions, repeating them so that she can understand: "Where are you from?"

She's thrown off, but answers, "Village, north, Chiang Mai? You know?"

I nod, but can't think of anything else to say. So we sit in a kind of dumb silence. I fixate on the rainy street. So she brings out some silly game with tiddley winks, one of the tricks to make it easy for men who are shy like me. I can barely move my fingers to play. It's excruciating. Finally she leaves. Another is offered the chance, but I can't speak or even look at her. She gives up, too, and I'm left alone.

I finish my beer and bolt, relieved but concerned. Back in the dark street, I convince myself that my odd behavior is due to hunger and jet-lag. I stumble down a street looking for a restaurant, but find myself turning a corner onto another strip of go-go clubs. Before I can turn back, a rush of women shriek and surround me: "Where you go, cowboy man? We got fun time for you." It's like a swarm of cheerleaders from my high school have broken out of my past with their go-go boots and short skirts. Playful but aggressive, these working women see a lonely man with dollars hanging out of his pockets. Two women grab my arms and drag me toward the door, their petite bodies pulling with all their might. Hanging out the bar window, a clutch of their co-workers cheer them on. I fight them off, jerking my arm a bit too hard, shocking them. "Oh, you no fun! No fun, you!" They pout and playact like they are disappointed, trying one more tactic—guilt. But I'm off and down the street before I turn to look back.

Sweet, acidic rain brings out the smell of cement, rotting garbage and diesel fumes. I flag a taxi but can neither remember the name of my hotel nor how to pronounce the name of the street it's on. I'm relieved to have to walk. At each tuk-tuk that slows to my side, I wave the drivers off with disgust, as if they are responsible for my humiliation. Rain drips off my nose, sweat stings and sticks to my back, my arms hang as if still being dragged by the go-go girls in their white blouses and boots.

❋

I have an appointment with Paul Toh, the coordinator of the UNAIDS prevention program for Southeast Asia. I'd met him in South Africa at the AIDS conference through our mutual friend, Charles Chan, the gymnast and activist from Hong Kong. Thankful to have something to do, I travel across the city, passing the stately temples and Thailand's government ministries. The UN building, a massive bulwark with a stone façade, is a monument to the ugly Bauhaus block design that you find all over Bangkok. I have to go through several layers of security before climbing aboard an elevator full of UN personal in their chic multicultural wardrobes.

After two hours without the slightest assistance by anyone in the office, I'm ready to give up, when a Chinese man in a suit that seems to swallow his short, thin frame quietly speaks from around a corner, "Michael?" My annoyance from having to wait is eclipsed by concern with how his work and HIV infection is affecting his health. I'd hoped Toh would help me make some contacts with NGOs and activists, but he looks pallid and too sick to be bothered with any extra work. I try to impress upon him the importance of my project, hoping to spark some change in his weary face. "I just got back from China and I'm still a bit tired." As he tells me about his recent meetings in China with government officials, his face is blank and his eyes look down at the piles of paperwork on his desk.

We go for lunch at the UN's cafeteria, but there's no change in his mood and he barely eats, making me feel uncomfortable about my own appetite. He gives me a name of an American at the Red Cross and says he'll compile a list of other names. As he stares vacantly at a glass-encased waterfall, I ask him about Buddhism's role in Thailand's success in countering its epidemic. He toys with his food in silence. I mention yoga, wondering if he's thought of trying it. Nothing. Other questions from my notebook fall flat on the table. He apologizes. I fold up my notebook. We shake hands. Toh goes up back to his work, and I wolf down my chicken salad.

I spend the rest of the afternoon in a melancholy mood, preoccupied with how thin and sickly Toh looked, catching myself stopping at windows to check for signs of my own physical decline. Toh's sad eyes haunt me. There he sat, a sick man, in the great hall of humanitarian hope—the UN. All that talk and paper, all those initiatives and plane trips, all those conferences and meetings. I wondered, how anyone, HIV positive or not, working in a bureaucracy like the UN could keep their spirit from scattering into a million pieces of email and memoranda.

I'd hoped that visiting temples would soothe and offer inspiration, but their classic Buddhist architecture is designed to cool the passions and prepare the heart for the teachings of the dharma. I visit Wat Pho, the oldest and largest temple in Bangkok, and meander through cobbled grounds staring up at the steeply pitched, tiled roofs that direct the eye ever skyward into the gray clouds. For a long time, I sit on a bench and contemplate these roofs and the mythical dragons flying up like flames licking the wooden gables.

Walking to the gate, I notice a large canvas tent, maybe sixty-feet long by forty-feet wide. A couple floats out with their faces aglow and mouths so relaxed they hang open. The air inside is warm and wet with a soothing whiff of eucalyptus, but before I can open my mouth, a woman announces: "No more, closed now."

I plead.

"Okay, only half hour."

Bodies lie wrapped in blankets as if dead, while on other cots the masseuses rub and twist limp legs and torsos, prying out the dormant demons. My masseuse is all business and not at all gentle. With gestures and grunts, she instructs me to lie just so, then goes to work. Kneeling on the cot, she digs her hands and elbows into my body, limbering my flesh and muscle, until its just right for her to pull up my shoulders with her knee firmly in my back. She folds and presses and wraps, handling my body like a sponge in need of being thoroughly wrung out. Warm shivers echo down my spine, reminding me of dead zones in my body where I've lost feeling. I'm struck by the simplicity of this ancient Thai tradition: essentially it is a woman holding you, squeezing and bending your muscles and viscera, and, in the process, naturally assisting the body to purify itself while bringing the spirit to the surface.

❋

Today both of Thailand's national dailies have headlines that refer to a "miracle cure" for AIDS, the V-1 Immunitor. "Fact or False Hope?" reads the *Bangkok Post*; "Drug Furor Grows" reads *The Nation*. On the front page helmeted police carry a sick man in a crowd of people. Apparently, this mysterious drug, created by a Thai pharmacist, serves both as vaccine and as treatment. The paper states that, the day before, over five-thousand people gathered in a soccer stadium to get free doses, creating a near riot. Today, to secure order, the drugs will be handed out at a police headquarters. I underline the name of the police station, find it on my map, grab my camera, and head out to flag down a taxi.

Three hours later, after stumping two taxi drivers and having to ask at another police station, I find the Narcotics Division of District One, Police Headquarters of the City of Bangkok. Military trucks and jeeps roll through the parking lot while police with semiautomatics wave families and the sick toward a three-story white stone municipal building. Families cluster under trees with their sick under trees, others sit alone, slumped on newsprint, their pasty faces haggard and blank. Many have been here all night waiting.

I spot a Red Cross truck and introduce myself to the nurse handing out water and snacks. "What is this V-1? Does it work?"

She hands me a cup of water and a few cookies. "Some say it cured them. We come because not good for these people to be outside. Heat is bad. Yesterday someone die."

I walk among people wearing white masks or scarves, fearful of contracting tuberculosis or pneumonia. Whenever I think I've found someone to interview, people drop their eyes or turn away.

An official with a bull horn calls out numbers to a throng of people waiting on the steps of the headquarters. There's a push and few souls squeeze through the barricade. "Excuse me?" I call through an iron fence to one of the white-shirted officials with a walkie-talkie. He squints and points to someone else: "No English." Another man comes to the fence and before he can speak, I bark out: "I am an American—a journalist. Can I come in?" The words that issue from my mouth sound more like a command than a question. Five minutes later, a woman walks out from the fortress.

"You are journalist from America? You have card?"

Thankfully I have a card from my university in my shoulder bag. While she looks at it, I blurt out my other identity: "Look, I am HIV positive. I'm writing a book."

She says something to the police, and the gate is opened. Wearing a bland blouse, a gray skirt, and overly earnest smile, she turns and asks, "Do you want to meet the General?"

It takes me a moment to realize that she's referring to General Solang Bannag, the former Head of Police, whom I'd read about in the newspaper. "Oh, yes, the general, and the people, and the doctors. But, the general—if he is available, yes, of course."

Inside the police headquarters, she takes me into what looks like a command center, where she introduces me to a Dr. Bourinbair. Bourinbair, a tall man with wire-rimmed glasses, announces in his best, relaxed English that he is an American-trained doctor, but originally from Mongolia.

"What newspaper do you write for?"

I hesitate, then mumble something about Chicago.

"Oh, the *Chicago Tribune*?"

I don't correct him and quickly switch subjects: "You see, I'm writing a book, I'm HIV positive. I read about it in the paper. What is this drug, the V-1 immunator?"

Confused he looks back at the woman. "HIV Positive?"

"Yes. I'm positive."

"Then you are here to try the V-1?"

"Uh, I'm here to write about AIDS in Thailand. I have my own drugs, but, well, I don't know, maybe."

His voice changes, "It's been proven to be effective, completely curing several people, you know that don't you? We have proof. We have the medical reports from our patients who have been retested and they test negative."

The articles I've read questioned the drug's efficacy and inventor, Mr. Vichai, who claims the drug is a combination of magnesium and calcium and something called a crystal carrier. This compound contains a model of the HIV virus that conveys a message about the virus to the immune system. Bourinbair met Vichai over the internet and together the two scientists believe they have done what thousands haven't been able to do, create not only a cure but a vaccine as well. I feel like I'm in a bad sci-fi movie.

Bourinbair leads me into a conference room and launches into a powerpoint presentation explaining that after a patient swallows the pill, it remains intact until it is broken down in the digestive tract, where it activates killer cells in the intestinal wall. Here the virus is detonated by the combination of the substances and the mysterious crystal carrier, thus blocking the HIV virus from latching on to the other immune cells (CD4 cells) and replicating. While he rattles on, I lose the train of his thought, staring into the black and white photographs of the shadowy gray HIV virus.

"This is what an HIV cell looks like, right?" I ask, trying to show interest.

"Yes, this is it. You see how it attaches onto the epithelial cells?"

This all begins to seem ridiculous. I ask again how many trials they have performed and where. He admits that they've not done as many as they would have liked, "only nineteen."

"Only nineteen?" I nearly shout, "and you're giving these pills to people?"

"We are in the process of doing more, of course." When I repeat the criticism that I'd read in the papers that they were not submitting the drug to governmental testing, he begins to speak faster and faster. "But you must understand, part of our problem is that if we submit our drug too soon, we can lose our patent. It can be stolen. Do you realize how much money there is in this kind of breakthrough drug? Drug companies have their spies everywhere. We have to be very careful what we show, and to whom. We want to make the drug ourselves. We want to help these people out there," he points out the window, "that's why we are letting them try it now."

I can hardly believe what I'm hearing from a doctor. "But you have to, this is the law, right?"

"Of course, oh yes, we will soon, very soon. They have it, it's not like we are hiding anything."

A mysterious-looking American man, perhaps in his late thirties with a bushy, blond moustache, stands behind me viewing the presentation. "They have to be careful," he explains in a soft-spoken Texas drawl, as he pulls me aside while the doctor takes a phone call. "There are a lot of people wanting to stifle this, as it would mean a lot of lost money for major pharmaceutical companies. You're probably asking what I'm doing here. My name is Jason McClain. I work for the foundation."

"The foundation?"

He explains that the general has a foundation that does charity work. "General Solang Bannag understood that V-1 was a real hope for people with AIDS. All we want to do is help sick people. People are attacking us; you've probably read about it in the papers."

"Yes, I have. But how did you get involved with all this?"

"I grew up here. My father was a missionary. I've worked with different organizations—working on health care and education." He turns to say something in Thai to the woman who brought me inside. "Do you want to meet the General? He is a remarkable man, he would be someone to write about."

"I'm not really dressed to see—"

"You'll like him. Ask whatever you want. Follow me."

Next thing I know, he opens a door and asks me to wait outside. I hear loud laughter.

"Come on in," he drawls, opening the door with this eerie, idiotic smile. When he introduces me as a journalist from Chicago with the virus, the boisterous group quiets. The general is sitting on a couch surrounded by three attractive young women, "daughters of one of his army buddies," McClain adds. Behind the general, and now closing off the door, are apparently his body guards, men in black pants and windbreakers with the foundation name on it. A healthy looking man of about sixty in a white short sleeve shirt, General Bannag breaks the silence and shakes my hand, exuding the confidence of the powerful.

"My English is not good," he tells me, so he asks McClain to translate, but I don't get the feeling that he really wants any questions. I mention what I'm doing and talk about how impressed I am with Thailand's efforts. I play politician with the politician. He wants a picture taken of us, and I oblige. But before I leave, he says he has one question. "You take the drug? Why not try?"

"I—I just got here. But, uh, maybe."

"You want to be cured, don't you?" Everyone in the room looks at me like the poor sap who can't see a good thing when it's given to him.

"Thank you, yes, let me learn more. Thank you." And I bow, obsequiously.

The general smiles with his big teeth, as if I've agreed. I fake a big laugh. Then they all follow with nervous laughter.

McClain takes me into a large gymnasium-like room where doctors sit at long tables meeting with those with HIV. "First they see a doctor, then we give them the pills." We are joined again by the woman I'd met earlier. "She will help translate for you. We can get some patients to talk to you. Okay?"

A woman hobbles over to us in the body of an old man. She can't be more than twenty-five years old, and yet she walks as if her bones are made of stone. She breathes with difficulty, clutching her packet of pills. Next, it's a tuk-tuk driver with a gray, forlorn face; then a young woman with her little boy, who is infected too.

I ask them a few standard questions: where they live; what they do; how long they've been infected; what they take or do for their conditions; how well the V-1 is doing. They are mostly poor and from the northern provinces where the epidemic is most severe. When I admit that I'm HIV positive, they have no response. They are scared, looking around, holding on to their paperwork as if it is their only hope. My translator tells me almost the same thing no matter what I ask, so I quit trying to think up different questions. She wants to make sure I hear how grateful they are. And they are, they speak as if in a daze, believing they've been saved. I want to push them, test just how well the drugs are working, but looking at their frail bodies with hope on their faces, I just can't.

A man comes up to us wearing a mask and old gardening gloves. When I ask him why the gloves, my translator explains: "He doesn't want to infect." Then he takes off his gloves and rolls up his sleeves to show me the fungal infections. He tells me he has come for his wife. He knows he will soon die. When he stands to leave, he bows deeply with dignity, then departs, walking one way then another, totally confused until he is told where to go.

Between interviews, I watch the patients as they meet with these doctors. The patients are docile, as with me, nodding their heads and agreeing with whatever is asked of them. The sick and dying know their role. They are beyond pride, it seems, forced to travel all day and stand in the sun begging for pills that are no more than some money-making scheme, because they have very little else to believe in.

I'm exhausted, wondering how smart it is for me to sit face to face with sick people. After a few more interviews, McClain comes over. "Do you want to talk to the young man who has reverted from positive to negative?" And just like that, the young man appears as if he were waiting in line with everyone else.

He is a poor man with dirt-stained pants and an innocent, big smile. He proudly presents me with the papers he carries. They are copies of copies. One says positive with a date of a few years ago and the other reports a negative diagnosis with a date of only last month. McClain speaks to him, making his already shining face beam that much brighter. He shows us the photo of himself in the national paper. I smile for him, for his innocent faith that this could all be true. All day I have mingled among hundreds of sick people, anyone of whom could have given me the flu or a cold or, worse, tuberculosis. But it's the front man for the foundation, the preacher's son from Texas, who has finally sickened me and made me want to escape this cruel charade as fast as I can.[2]

❊

I spend the morning at an internet café in front of a computer, transporting myself from the streets of Bangkok into the false sense of connection one gets by tapping out email emotions. Looking up from long letters of complaint about the heat and Bangkok, I'm reminded of those mornings in my little Senegalese hut when I first learned this trick of pretending to be deeply involved in another culture by describing it to others. From time to time, I'm brought back by the sight of the youthful bodies of women and men who sway and swagger in playful, psychedelic clothes with spiked hair.

Back at my hotel I practice my yoga only to find myself that much more restless and lonely. I contemplate going north to find one of the Buddhist monasteries that cater to Westerners. Or south to Phuket, the gay Riviera, or to the wild tropical islands where ravers dance under the influence of the full moon and ecstasy.

Later at a restaurant, I sit alone, surrounded by those forty-five-year-old playboys from the Western world, who seem to be everywhere I go. They politely pull out chairs for their diminutive, long haired, daughter-like dates whom I imagine suffocating under expanding, sun-burnt bellies as these men grunt and grope their way back to their "glory days."

Determined to break this downward spiral, I take out what I have left of my hash from India that I was saving for an emergency. I empty a cigarette, fill it with a few bits of pungent hash, tap back in the tobacco, and open my guidebook to the section tabbed for gay clubs. I see a circle around Club Babylon.

With the hash, the city opens and I feel like an arrow shot into the night. Inside a tuk-tuk breathing dust and diesel fumes in the midst of a traffic jam is no place to experience any high. I pay and exit. At a service station, a gang of motorcycle taxis lean against their bikes in ripped jeans, with cigarettes poised on their thick, youthful lips. I show them the address. The tallest and most aloof takes it, nods, points to his bike, throws down his cigarette and hands me a helmet.

With a jerk, we enter the clogged expressway. I'd seen these daredevils in traffic and read about how the police were trying to crack down on their recklessness. But in Bangkok's traffic, where people are trapped in their cars for hours, these urban cowboys are in high demand, and there are plenty of poor, young men willing to take the risk in order to make the money and enjoy the macho image. Somehow I'd imagined my pony-tailed dude had more of a laid back personality. I'm wrong. Faced with nowhere to go, he rockets down a narrow strip between a cement embankment and the outer lane of cars. Seeing an opening in front of a truck, he down shifts, jerking me forward into his back and then bursts through, cutting into the next strip between lanes of traffic, and then opens it up. My hash high is gone and replaced by adrenaline. Over his shoulder, I watch as the odometer goes from 90 RPM to 135 in seconds. Terrified that I might fall off, I adhere to the understood rule that governs how men should ride together on a motorbike: hands placed on the back bar or the seat and off the body of the driver. But my driver pats his ribs to show me that my hands belong there. My body follows, leaning in, my legs hugging the seat and him. The slightest mistake—an oil spot, a car inching over at the wrong time, a hand popping out the window—and we'd fly head over heels to our certain death. I scan the road ahead, wondering if there might be a stop light where I can jump off.

Suddenly, this cowboy darts down an off ramp, and we are on a darkened side street in a residential area under a canopy of eucalyptus and banyan trees. I'm relieved to be out of danger but at the same time miss the recklessness of speed that held us together. I swallow hard at the masculine energy that ripples through this man's body. His triceps are still flexed, his shoulder blades stick out of his t-shirt, even his woven braid of black hair is firm and smooth as it rests inches from my face. When he pulls to a stop, I don't want to get off. Something isn't quite finished. I don't understand my emotions nor how this cyclists has provoked them. It's not the hash. It's that image of flying, full-throttle, head over heels, red lights spinning, the sky peeling open as he and I are thrown together into mutual death, our backs breaking, our bones and bodies blissfully crushed into the asphalt earth. I dismount, reluctantly take off his helmet, and hand him some money; refusing to take off his helmet, he remains faceless. He folds my money into his tight jeans and disappears back into the city.

Club Babylon stands before me, partially hidden among the trees. A torch-lit path, flanked by faux Romanesque statuary of male nudes, leads up to a mansion with pillars and a portico. The club looks new, painted gold and ochre with tiled floors. Fountains and leafy plants decorate alcoves. An androgynous young man slides me a towel with two condoms, smiles shyly and points up to the dressing room.

There's none of that back-alley quality of adult book stories and gay bars that were the first establishments I associated with meeting men. The club resembles a spa more than the American cave-like bathhouses. There is a sense of health and that Thai penchant for cleanliness and simplicity. Walking up to the locker room, I get an idea of who comes to a place like this—young Thai men who have the five dollars to spare along with a smattering of Western tourists like me. Ironically, Thai men undress discreetly, shyly wrapping towels around themselves before slipping off underwear. Descending an open set of stairs onto a patio and restaurant, I'm struck by how carefully the place is designed, so that in every direction men have a chance to do what all men do in places like this: parade and peruse.

For me, there is always a reluctance and relief entering any so-called gay club or bar. Tonight I just want to embrace the contradictory elements that define my life. After wandering this city for five days alone, I want to meet people, hear stories, talk about the trivialities of everyday lives. Sometimes in gay bars you can see behind stereotypes and exaggerated masks and see nothing more than men needing to be in the company of other men—no different than men who gather anywhere else. A man buys me a drink just to be polite, asking me simple questions, nothing intense.

I befriend a young man somewhat off to himself but not alone, thin with handsome features. He is from Myanmar. He tells me, in a rather tired voice, of the chaos in his country and the problems he has had with his family accepting his desire to have a boyfriend and live outside the norms of his culture. He has snuck across the border to avoid conscription and the brutality of the army. He is reluctant to talk much about the AIDS epidemic there, which is far worse than in Thailand due to drug use and the government's open participation in trafficking.[3] He is here in Bangkok to find some happiness, he says. He is also likely looking to find some work in what has become one of the few options for poor, young gay and bisexual men—commercial sex work. Trying to tease a bit more out of him, I realize, as he looks away, that I have broken the unspoken taboo: one does not bring up such subjects as AIDS in a place where people come for comfort and escape from the harshness of the world in which they live.

In a carpeted, glass-enclosed gym next to the pool, men work out while pausing to watch a tennis match on a mounted TV. They are serious about their workouts but glance my way to size me up. There is a marked difference in the attitude of these men from those around the pool. Here, there is silence and dedication to the regimen and rules of bodybuilding. As I try to do my own blend of lifting weights and yoga-like stretching, I can't help but admire these men's disciplined bodies and sleek sensuality. Men here prize a softer, subtler physique, unlike the beefy bodies of American men; no bulges and bulk, but tapered torsos that accentuate the smaller frame and the smoothness of skin and muscle. As they move from machine to machine, exercise to exercise, I admire their cool, catlike demeanor, their towels tightly wrapped to reveal their thighs and taut glutes. No matter how I wrap mine, it continues to sag and slip. What most attracts me to these men is how relatively free they seem from the need to project themselves into something bigger than their true form. Perhaps it's all attitude, or my own skewed perception filtered through desire, but strangely, as I move about among them, they seem to become larger, taller, their chests and shoulders broader. Or is it me, shrinking?—accepting my truer form and size?

I buy some orange juice and slip into the pool on the dark side, conscious of how their modesty works. Under the cover of the translucent water, my body is but a moving shadow, yet I feel its fullness, its completeness, as it has come back together here under the moonlit evening: arm connected to shoulder connected to chest, each stroke and flutter of my feet, like the orchestration of music, echoing forth, muscle by muscle, stemming from one inner chord. After five days in this country, I'm no longer just a walking wallet from America; I'm someone with a body full of warm blood, a breathing intelligence living inside skin. This, after all, is why I came here: to belong in some basic human way, to be seen and identified as man with a past and future, something other than a farang, a cock with blue eyes and blond hair. Desire, for all its destruction and delusion, is also the great humanizing instinct which recognizes no language, no class or race, no gender, no form.

❋

By day, Bangkok's red light district, Patpong, is just another crowded collection of stores, eateries and businesses. In the late morning, all of its glitter and raucous night life is packed away and, like the rest of Bangkok, shopkeepers are meticulously sweeping off their sidewalks and rearranging their wares. Turning onto a narrower side street where tourists will later throng to gawk at the girls and paw over millions of knock-offs at the Night Bazaar, I see the go-go club, Pussy Galore. Above this famous bar are the offices of EMPOWER (Education Means Protection of Women Engaged in Recreation), where I'm headed to meet its director.

After my awkward attempts to learn about the world of the commercial sex industry on my own, I'm eager for a more formal introduction. Founded in the eighties, EMPOWER is a grassroots organization that advocates the rights and safety of women working in Thailand's growing entertainment industry. EMPOWER's office is cozy and warm with yellowing wooden floors and wood-framed cubicles of frosted glass that surround a main room, which is decorated with posters and homemade wall hangings touting the power of women. There is also a glass case with t-shirts and other handicrafts for sale. EMPOWER has offices both here and in the northern city of Chiang Mai as well as a mobile classroom offering information, condoms, and dramatic street performances to promote safe sex and sexual health. There is also a resource library for sex workers to consult for employment, educational opportunities, and legal services. It all seems light years ahead of India, or America, for that matter. As I can see and hear from a classroom off to my right, EMPOWER offers language classes for women who want to improve not only their Thai reading and writing skills but also, and perhaps more importantly, their English, German, and Japanese—the three most common languages spoken by their clients. It's not lost on these women that those with the best language skills make the most money. Not all men are looking strictly for sex; companionship is also a commodity.

The director of EMPOWER, Chantiwapa Asmisk, is a diminutive, vivacious fireball of a woman, who asks me to call her Noi (a nickname, which means small in Thai). In another example of the worldwide AIDS network that has propelled me from country to country, it's Sunil and Khan who suggested I meet with her once in Bangkok. When I'd called a few days before, she invited me to a benefit at a plush hotel, where she and her partner, Chumpon, introduced me to other activists and artists who'd come together to support various HIV/AIDS organizations. Today, she steps out of her office wearing jeans and a t-shirt that reads "Bad Girls Are More Fun." She opens her arms and smiles. "Michael!"

"I like your shirt."

"You want to buy one?" Ever the promoter, she sells me three.

Noi's relaxed and warm demeanor reflects the philosophy of EMPOWER's advocacy work. When we sit down to talk, she is nonchalant but direct: "I don't do much. The place runs itself. It's not our role to make choices for these women; many women use these jobs in the entertainment business to find better jobs." She sighs, having to spell this out to me as she has done for an endless stream of media types who have preceded me. "It's a chance they take. It can give them a better future. We know it's not so good, but it's not so bad either."

She tells me they come from everywhere, but mostly from the rural areas outside of Bangkok, where they can only hope to work in poor paying agricultural or back-breaking factory jobs. "They could never have this kind of life, meeting other girls and people from all around the world. It's hard work, but it can be an exciting life. We don't keep track of the numbers that go on to other jobs. But when we have our yearly festival, many of our old members come back with their children; some come from as far away as Europe and Australia."

Noi says over one thousand members participate in their programs or use their many services. Primarily, they serve the women working in the eight-block area of Patpong, Bangkok's highest concentrations of sex clubs, where at any one time more than five thousand women work. EMPOWER works with the bar owners as well as the police, training the officers who work in Patpong. Noi tells me that they also work with the pimps, or as they are called, "uncles" or "brothers." "Sometimes the bar owners bring new girls here so that we can help educate them on how to protect themselves." The fact that EMPOWER is given nearly free rent by the owner of the building is a testament to the degree of community support they receive.

When Noi first uses the word "industry" to describe the world these women work in, I naïvely think she's misusing the word, but I soon learn that's precisely what it is. All the businesses surrounding these bars depend heavily on this sex business as does the entire city of Bangkok. The more I hear Noi's description of how EMPOWER has come to work with these bar owners, the more I understand how their effectiveness in caring for the health of the women is linked to their pragmatic approach. Behind the sex industry are the forces that run all of Thailand: big business, the police, the Thai government, and the infamous Thai mafia that permeates all of them. Officially, prostitution is illegal in Thailand, but the bar owners get around this by providing only entertainment and opportunities for women to meet their clients. Unlike in the U.S., those seeking sexual services cannot be arrested. This way the women are dependent on the bar owners to find clients and the government can take their cut via the bar owners.

Every part of the sex business has been scrutinized for cost-effectiveness. Keeping women healthy is seen as good business. Consequently, sex workers must be tested for STDs including HIV every month, or in some bars each time they see a client, and they must pay for it themselves. If she fails to do so, the woman can be fired or fined 200 baht ($5). Noi explains that the women must abide by a long list of such bar rules set by the owners. Each night they must sell so many drinks, arrive on time, dance so many times, and wear certain clothes. The women aren't forced to take clients, but if they don't, they have to pay for it with a fine of 350 baht ($7). They must go out with clients three to four times a month. Generally, they work ten to twelve hours a day, getting only two days off per month. On average, those women who work in the go-go clubs make anywhere from $400 to $800 per month. The cost to clients varies, generally they pay around $10. The money is paid to the bar owner. Whatever tips the women make are, of course, theirs. It's not surprising to see why a woman would want to find a client to take her for several days, serving as a kind of glorified tour guide. Noi laments that with all of these rules and penalties, the women fall into debt with the owners. Debt bondage, in fact, is very common, as bar owners can charge extraordinary rates of interest to the woman. By including math in their language classes, EMPOWER teaches women how to manage their money and avoid being cheated by owners and clients. Even so, Noi sighs, "sometimes we have to help our women get out of debt."

It so happens that I've come on the same day as a BBC filmmaker and his assistant; consequently, we are joined by Noi's partner, a pony-tailed sculptor and activist, Chumpon Asmisk, who I'd encountered at the benefit a few days before. When we'd first met, I'd just come from the surreal episode at the police station with the V-1 Immunator. My attempt to explain my take on what I saw amused him so much that he told me to stop so that he could fix me his favorite drink, a concoction of liquors and rum that nearly knocked me on my ass. "Here, this will make you understand this place," he smiled, patting me on the back. I liked this guy.

When the BBC filmmaker proposes a rambling idea about following some women from Northern Thailand into the night life of Patpong, Chumpon responds with a suggestion: "I got an idea. How about you teach these women how to film each other? Huh? Why don't you give them the camera? Excuse me, but what these women need are skills and experiences. So we are always thinking how people can help them." Then he laughed this glass-shattering laugh that sent chills down my back. "Maybe then they can become documentary filmmakers like you?"

The filmmaker, an award-winning veteran who's been all over the world, can't do anything but laugh like everyone else. Earlier, while waiting for the filmmakers, he'd asked me pretty much the same questions: "Well, I was thinking that if you really want to learn and write about what these women's lives are like, you should just teach them English? Perfect, huh? That's what you do, right? You said you teach writing. Well, then?" I'd thought about this, of course, but thought I didn't have the time. "We can find a place for you to stay. That's not a problem." He was serious in a cajoling sort of way. He admitted they'd learned a long time ago to get what they can out of journalists: "You guys are always coming here with all your good ideas on how to help these women, but you don't really do anything but take up our time and leave us with very little." Then he laughed, as he could see in my face that something was wrong. This was the third time, the third country where someone had asked me to put my money where my mouth was. The expression on his face became quizzical and almost mocking: "What's the idea being so serious? Who are you trying to impress? Relax, man. You've got to just live your life." For a moment our eyes met, then his eyes softened and he was on to his next little joke: "You know why people laugh?" I shook my head, fearful of what he would say next. "People laugh because it gives them time—time to enjoy their life."

After Chumpon wrangles both a commitment to train a few of the women and let them do some of the filming, he and Noi invite us all out for drinks and a tour of the neighborhood. It's early and the bars are just starting to open. To give the filmmaker and me a flavor of the nightlife, Chumpon pulls us into a bar down the street from EMPOWER's office.

It's a bright, late afternoon, but when we enter, it might as well be midnight. The go-go bar is narrow, and the oval shaped bar takes up the whole room. A runway bisects the bar with two poles for the women to use in their free-style, semi-erotic dance. Five women in hot pink swimsuits dance to the pounding mix of rock 'n' roll and disco music, while one takes her turn on the pole, mechanically bouncing up and down. Others huddle on the other side of the bar talking. The place is almost empty. The soft, pink light gives off a warmth I don't expect. The warmth also flows from Noi and Chumpon, who are friends with the bar owner as well as the women, several of whom come and hug Noi.

Thankfully, the filmmaker's assistant eases my anxiety and her own by turning our conversation into an interview about my work and travels. But while we chat, the dancing women zero in on me and the filmmaker. I do my best to act like the worldly-wise freelance journalist, but I'm aroused even though the women seem bored and dance like spiritless dolls. I try to convince myself that I'm watching them as a kind of anthropologist, hoping I will somehow feel less discomfort. Yet, I can camouflage neither my appetite nor my awkwardness.

We are joined by the assistant director of EMPOWER, a tough former sex worker, who makes me feel uncomfortable the moment she sits down. When I bring up the subject of my work in India with Sahodaran, she doesn't buy it. "Who are you?" She turns to Noi and Chumpon, "The serious ones are the ones who scare me." She laughs. "You're full of bullshit. You talk too much. I think you need to get laid." At my expense, she's got everyone's attention. She stands in front of me and points. "Here, you want a girl? Just pick one. Go ahead, for fun!"

Chumpon smiles and raises his eyes as if to say, *why not?* "Who do you want? That one—number fourteen?"

My masculinity is under scrutiny, and I know I must choose fast to save face. Suddenly, now that I have to choose, the women all look too young and innocent and bored. So I choose the older looking woman, the one Chumpon suggests, number fourteen.

She slips onto my lap and puts her arm around me. Instinctively, my hands stroke her arms and legs, and my nervousness fades with her there, smiling and looking at me. I lose her name to the noise. She comes from Northern Thailand. She says something about her family that I can't understand. But when she asks if I want to go with her tonight, I shake my head, "No, not tonight, maybe I come back?" She leans her head to one side and frowns in a girlish way as if genuinely disappointed. Thinking of her co-workers, she asks if there are any other girls I want to talk to? I shake my head. As soon as she rises from my lap, I feel relieved, but then feel the difference between the electricity of her skin rubbing against mine and the sexless contours of my khaki pants and my lifeless cotton shirt sticking to my body.

We saunter through the streets of Patpong to an outdoor restaurant and carry on drinking and eating off the top of the menu, thanks to the good people of Great Britain, who bring the world the BBC. In that liminal space of early evening when you've had too much to drink and have no place to go, I leave the party and wander the streets of Patpong. Half-thinking I'll find my way back to the bar and pay a visit to number fourteen, I meander in that direction. Even though I walk with purpose, I know I will not walk in that bar, or any other on that street. I can't will myself to believe that there's any passion or pride involved in fucking a poor woman who needs my money, just because I'm lonely.

So, I head to the only place I can take this emptiness. In another corner of Patpong, the other half of the sexual underworld plays. I find one of the gay outdoor cafés and pull up a chair. I take out my notebook. Couples, Thai and tourist, gay and straight, float by. Here there are no boundaries. Thai guys half my age walk by, turn back and smile. It's all a game that keeps my ego bathed in its little dreams of desire.

At a table not far away, two Thai men and a woman are drinking and enjoying themselves. One of the men smiles and I smile back. Soon I'm sitting at their table with a new drink in front of me. They've stopped for a drink after work. They are youthful, smart, and fluent in English. Emboldened by drink, I tell them what I'm doing, adding some ramble about Buddhism and its effects on Thailand's response to the epidemic. They have some opinions but aren't too interested. In fact, having never met anyone with HIV, they are uncomfortable and we quickly switch to another topic. After a while I get up to go, but the tall thin fellow who initially invited me to the table pleads with me to have one more drink. His friends take their cues and say goodbye.

He works as a desk clerk at an upscale hotel and is infatuated with a man from Boston he's met on the internet. "He's coming soon to meet me. I am dreaming of this every day," he says, his face brightening. From there it's not long until we disappear into the city only to emerge in front of a hostel on the end of darkened, narrow street.

His apartment is little more than a cubicle, with a fold-out bed that takes up half the room. His bathroom is the size of an airplane toilet. The kitchen is a hotpot and some glasses on a shelf along with a cooler on the floor. An entertainment cabinet with a TV dominates one wall. He proudly turns on his stereo and fills two fat tumblers with ice, emptying a bottle of Johnny Walker Red into them. Tacked on the wall are photographs of a middle-aged, balding, happy-looking white man: the internet dream.

My new friend talks about his future and the man from Boston, hoping he will take him back to America so he can go to school. I try to listen, but I'm tired and sickened by the scotch and the memories of situations like this that I know, in the end, produce only bad headaches and bouts of depression. The room gets smaller and smaller, until we finally fall onto each other. He is so thin and long, his bones so sharp, I feel they might pierce through his skin into me. He gets up to get a condom, turns off the light and turns on a sparkling string of white Christmas lights, as the man from Boston dances on the wall to Janet Jackson.

❋

I'd heard about the "AIDS Monk" from Greg Carl, a former Peace Corps volunteer who'd followed the epidemic from its infancy in the late eighties, working in one AIDS-related development job to another until he now ran HIV/AIDS programs for the Red Cross in Bangkok. I'd gone to talk to Carl about attending a program called "Wednesday Club," a self-help group he facilitated for men with HIV, but he felt the men would be too nervous and not respond well. However, he agreed to talk with me in his cramped office over breakfast, as he sat hunched over some coffee. Tall, sandy-haired, and soft-spoken, Carl was shy and somewhat suspicious of me, despite my HIV status and our shared Peace Corps experience. But like a good Midwesterner he greeted me with an apology: "I'm sorry I can't spend more time with you, but I've got to finish writing this manual on at-risk youth."

His sad eyes and slumping body suggested a man who'd martyred himself to his work. "I can't believe I've stayed this long. I've tried to leave but . . ." He shrugs. His face told the story I'd heard many times now. He spoke with passion about the young men he was trying to help, particularly the growing numbers of male sex workers (well over five thousand, he said, both in Bangkok and in the beach resorts of Phuket and Pattaya). "A lot of what we do is basic life skills training, that's what this manual is," he said, picking it up and tossing it down. "They come to the city without any social network and are totally unprepared. They're used to a whole community of people they can rely on; here they are very vulnerable." I asked him about Buddhist organizations I've heard about who have contributed to Thailand's successful campaign to stem the epidemic. He disagreed with my theory that monks were a critical part of the dramatic turnaround in infection rates in the nineties. But he mentioned a monk in the town of Lopburi. "Yeah, you ought to take a train up there for the day. I used to go up and see some of the patients, take them fruit and things. Nobody goes to visit them. They're left there to die by their families. Yeah, go see Phra Alongsit in Lopburi."

What I didn't reveal to my fellow Midwesterner and Peace Corps alum was that I had perhaps more understanding of his work with those at-risk young men than I let on. My *research*, if that is what you want to call it, had begun to lose all objectivity and was perhaps, more honestly, a lonely traveler's excuse to hang out in the side streets of Patpong, where Bangkok's booming international gay scene erupted each night. It was impossible to sit at those outside tables and not be swept into the seduction of youth and desire; I barely had time to order a drink before what Carl would call a "freelancer" would pull up and introduce himself, or perhaps a flock of them would land all at once as had happened two nights ago. Before I knew it, I was invited to a club by a fierce-looking, athletic, young man who wasn't going to take no for an answer, squeezing my biceps until I nervously agreed.

I tried to tell myself that they were only being friendly, but I knew where this was going. These young men befriend men in hopes that a night of "fun" becomes a contractual relationship whereby in exchange for companionship, sexual and otherwise, they are afforded certain payments such as room, meals, travel, gifts, clothes, spending money, etc. These relationships also mean prestige and free nights out on the scene, a way to finance the party life these young men find so alluring. I had no objection to the flattery and soaked up every glance and drink that came my way, infuriating my fiery, young date, who threatened an architect I struck up a conversation with at the dance club.

Bangkok is full of cheap drugs and eager young men. My desires were real, but so was my history of addiction. I knew I couldn't distinguish them in the state I was in. The challenge is to get close enough to the reality of the lives of these men and women in order to observe and write about it. But after a few nights, I knew if I didn't find a way to break out of the seduction of this scene, I'd be in trouble.

The next day, I roll out of my hotel determined to catch the early train to Lopburi to find the AIDS monk. My taxi driver, aware I've no idea how far it is to the train station, suggests he could drive me to Lopburi, but I'm know how that will turn out: what costs $25 here, will cost $50 or $100 later when I'm stuck in the middle of nowhere. When I get to the train station, the train has already left. Old guidebook, old schedule. So, I head for the bus station across town, buy my ticket and promptly fall asleep. When I wake, it's just me, an old woman, and the bus driver.

Five minutes later, we pull into a little town that doesn't seem at all like what I'd read in the guidebook. Stepping off, I am surrounded immediately by a pack of cyclo drivers happy to see my white face and eager to bike me to a hotel. I knew I'd never be able to pronounce the name of this temple or the Buddhist monk, so I'd asked Carl to write down the name for me. "All you have to do is ask for the AIDS Monk and they'll take you there," he'd assured me. So I hand the piece of paper to the first driver who approaches and ask: "AIDS monk? AIDS monk?" A crowd of young men huddle around the driver with the piece of paper. A debate ensues, then another driver takes the paper and breaks out into guffaws. All the while I continue my mantra: "AIDS monk? I'm looking for AIDS monk." The man with the piece of paper points to the ground. "Here, Ratchburi," then lifts his hand and points back in the direction the bus had traveled, "Lopburi, there." Then they all start to laugh, slapping me on the back. I am 150 kilometers in the wrong direction.

A day later I am up early, determined to find my way to Lopburi. I stubbornly stomp by the taxi driver, who makes the same offer as the day before, and find my way across town to the right bus station.

On the bus sitting across from me is a smartly-dressed, young, professional woman. I watch her unwrap her perfectly packaged Thai snacks tucked into her stylish, imitation Gucci handbag. Her orderliness and youthful brightness soothe me, but when she smiles, flattered by the attention, the pleasure turns into emptiness. I look out the window into the landscape of organized rows of vegetables and square plots of rice next to neat narrow roads, but the land only intensifies my melancholy. I try to think of what I will ask the AIDS monk, but images flood into my mind of the freelancer of two nights before with the kick-boxer body whose idea of sex was not so much different than this Thai national sport. My body is still sore from his pummeling bursts of passion. Closing my eyes, it is impossible not to feel the grip of his mouth, the hard hairless legs, the force coming from each heave and hiss of his breath. The guy was a good ten inches shorter than me, but he fucked me with a mix of visceral hatred and boyish envy that made it impossible to sleep afterward, not sure what he might do in the middle of the night: pull out a knife or demand that I do something to him that would force me to have to tell what I should have told him in the first place. I didn't have any reason to think we'd done anything unsafe; we'd used a condom. But it didn't matter: I'd not told him and I could have. What was the point of sitting across from AIDS experts and asking questions and noting statistics and strategies on how to work with those at-risk, if I didn't have the guts to do some peer counseling on my own when given the chance? Why didn't I tell him that he should always ask every partner—especially foreigners? And if he didn't speak English, then why not teach him the phrase? That morning I'd thought about it all through breakfast, trying to tell him that I was a journalist and writing about HIV, hoping at least to tell him after the fact, but he could barely understand me and was much more interested in wolfing down his third helping from the buffet. When he finally left after I feigned that I had to go "do my work," I walked into my room and felt like packing my bags and heading to the airport.

Finally, three hours later, our bus rolls into the town of Lopburi and I want to stand up and cheer. But it's now well into the afternoon, and I still have to travel some fifteen kilometers outside of town, find this monastery, and then get back to town to catch the last bus back to Bangkok before nightfall.

First, though, I have to eat something, since all I have had today is coffee and a banana. I find a nondescript restaurant, go in, sit down, open the menu that might as well be blank. No pictures, no English, just the indecipherable set of squiggles and little circles of Pali. The old Thai couple, who run the place, don't speak English either. The café is empty except for three soldiers, merrily eating and drinking beer in the corner. From experience, my rule in traveling is always stay away from men with guns in fatigues and black boots. The owner sheepishly approaches with that ubiquitous broad grin that is the default facial expression of all Thai. I turn around looking for something in the café: a coffee maker, a candy bar, anything to point to, but there's nothing. I am about to get up and bow my way out, when one of the soldiers stands up, beer in hand, and speaks to the owner, then to me once he realizes the situation. "I help you."

I tell myself, just order a coke and get out of here. In three boot strides, the soldier is at my side, towering over me with his buddies looking on from their table.

"What you want? I get it."

"Uh, noodles, just noodles. Well, could you get them to put in some vegetables, too?"

Soon the smiling owner brings a bowl of noodles and broccoli. I nod to the soldier who waves, smiling. I eat and study my map with no idea where this monastery might be. Meanwhile, the soldiers keep watch, shouting over, "Okay? You like?"

I give him the okay sign, wondering if I should ask him how I might find this well-known Buddhist temple that serves AIDS patients. But I decide, better leave well enough alone. I get up slowly, pay for my meal and look over one more time, thinking I ought to at least thank them again. The soldier who'd helped me immediately stands and comes to attention as if I'm his superior. He can't be more than twenty-five years old and now standing he's actually smaller than me. I pull out my map.

"Do you know the AIDS monk—where they take the AIDS patients? That's where I'm going. I'm a journalist."

"Yes, yes, the hospital. I know. Near our base. We take you there."

"Oh, no. You're eating."

He points outside to his motorbike and those of his friends. "We take you there."

Before I know it, I'm motoring through town with a military escort. Though it's loud and difficult to understand him riding on the back of his motorbike, I learn that he is a sergeant who is on his day off, waiting to pick up his girlfriend later that day at the bus station. Proudly, he tells me his platoon has done maneuvers with U.S. forces in Northern Thailand near Myanmar.

Out of the valley of rice paddies and ochre-colored farmland rise dramatic rocky hillocks. The sergeant points to a cluster of buildings at the base of one of these small mountains, and among the tall pines surrounding them, I see the steep triangular roof of a temple—Wat Phra Baht Nam Phu, home of the AIDS monk.

We enter through an arch and park the motorbikes. In the parking lot, school boys in blue pants and white shirts run to get in line to board two large buses. I pop off the bike, ready to thank the sergeant and his buddies, but the sergeant dismounts and says something to his friends. "We take you," he says pointing up the hill. "Later I take you back to bus station." Reluctantly, his soldiers follow us as we set off toward the monastery. Further up the hill, monks and laymen work in terraced gardens, others are directing workers building cabins. Then three men approach, talking and laughing. Though I can't see them clearly, by their ambling gait and clothes, I suspect they are patients. They greet the soldiers loudly, almost defiantly, "Sawdee Kaa!" I wave back unfazed by their cancerous, freckled skin and sores on their arms and legs. The soldiers move off the narrow road. One flinches, hunches his shoulders, as if to duck for cover. "AIDS" he squeals, after they pass.

Ten-foot, silver-painted dragons, weathered but ferocious, dazzle in the afternoon sun as they guard the steps that lead to the temple. Several buildings, old and new, surround a garden with a wading pool. Carl had told me that the monastery not only treats those with AIDS but educates the public as well, hence the school boys. We spot a single-story, modern-looking building with a large picture window and a long Thai name printed on it.

An older monk sits at a table outside, handing out brochures. "AIDS monk not here, traveling," the sergeant reports, handing me a brochure. Hoping to find some information on what goes on here, I scan the brochure, but it's so over the top I have to conceal a laughter of nervous incredulity. A collage of horrific images stare back at me: men eaten by fungal infections, emaciated with protruding ribs, children with heads too big for their wrinkled, shrunken bodies. On the back, flames lick the black-haired head of man buried under a mound of flowers.

The sergeant looks at his watch and decides to show me around. "We go to hospital?" I look across the garden to the clinic, where he points. Through the windows, nurses and a white man walk purposefully among beds. His soldiers are reluctant and so am I. I try to convince the sergeant that I will be fine on my own, he doesn't understand and walks ahead. Every time I've had a chance to see an AIDS clinic, where I know I will have to see a room full of dying people, be it in KwaZulu-Natal or at the government hospital in Chennai, I've found excuses not to go. Now I don't have a choice. It's hard to see if there are any patients at all, but as we approach, I can see the bent brown knees of the dying in beds. The sergeant has already gone inside and approached a nurse in the foyer. The other soldiers have followed and look back wondering why I'm walking so slowly. Through the window, I see ten, maybe twelve, patients. Wrapped in diapers, they have pulled themselves into a fetal position, regressing toward their final release. One patient is sitting up, but his body slumps, held up by a nurse's hand. Some are given sheets: the healthy, perhaps. Most lie only on plastic-covered mattresses, no doubt easier to clean. My feet are heavy. The air feels thick. It's as if my body is being squeezed so tightly I can't breathe.

"Do you want to go in?" The sergeant asks. "See inside?"

My motto should be: do everything, go everywhere, meet everyone. But I'm not moving another step: "No, no. I can see from here. "

The sergeant, wanting to help, calls another nurse over. The sandy-haired doctor intervenes, clearly annoyed. "You want to talk to the monk?" He barks, revealing either a French or Belgian nationality. "He is not here so you come back." Walking away, he shakes his head in dismay, but then turns and asks: "You come from?"

I'm almost afraid to say, but it doesn't matter, as soon as I open my mouth, he sighs, eager to offer commentary: "Why do you people come here? You come and stay one, two hours and think you can write something; you know nothing. You must stay two days, a week. We have two hundred people die. We serve many, many people; they bring them and drop them off. Please, I don't have time to talk to you."

I consider defending myself in my bad French, but know that will only annoy him further. And what would I say? If I'm not prepared to spend time there to understand more fully the work they are trying to do, why should they take time away from caring for dying people to answer my lazy questions? The doctor looks haggard, yet his body moves with urgency and purpose.[4] I apologize, telling him I'd come today only to find the place so that I could come back later. I want to believe this is the truth; but even as I tell him, I know I can't spend the night or come back the next day, not because I've planned to fly to Vietnam in the next couple of days, but because I don't want to face what these patients represent.

The sergeant suggests we see the museum. I follow them over the stone walk, past the shrubbery sculpted into shapes of animals to a white stucco building next to a wading pool. A sign over the door reads "After-Death Room."

"Are you afraid of dead bodies?" The sergeant asks. I peer into the first room and see what appears to be some tanks filled with water. Drawn by a curiosity for anything that calls itself a museum, I enter. The smell of formaldehyde poisons the senses. The faces of the soldiers seize and twist with displeasure at what is before us: three corpse in tanks of formaldehyde and four more lying on wooden tables preserved like mummies.

Out of nervousness, the soldiers smirk, one laughs. My face becomes hot like someone has slapped me. I try to maintain the image of the journalist, by pulling out my notebook and surveying the room for some signage to explain who these people are and why they are on display. The soldiers approach the first tank. The glass tanks are discolored, stained by a greenish-yellow film. A man's body, whitened by chemicals and time, rests just below the bottom. I blur my eyes, hoping to keep the details of its humanness fuzzy, yet the brain can't help itself and brings the body into focus: scars of skin lesions dot his forearms, pelvic bones protrude through his emaciated torso, his dangling penis floats in the still liquid. I turn to the next tank, avoiding the face, striving to see without seeing, until my mind can find an idea, an emotion to transform them from what they are: people who have died of AIDS.

The soldiers move on to the next tank, silent, transfixed, their faces softened by disbelief. They lean over the tank, hands firmly clasped behind them. Encased in its watery tomb, the body of an adolescent boy floats there, whiter than the others, as if he is the ghost of his former self, caught moments after death, before he flew up through space.

Further into the room, four, dark-skinned corpses lay on wooden tables. They remind me of mummies I've seen in the storage rooms of the Field Museum of Natural History, where I once worked as an educator. Like those lost Egyptian souls and Inca soldiers long ago entombed, these bodies have been denied their burial to indoctrinate the living. Here, faces are frozen in death, mouths slightly open like fish, eyes sealed shut, shrunken bodies boiled down by man-made potions. No robes, no consecrated cloth binds them for their passage to the next world. They remain robbed of identity save a yellowing card that tells of their shameful lives as sex workers or drug users. Their meatless arms and legs wrapped in iodine-colored skin look like fallen branches, charred by lightning, twisted and tossed by the violence of weather. But unlike severed forest limbs, these remains are cruelly kept from the comforts of the warm earth.

The display sickens me, which is its aim. The soldiers gawk at the body of a female sex worker, a tiny frame, shrunken to four feet, her fingers and toes and face that of a child's. To my horror, stuck in the lips of her vagina is a wad of cotton. A touch of modesty, no doubt, from monks who have no idea what the lives of these women are like. I am sorry the AIDS monk isn't here, because I no longer feel only fear and sickness, but outrage. These bodies have been desecrated, reduced to curios in specimen jars and tacked onto wooden boards to serve as moral lessons.

The soldiers lead me next to the "Bone Room." Here, stacked in shoe-box-size containers are the cremated remains of the dead. Another mummified corpse lies on display in the middle of the room, but I've had enough and walk out of this dharma house of horrors.

Beside myself with anger, I look about the courtyard for someone—anyone with whom I might vent my disgust. The sergeant points to a newer building next to the clinic. I march over. Inside this two-story dorm or part of the clinic, a young man stands behind a desk flirting with a young woman. Both are volunteers, healthy and seemingly oblivious. I bark out the two Thai words I know, the greeting, "Swadee kaa!" They smile innocently, return my greeting, then go back to their tryst. I turn to walk out, but a photograph of Michael Jackson on a bulletin board catches my attention. He shares the stage with Madonna. Everything is written in Pali. The only symbols I can understand is the question mark and the word "AIDS." Since the After-Death Room, I don't need to be able to read Thai to figure out what these two icons of American popular culture personify: the seduction of desire and its ultimate unhinging of dharma.

There he is, Michael Jackson, the name the young men in the gay bars of Bangkok repeat when I tell them my name: there he is, dancing backward on the bulletin board, the littlest brother of *The Jackson Five*, who sang their way out of Gary, Indiana, the Soweto of the Midwest; Michael Jackson, the hero of Ryan White, the teenage hemophiliac who contracted HIV from the blood supply of Central Indiana where I grew up. Yes, it was Michael Jackson who sobbed in Ryan White's hospital room, after Jackson, frantic, flew across the country to be at his bedside. The ironies of this disease are no crueler than the ironies of the world's response. Later, it would be a pencil-thin Ryan White who would testify before Congress to demand funding for health-care and housing for the thousands who live with HIV and AIDS in America.[5]

Before the soldiers leave, they ask a taxi driver, who has just pulled in, to take our picture in front of the After-Death Room and the wading pool, which now has a tiny white poodle swimming in it. Waving goodbye, the sergeant reminds me he'll be back to take me to the bus station. Watching them leave, I wonder why I don't go with them. There is nothing more I want to see here. I think about hiking up the hill to see the temple, but I'm in no mood to slog up a stone path in a swarm of mosquitoes to see another peeling, gold Buddha on a tacky bright red enamel throne. So I stumble over to a tree, plop down and lie back in the grass, my hands unconsciously ripping out clumps of grass.

Weary and hot, I close my eyes, but there's no escape. In my mind are the images of the nearly naked patients only yards away, rotting on their plastic mattresses, their sores oozing, their eyes fixed on the eternal churn of the ceiling fan.

V

Ho Chi Minh City, Vietnam (June, 2001)

In the sixties, Vietnam was a game we played in the yard with BB guns. In the field behind our house, we dug foxholes, threw dirt-clod grenades that exploded against the back of the garage, and used the poor kids who lived in the run-down houses behind the bowling alley as the Vietnamese—from a distance, anybody can be the enemy.

My cousin's husband was over there and a few neighbor kids had an uncle or brother who'd been drafted. But the war was far away, except at six o'clock when my parents sat like stones in the family room and watched helicopters hover over rice paddies carrying away the dead.

Years later, I got a job teaching English to immigrants at a college in Chicago. My images of Vietnam now came from the personal essays of students and the memories transcribed in them. Hundreds of images, written in an awkward but often poetic prose, created a composition of its own. Or sometimes, a single image came to represent them all.

One such image is of a student's face, a young woman who spoke very little and kept to the back of the room, a shy but intelligent woman with a long scar that began below her right eye and ran down her cheek, disappearing under her chin. She had a delicate face with long shiny hair, and yet the reddish, worm-like scar saddened her beauty. She often walked with her head down. And when she talked to other students, she'd turn her head this way and that, constantly keeping it in motion. After several weeks, I assigned students to write about something that had happened to them that they would remember for the rest of their lives. In a stack of papers, I'd learn what it was like to be hunted at night by marauding soldiers while crossing the Sudanese desert, or what it was like to watch drunken, gun-toting Haitian police rip apart your house and carry off your uncle. Students wrote their first drafts and I read them quickly until I came to the essay written by the Vietnamese woman with the scarred cheek. She described how her father had arranged her future marriage with a businessman to whom he owed some money. The man came to her house, and she was so disappointed when she met him that she ran crying out of the house. After pleading and pleading, the parents could not change her mind, and the father had to break off the contract to the fury of the businessman. Some days later, she was walking home from school in the streets of Saigon when she was suddenly grabbed from behind. She turned, and it was the businessman with a knife. "If you can't have me," he told her, "then I'll make sure no one will have you!" He then grabbed her face and slashed it open.

It was in that class, too, that I heard other stories about life along the Mekong Delta in post-war Vietnam, from a student who, five years later, would end up taking me into a world he'd been forced to flee.

Mekong Delta, Vietnam (June, 2001)

Tuong Nguyen finds me standing in the late morning sun in the parking lot of Tan Son Nhut Airport. He looks the part of the American "Vietkiew"[1]—stylish shin-length jeans, Nike shirt and baseball cap, sunglasses, and flip-flops. He's so excited to see me that he nearly tackles me: "You finally make it!" He throws down his cigarette and takes my bag, then stops: "Wait! Let me take your picture. First picture, right?"

Indeed that was the plan we'd discussed in Chicago. He would translate and photograph, as I explored his country to learn how Vietnam is facing a spreading epidemic of HIV that has doubled every year since 1994.[2]

I'd met Tuong Nguyen in my second year teaching at Northeastern. He would have come and gone like other students, if he hadn't had such trouble with his essays that I'd asked him to retake the class. When the class was over, I gave him an A and thought I was finished with him, but then the next semester he was back outside my office, asking me to take a look at an essay for another class. Sometimes, I must admit, I'd look down the hall, see him hanging outside my office, and I would turn around and go get some coffee, hoping he'd be gone when I got back. One day, he showed me some of his photographs. Flipping open his portfolio, I thought I'd see the photographs of a beginner, but they were poignant close-ups of the wild and weathered faces of street people in Uptown, one of Chicago's poorest neighborhoods and the home of the Vietnamese community. There was more to Tuong than met the eye.

❄

The streets of Ho Chi Minh City at midday are clogged with motorbikes. Businesses and street vendors buzz with activity. Having lived in West Africa, I thought I knew what heat was, but here in June the heat penetrates the skin and makes you feel as if your flesh is evaporating. The city stretches out into farmlands overtaking rice paddies. Polluted pools of stagnant water run along crumbling roads. As peasants migrate into the city from the poorer regions of the north, Ho Chi Minh City has doubled in size since 1988, swarming now with nearly 6 million people. Tuong and I pass four or five-story cement apartments with iron grating over windows and clothes hanging from lines, not to dry, but simply because there is no other place to hang them. Children and young people are everywhere. With nearly 80 million people, Vietnam is one of the world's most densely populated countries with 60 percent under the age of twenty-five.

I check myself, mile after mile, anxious and exhausted from traveling for three months through India, Thailand and now Vietnam. I am glad to be in Vietnam with Tuong and his family, who have gathered together, for the first time since they left Vietnam in 1990, to prepare for Tuong's arranged marriage. Here, at least, if I get sick, I know they will take care of me.

Tuong, after all, had the guts to come into my office that day four years ago and ask what few faculty members would. "Are you okay? You look so sad all the time." The directness of his words and his open face felt like a push that knocked me backward down a flight of stairs. I'd had to pay a therapist to finally find someone to ask questions like that. But I recovered and offered the all-American, all-purpose defense for ill feelings of the spirit, "Oh, I'm just a little tired is all." It took every ounce of will to make it into the safety of my car before letting my body wail, and another three years to tell Tuong and my colleagues that I was living with HIV.

We finally arrive at one of the tributaries of the Mekong, albeit after our taxi runs out of gas, and board the ferry at Mytho. The sun begins its decline, giving the land and the river a glow that suits its name: *Cuu Long*, which Tuong tells me means "Forever Life of the Dragon." Originating in the remote mountains of western China, three thousand miles to the east, the Mekong traverses the borders of Myanmar and Thailand, crosses Laos and Cambodia, then empties into tributaries that make up the delta of southern Vietnam.

The ferry fills and we head at a diagonal across the muddy river. I look around as the children stare at me, reminding me of how mesmerized I was as a boy when I saw Korean students from the local Methodist college walk into the drug store, surprised that their eyes were really eyes and their hands really hands.

In Vietnam, as elsewhere in Southeast Asia, children are often used to fuel a struggling transitional economy, sent off to cities by parents to be sold into brothels or to sort through trash to find scraps of metal to recycle. Though Vietnam has made strides, well over a third of its people remain in desperate poverty, severely affecting its public health.[3] I notice passengers' baggage: baskets of fish, a tub of soap lard, spilled blood running in a rivulet from a package of meat, a new TV in a box, and a cage of young dogs on the back of a motorbike going to market.

❈

Tuong's brother, a meat wholesaler, has a new house off a little highway. Airy and bright, this two-story house with several bedrooms is a palace compared to most. His family has reunited for the wedding, both those who live here and those who immigrated and work at Motorola in Atlanta or give pedicures in hotels in Chicago. In the background Tuong's brother and his Vietnamese nephews are blasting hip-hop on the stereo and playing a video game on the TV. In the kitchen, a pot of meat is steaming while Tuong's old buddies and brothers sit around the table and drink rice wine and sing Beatles songs in Vietnamese. Tuong's father, a former officer in the South Vietnamese Army and a prisoner for eight years, sits quietly without expression in the other room.

After I meet his family, eat a noodle dish, and force down a few toasts of rice wine, Tuong takes me to my hotel. The hotel is on Coconut Island in the middle of the river. The island was made famous by the Coconut Monk, a former priest educated in France, who is said to have meditated on the island for three years eating nothing but coconuts. Before his imprisonment after the war for supporting reunification, he'd created a devoted following for his cult, which blended Catholicism with the spiritual traditions of Vietnam: ancestor worship, Confucianism, and Buddhism.

At the dock, which is part community bathroom and part dump, Tuong procures a motorized skiff and we cross back through the muddy river to my lodgings. Remnants of the Coconut Monk's religious sanctuary appear as we approach the island: a thirty-foot-tall stone grotto, dragon-like lamp posts made of colorful tile fragments surround a ceremonial patio, and, strangest of all, a steel structure of about fifty feet, from which a series of cables and pulleys suspend a globe of the Earth and other planets. Tuong points at the structure, "See the spaceship?" At the base of this bizarre religious icon, ready for take-off, is a ten-foot long rocket with "Apolo" [sic] painted down its side. "It's been here for years," Tuong laughs, shaking his head. "This priest was kind of crazy." Once on the island, Tuong takes my things to the office, where he meets an old friend who runs the hotel. I'm a bit nervous as the place is quite run-down and seems empty. But then, in the gift shop, I see a few shoppers pondering postcards and bottles of rice wine with little brown snakes floating in them.

Tuong, anxious that everything go well on my first day, keeps asking if I'll be alright, but I don't want to tell him that the place gives me the creeps. "I pick you up tomorrow morning." I tell him I'll be fine, but I can feel that I'm beginning to be sick. I'd felt feverish on the ride from the airport, and now knew it was more than the heat and the two shots of rice wine. Being off medication and not having any problems, I have begun to forget just how vulnerable I am. Light-headed and nauseous, all I want to do is shower, read, and hope that restful sleep will cure whatever illness is coming on. The room hardly gives the feeling of comfort. Three single beds with thin foam mattresses are pushed together. A rickety wooden armoire takes up a whole wall. When I open it, the cabinet door falls off nearly severing my toe. Under a window rests a Soviet air conditioner the size of a small car engine, only louder. A single bulb over the bed emits a gray dull glow that erases any idea of reading unless I use my flashlight. I lie on the bed and begin to feel chills. The air conditioner proves impossible to turn off. Huddling under my thin bedspread, my bowels gurgle, and I flee to the toilet. This repeats itself. So I sit in a nest of bed sheets, towels and my clothes, trying to read an Indian edition of *Gulliver's Travels* with print so small I have to light a candle and put the book so close that I nearly burn my hair. Just as I begin to feel that the diarrhea has subsided long enough for me to fall asleep, I hear that telltale gnawing. Rats.

I try to ignore them, but when the heaviness of sleep comes, there they are on cue. One darts from behind the armoire, another wiggles through a hole under the air conditioner, a third appears from under my bed and boldly jumps on to a chair. I throw a shoe, then another, cursing them. The diarrhea returns. It goes on this way much of the night: running to the toilet, throwing shoes at rats, and reading strange passages of *Gulliver's Travels* by candle light.

✸

The next day Tuong picks me up to show me the countryside where he grew up. I can't bear to tell him, but there's no way I'm staying another night on Coconut Island. My bags are packed when he knocks. Mortified, he takes me back to his house, where his sisters roll their eyes at Tuong's idea of having me stay there in the first place, then order me to take off my shoes and socks so that they can give me a pedicure. "Rats! Why didn't you stay here? My brother is crazy." They are displeased with Tuong as he is ignoring his bride-to-be, who has been cooking and cleaning for the family to show her loyalty.

Tuong finds another hotel in the town of Ben Tre. In the lobby of this drab, cement-block, two-story hotel are a group of bored, young women in the floor-length, traditional, brightly-colored dresses Vietnamese woman wear. They perk up when Tuong pushes through the door with my duffle bag. Flattered, he jokes with them. Outside, however, he whispers: "I think they are the sex workers for the hotel. This place is only for the government people; nobody else has the money except tourists. You better watch out for them."

With a couple of his old friends, we motorbike through the countryside to meet rice farmers he'd befriended when he trained to be a veterinarian before he came to the U.S. Passing through the town of Mytho, I spot a rather large wooden sign posted next to a school that says something about AIDS. I've seen these billboards already on the highways, sometimes three or four posted together warning people (mostly youth) against drug use, sex work, and gambling. Here there is a silhouette of a woman lying in a suggestive pose with a red syringe dripping blood. Underneath there is a reference to SIDA (AIDS). Tuong points out the fact that if the posters really wanted to help people, they should at least have a phone number or address for more information. "These are just propaganda," he snorts. Another billboard looks like a red monster, which apparently, according to Tuong, depicts what happens when you become infected with HIV.

As we leave the city, turning onto red dirt roads that parallel the irrigation ditches, we pass rice farmers in their fields, some with old tractors and others working by hand as they have for centuries. In the middle of one field, chalk-white stone monuments hold the cremated remains of the dead. Along a small river, a large eye, painted atop a door of a wooden house, looks out at us as we pass. "Cao Dai temple," Tuong shouts, pointing. The Cao Dai blend Buddhist beliefs with that of ancestor worship and other ancient folk traditions of the Vietnamese. It's never far from my mind that I'm passing through a land that was once a battlefield where thousands of Vietnamese and Americans were maimed or killed. Even in the brightness of this sunny day, with emerald rice fields and smiling young people riding motorbikes on their way to school, I know there are shattered bones, land mines, and wandering souls under the surface.

Tuong suggests we stop at a famous Buddhist temple. It has the feel of a colonial estate, with a neoclassical, terra-cotta façade, a red tiled roof, columns, and a crumbling stone fence with a wrought iron gate. A sign says that it was built in the 1800s and rebuilt several times. The last time after it was bombed during the war, killing over a hundred civilians, mostly women and children. Whether the bomb was dropped accidentally or not, it doesn't say.

Inside the damp and dusty temple an old monk lies on a lounge chair, his belly rising and falling as he fans himself in the midday heat. On the wall above him is not a portrait of an abbot or the Buddha but of the goateed Ho Chi Minh. A few worshipers make offerings at an altar cluttered with candles, urns stuffed with scrolls, and framed photos of the dead. Most of the photos are of clean cut young men with eyes staring out into futures they never lived to see. Tuong stops photographing to tell me that the photos are given to the monks with payments so that they will pray to release them of their karmic burdens for the next life. Why so many young men, I ask him. Could it have something to do with drug use and the growing AIDS epidemic? He tells me its more likely that they have died because of drug use or accidents. In Tuong's own family, his sixteen-year-old nephew was recently caught stealing from his parents in order to buy heroin, which for young people is easier to get than alcohol. Like in Thailand, China, and other parts of Southeast Asia, heroin use among the young continues to drive the AIDS epidemic. Earlier, Tuong told me that his nephew has been depressed because in the last several months one of his friends overdosed, another was beaten to death by farmers who caught him stealing dogs to pay for his habit, and a third was killed when his motorbike hit a tree driving home drunk after the boy's funeral.

We move on to the little rice farm where Tuong's old friends have prepared lunch, or the farmer's wife has, as she slaves in a smoky kitchen with three walls and a dirt floor. We sit in an outdoor porch under a low hanging awning of thatch that connects three wooden cottages. I stuff myself with fish and try to keep up with their rice wine toasts. Two neighbors join us. After more toasts, inevitably, the subject of the war comes up. I ask them if it was true that the Americans bombed the temple we'd just visited. They all nod emphatically. One neighbor points behind us, and Tuong says that the man shot a GI over there through the trees. "They were cowards," Tuong whispers translating, as they drink and laugh nervously, glancing my way. I don't want to argue with my drunken hosts, but I have to defend young men from my own high school who probably died within miles of where we're sitting. "They were not cowards," I whisper back to Tuong. "They were young, they were lied to, they didn't want to be here." Tuong translates. The men nod and we raise our glasses again. At what, I don't know.

❋

After only four days in Vietnam, the weariness and anxiety which I thought I'd put behind me in Thailand is eating away at my sanity and patience. The night before, thinking I might learn more about the lives of Vietnam's youth, I'd met some young people outside my hotel and let them take me to eat only to find myself in a drunken party. I demand to be taken home, but then have to fend off the advances of my driver, a young woman, who begs me to take her up to my room.

I try to make it clear to Tuong that I can't stay in the countryside long and that we have to travel to Ho Chi Minh City and set up interviews. "I've got to work." I tell him. "I'm almost out of money and very tired."

Checking my email, I see that an editor at Salon is interested in my pitch on doing a piece on the AIDS clinic in Chennai, and a newspaper in Bangkok has taken a commentary I wrote about the V-1 Immunator controversy. Fixed with a sense of purpose, I bury myself in work in my room.

Breaking for lunch, I take a walk to look for something to eat. To my surprise, I come across an Olympic swimming pool in a park near my hotel. I lean against a fence and watch a coach drill eight- and nine-year-old athletes. Watching their thin, fish-like bodies slice through the inviting blue pool, I can feel my sluggish body, the tightness in my shoulders and back. It's been days since I last practiced yoga or done any form of exercise. When I turn to go, a group of children block my path: they start to chant something in Vietnamese, pick up stones and throw them at me. They can't be more than five or six, but their angry faces make my legs wobble. I want to stop and scold them, but the stones are not small. Quickly, I head toward a wide boulevard, which leads to a round-about with a large stone monument in its center. Behind it, taking up a whole city block is an enormous mural of Ho Chi Minh. Even though the sky has darkened and it looks like rain, I cross the wide street to get a better look at the monument. It's a war memorial, honoring the bravery of Vietnamese women. From left to right my eyes follow a stone frieze of fifteen or more fierce-looking women with bayonets and sticks trampling the bodies of American GIs as they march to victory over the imperialists. Overhead, clouds churn and rumble, the sky turns black, and I run to my hotel as it begins to pour.

All afternoon I write, as rain pelts against the windows. The lights flicker on and off and eventually go off altogether. Engrossed in my work, I light a candle and continue writing by hand until a strange feeling makes me stop. Outside it's dark. Something is wrong. I must be getting sick again, I think, so I decide to lie down. But lying there and looking around the room, suddenly I can't remember where I am or how I got here. My mind is blank. It feels like some unknown force has sucked out my memory. I jump up, as if this feeling is a living thing, sharing my bed. But it's *in* me, it's not *on* me. I grab the armoire in an effort to connect to something real, something I know won't change. *This is an armoire,* I think with my fingers. *I am in a hotel room in Vietnam. I came here yesterday with Tuong. This is the door. It's made of wood.* I drop to my knees, stretch my arms out and try to calm myself with breathing.

Outside, it has become darker. I take off my clothes and roll out my yoga mat. Put the candle on the floor and try to concentrate on my body and breath. Sweat pours off my body into a pool on my mat. The sky lightens. I walk to the window. It's still raining. Then I remember, today a solar eclipse is to blanket all of southern Asia.

❄

The next evening Tuong takes me to meet one of his childhood friends, a Buddhist monk who now presides over a local temple. Hidden in the thick trees off a dirt road near his brother's house, we come upon a garden of Buddhist statuary surrounded by flowering trees and shrubbery sculpted into the shapes of deer and elephants. We climb the tile steps to a modest, white temple, where a statue of a fat, laughing Lucky Buddha greets us at the door.

Inside, there is an altar with a golden Buddha and two poorly-painted portraits of monks. A large bell hangs from the ceiling. Landscapes of rivers and mountains are painted on the walls. Without a sound, out of a back room appears Tuong's friend Le Hong Thai, wearing a long, simply sewn, white shirt with brown pants. He is small and birdlike, with a translucent quality to his skin and his whole presence. He studies me as he takes the gifts of fruit from my hands, places them in a bowl before the Buddha on the altar and slowly bows. We follow him to a small room, painted in a soothing light shade of lime green. The room is polished and clean, simply furnished and fresh. A bowl of jackfruit awaits us on a sturdy wooden table. Le Hong brings us iced tea, and Tuong explains the purpose of our visit.

The monk folds his hands as he listens to Tuong's translation of my questions and then waits in silence until he composes his answers, which are delivered in crisp, diphthongal phrases. "We have a Buddhist Association that helps the poor, the sick, and the old," Le Hong informs us. He explains that people are dissatisfied and that is why they turn to drugs and destroy themselves with desire for money and sex. Over the years Buddhism has been weakened in Vietnam by one after another of the great powers of the world: China, the Colonial French, the Catholic Church, the Japanese, and then the United States. But perhaps its greatest and oldest challenge is globalization: the seductions of wealth and the material world. Falling away from the practice of the *dharma* brings suffering, he reminds us. "Right thinking brings right action," he says with a smile curling his lips ever so slightly. Then he says something that intrigues me, or this is how I understand Tuong's translation. He says that HIV doesn't come from a scientific cause but from superstition. After listening to him a bit longer, I think I understand what he means. Superstition is false belief or delusion, and this is what perpetuates suffering.

"People are afraid for the future," he says. "They are confused and seduced by the new materialism that is coming with the money and the culture of foreigners." Le Hong's mouth is pursed with emotion. Tuong, who has filmed part of our conversation, now has his camera on his knees and is deep in thought. I wonder what he thinks about his friend's explanation of how karma creates its own endless cycles of suffering. I wonder, too, how this explanation would help Tuong's nephew as he struggles with drug addiction, or how it would have helped his dead friends.

Le Hong leaps up from his chair and disappears behind a curtain into his tiny sleeping quarters. When he returns, he carries a bracelet of dark orange beads in his delicate hands. "Eighteen Buddhas for you," Tuong explains. "These are prayer beads for good luck and protection."

A boy appears in the doorway and the monk rises and leaves with him. We follow. A bell rings three times and the boy's chanting voice echoes in the temple and floats out into garden, as he shakes three burning sticks of incense. As the ceremony ends, I am filled with an overwhelming sadness. I want the boy to keep singing; I want to stay in this little temple and not think or do anything until I can understand what's happening to me.

Ho Chi Minh City, Vietnam (June, 2001)

That first morning in Ho Chi Minh City, Tuong leans against the railing outside our hotel room, looking out at the stream of humanity, as motorbikes and bicycles pour through the city's grand boulevards. "Let's just walk around," he suggests. The sidewalks are thick with entrepreneurial energy. Mobile markets arrive with the sun and by night are pulled home: noodle carts, make-shift kitchens and cafés, vendors selling cigarettes, vegetables, fish, books, papers, flowers, children's clothes. A truck bedecked in flowers and painted in gaudy lacquered reds and yellows slowly rolls through the streets. An old bus plugs along behind it half full of people all wearing white. A placard-sized photograph on top of the truck announces the death of the man buried under a mound of flowers on the truck bed.

Tuong seems conflicted, excited by the modern feel of the city yet troubled by the young women lounging in the windows of the so-called hair salons. "Look, Michael, they are too young to be the haircutters, they are the sex workers." After Bangkok, this is nothing, but I nod and tell him that he's probably right. Small children follow him, trying to sell him fists full of lottery tickets. This glorified form of begging employs thousands of children and the elderly as they hustle dreams to those with not much more, while businessmen and the government haul in the profits. Back at our hotel, Tuong makes a few calls and sets up a meeting with a government doctor at Friends Meet Friends, a half-way house for drug users and people living with HIV, and also with Mr. Thanh Van Pham, a social worker recommended to me by Noi and Chumpon Amisok at EMPOWER.

After a grueling morning at Vietnam's War Remnants Museum, viewing hundreds of gruesome photographs of bombed villages, children deformed by agent orange, and the stricken faces of both the war-weary Vietnamese and the baby-faced boys of America, we set out to find this government doctor and his HIV group. But when we arrive at this community center, the doctor is not there and the two HIV-positive men, who apparently work there, are so fearful of the police that they refuse to talk to us, whispering to Tuong that the doctor is at the government clinic a few miles away. Undeterred, we head to the clinic to find Dr. Dung. But the doctor isn't so happy to see us either. Frowning, he takes our gift of fruit and hustles us to his dusty, cluttered office, which is heavy with the odor of cigarette smoke. Dr. Dung, a handsome man with long, delicate fingers, barely gives Tuong a chance to explain why we have come before he lashes out at us for coming without papers. He lights a cigarette and sighs, turning to me to apologize, "No English, sorry." He picks up a stack of papers, pantomiming the need for official papers, trying to get me to understand. Tuong explains that we need to have papers signed by the ministries of health, culture, and information before he can talk with us.

Back in our hired car, I whine that this day has been shot.

"No Michael, Dr. Dung wants to help us but not here. He will meet us for lunch. He told us not to go back to the center or this clinic. He said they could be watching us."

"Who's they?"

"The government people."

At lunch, Dr. Dung is more friendly, laughing at our innocence, but warns us again not to go places without permission. Though he doesn't mention it, I know that the government could arrest Tuong and me if they discovered that we were here without papers as journalists, not to mention that as a carrier of HIV, I'm not even supposed to be in the country. Vietnam has opened up, but not that much. The doctor tells us that Vietnam is struggling to come to grips with its growing AIDS epidemic. Each month they have more cases, but he has no antiretrovirals to dispense; only those with money and power have access to antiretroviral treatment. Remarkably, he admits that as far as he knows only seven people in the entire country are using the combination therapy I take. I can't believe it when Tuong tells me. I have to ask him to repeat it. "Seven," he says.[4]

That evening, we traverse the city one more time, picking up Dr. Dung, who takes us to the brightly-painted Condom Café in a working-class neighborhood called Tan Binh. There we meet a shy, slight, HIV-positive activist with a shiny face and hollow cheeks. Bowls of colorful condoms sit on each empty table. Pop music pumps out the door trying to attract youth. However, while we're there, only one couple comes in and sits down. Dr. Dung in his Calvin Klein t-shirt and slick shoes does most of the talking. The doctor is pleased, thinking this is what I've come to see. I nod, trying to show how impressed I am, but I'm suspicious, feeling that this café is more to show foreigners how well the government is responding to the epidemic than a place to inform those at-risk. He says positive people feel comfortable here. He estimates that there are probably about five thousand people with HIV in Ho Chi Minh City.[5] When I ask him about MSMs, he really doesn't have much information. He knows that gay, bisexual, and male sex workers account for part of the at-risk population. They go to clubs which open one night a week for them, he says derisively. They have some organizations, but men who are infected by other men don't admit it. I'm surprised at how little he knows about MSMs, as one of the government's main experts. When a female sex worker—or perhaps she is a *katoey* (transgender male)—goes by the window, he points for me to look, smirking.

The HIV-positive man is silent, deferring to the doctor if we ask him any questions. When he does answer, he only looks at Tuong. He says they have special music and educational radio programs as well as other events to attract young people and disseminate information on HIV and the dangers of drug use. With no expression on his face, he tells Tuong that he knows he will die soon. We drink coffee in silence. I feel sorry for this man, the HIV activist; he too appears to be a prop in a stage set.

❀

Mr. Pham Van meets us at our hotel as he promised me on the phone. Van greets us precisely at two o'clock in our hotel lobby, motorbike helmet in hand, with a broad, warm smile. Not young, but energetic, Van brushes off his dusty khakis and sticks out his small hand. Hearing how good his English is, I begin asking questions at once. But he answers in Vietnamese, speaking quietly to Tuong. "He wants us to go someplace and talk," Tuong interrupts; "it's not good to talk here." So we take an elevator to the empty restaurant on the top floor. Here, overlooking the city, I tell him about myself and what I'm doing. Within a few minutes he has me saying more about what I've been through than I've even told Tuong. He also tells us about his work with "the poors," as he calls them in his mix of English and French. He works with a variety of groups: female sex workers, drug users, street children, and young people. In Van's varied career, he has not only been a social worker but a journalist, film reviewer, and theater critic. He returned to social work in the nineties when he witnessed the unprecedented social upheaval caused by globalization and Vietnam's opening up its markets.

The meeting is more of a risk for him than to us, as he is jeopardizing his own complicated relationship with government agencies. He tells us that he worked with Save The Children, but became frustrated with the endless red tape of the Vietnamese government, who kept tabs on their work and took credit for their successes. Now he has set up his own non-governmental organization, finding funds where he can but keeping a distance from international agencies so that he can move more freely to help the communities he feels are most in need. "I take you to see my groups, but we must be careful; government don't like. They want permits and it take a week, maybe two weeks."

Back downstairs, his assistant arrives by motorbike, a light red scarf around her neck, boots and long, white dress gloves. Underneath is a tough-looking woman with a lion-like face framed in dark hair. Tuong rides with her while I ride with Van. "We go see the sex worker community," he tells us as we mount.

We fly into the streets, pulled by the rush of thousands of cyclists and motorbikes. We cross over a few bridges, and before us is the vast expanse of the city where the poor live in cramped boxes of cement block and corrugated roofs. It is treeless, dangerously polluted, and, except for the clothes worn by women and children and the brightly painted Buddhist temples, almost devoid of color. How people can navigate through it without incident mystifies me until I watch as a woman tumbles from her bike and is buried under waves of cyclists. I am relieved when we finally pull off a main street into a maze of narrow alleys.

Van maneuvers around old men playing checkers with grandchildren, teenagers on bikes, and women selling food out of their homes. A crowd of children runs behind us. Inside the opened doors of these single room homes, I peer into the everyday lives of the Vietnamese poor: in one house, children sit on the floor eating lunch, in another, a family huddles around a large TV watching a women's ice skating competition, and in a third, a man lies in the lap of a woman as she extracts his whiskers with tweezers. In these homes, a single room serves as kitchen, playroom, workroom, and bedroom.

When we arrive, women and children gather around Van's assistant, Hong, who greets them as she sheds her bike gear, revealing an attractive woman with dramatic eyebrows drawn on a large brow. She motions for us to enter one of the women's homes. The lane is no more than eight or nine feet across. The children try to push in but are shooed back. Van introduces each woman to Tuong and me, yet they refuse to shake our hands as they are all peeling skins off of red onions. He explains that the women, under the leadership of Hong, have formed a cooperative of sorts, working collectively and investing a small amount of money to use for emergencies. In this case, they have hired themselves out to a company that buys onions to make soup. "Little by little," he says, pointing to the pile of onions, "They make about a dollar with the onions. We work with the children, too, take them to the zoo or to the park. But they have to make the money." He turns to a little boy and asks him if he has the money saved yet for the trip to the water park. "We don't give the money. Maybe pay a little, but they must work. We take them outside, the children and women, so that they can be more confident around other people. We want to show them that they have to take care of themselves. We tell them that they have the rights." His face is pained, he wants to get across how strongly he feels about how it can work. "They have rights. In the North they are used to the government doing everything for them. But here in the South it is better, government not so much control." He laments how communism went wrong: "Subsidize no good, people don't work. People need to do it for themselves and work. People change if they know the rights and laws."

He turns again to the boy: "No money? No water park." These boys, he says, can make 10,000 dung, about a 65 cents per day, sorting through garbage and scouring the streets for bottles and metal scrap to be recycled.

Where the men are, I have no idea. Van and Hong are trying to convince the women to depend on each other to find a livelihood other than commercial sex work. The real problem for Hong and Van are the teenage daughters of these women, who follow their mothers into sex work. Van explains that it's a difficult cycle to break. Sometimes drugs are involved or sometimes a policeman accuses one of the girls and has her arrested. "This is blackmail," he says. They then must pay ransom so that they aren't sent to work camps outside of Ho Chi Minh City. Often, this is how the police keep control, forcing women to resort to sex work to pay the ransom to save their daughter from these camps.

We move on to another woman's house. Tuong has disappeared. I have to climb up a metal ladder and carefully inch my way on a ledge to make it inside the second-story flat. From here, the row of houses below look more like rooms in a single corrugated roofed building. The houses make me think of the livestock shelters on my grandmother's farm. At the end of the alley shanties cling onto the riverbank. Van explains that perhaps two hundred people live in this space that can't be more than thirty square yards.

Our host seems happy to have us in her scrubbed flat. Two women enter and hand us bottles of soda. This second story flat is a bit larger— a twin bed, a small stove, cupboards, and shelves with a kitchen and household items arranged within easy reach. A woman rushes in and whispers something to Van. Suddenly, our quiet afternoon is cut short. "Stay here. We must leave now." He points to my host, "She will take you in a few minutes to meet us. Better like this, not all together. The police. One by one, better. Wait."

My escort watches me while we wait. Looking at her rugged features, her strong build, short-cropped hair, and man's clothing, I feel safe. She looks as if she could defend herself from anyone, and she probably has had to do so as well. I recall an observation Van made about homosexuality in my interview with him at the hotel: "With 'the poors' in the slums, the life is not easy. Some use the drugs, some are gay; the women who do the sex work, some are lesbian. But they, you know, do not judge. Down here, all people have struggles. They accept."

It's time to go. My host points to the door. Hurrying, I nearly trip on the tight steps. When I'm down, she grabs my wrist and leads me like a child through the alley. We run, my shoulder bag flapping and falling off, my feet stepping on toys and knocking over tubs of clothes until she pulls up at a corner. There she points, turning my shoulders in the direction of Van, Hong, and Tuong, who are sitting at a café on the sidewalk under a tin awning. She won't stay even though Hong asks her to sit and have coffee with us. Embarrassed, she steps back. I bow in gratitude. She nods, smiling weakly, and just like that, slips back down the alley and is gone.

Tuong is smoking and talking excitedly to Van. I ask what happened.

"The police, they wanted to know what I was doing."

"The police were watching us." Van says. "That's why we had to leave."

Tuong continues, unconsciously getting out his camera again. "They asked me what I was doing. I told them I was visiting. I thought they were going to take my camera."

"How many were there?"

"One, I think. Then a man came out of his house and told them I was his cousin." Tuong laughs, nervously, and orders my coffee, describing just how I like it, indicating with his fingers the amount of milk. "I didn't say anything," Tuong continues handing me coffee, "but just in case, I took out my chip." He shows them the thin digital wafer. Hong squints trying to understand.

"Old man save you," Van says, joking. "They all hate the police," he tells me, sipping his coffee.

Van says that once he'd had to rescue Hong from the police because they had jailed her. When I ask her a few questions, she says she owes her life to Pham Van. She began working with him in 1993. Before this, she'd had a very difficult life, growing up in a rural area and forced to marry against her will at an early age. She came to Ho Chi Minh City with no education or family support. When her husband began to beat and abuse her, fearing for her life, she had no recourse other than divorce. Like many of the women she works with, she had few options and began working as a sex worker in order to make a living. These women became her support as well, she says with pride. "We had to help each other." But her life was not easy, and when she met Van, she wanted to work with him. "At first, I volunteered," she says, "I handed out the condoms and talked to the women about their rights. Then he trained me to be a peer counselor and I began to work as a community organizer."

Hong chooses her words carefully, as if out of respect for herself and

Van. A hint of emotion lights her tough face, her lip purses, as she thinks back on her past. Van offers some perspective: "It is hard for the women and for her. They want not to do the sex work. But they need affection, too. They want a person to care for them. They need money. It's hard for someone to go back to a life like she does when she works with these women. She remembers."

She points to Van, "He helped me to return. I never thought I'd return to my life before I did this work. It took time, but I began to think about myself more seriously."

"How do you help—how do you work with these women?" I ask.

"'We are educators,'" Van translates. "She say, 'we try to help them develop their needs, the deeper needs, the need for understanding, the need for talk and confess.' She say, 'the human needs of the women are very great.'"

I take a sip of my hot, sweet coffee. I write down what Hong has told me. Lifting my eyes, I see that Hong is staring at my hands and the words in my notebook.

✻

The first thing I notice are the sores, open and wet from the rain, running down his left side from his face to his foot. He smiles. His name is Minh. Beside him, his friends sleep on the window ledge of a closed department store, slumped against each other, a girl and a boy. The girl has bloodstains on her pants. Tuong takes a picture. Van, who has set up this appointment after our day with the women's community group, pulls me aside: "These are street children and Minh is sick; he will tell you that he got the AIDS from some Japanese woman but he does the drugs. These young people are on the drugs, too. You must be careful."

The rain has let up. Van leaves to go home on his motorbike. Tuong is soaked. Minh eagerly leads us to a café across the street. Night is falling prematurely from the daylong rains. Behind the café is a tourist art gallery, with replicas of European masters—Van Gogh, Cezanne, Monet, painted meticulously from postcards. Minh has been waiting all day to tell us his story. He wears a blue fishnet shirt. Smiling, he reveals a chipped front tooth, like I had as a boy before it was capped. Two tiny girls, no more than four or five years old come up to sell postcards. He waves them away, and they totter back to a couple sitting on a bench, presumably their parents, who ignore them.

Minh describes his life on the streets as a shoeshine boy. His English is remarkably good. When he struggles, Tuong assists him. But generally Tuong is off, thinking to himself, conflicted by the calls he keeps getting from home wondering when he will be back to carry out his duties as the groom-to-be. Tuong is also suspicious of Minh, worried that he will try to take advantage of me. Minh tells us stories about encounters with tourists: "A Japanese woman, she just wanted me to come up to her room, have a drink . . . that Australian man, he was nice to me, but I didn't know he was the gay. I'm not like that. I think they gave me AIDS."

I ask Tuong to order food and drink, but Minh wants nothing. "I can't go home now. My father, he throws me out, he beats me when he is drunk. But I love my Mom and my sister. I sneak there sometimes and spend the night. I bring her my money."

I ask what his father does. He tells me his father works in a factory making Mickey Mouse dolls.

"Do you take drugs?"

"Not the bad drugs, just sometimes. I like marijuana. I like to listen to my music and dream. They call me Mr. Marijuana." He smiles, laughing at himself. Then to my surprise he asks: "Mr. Michael, do you know marijuana?"

"Yes, I *know* marijuana."

He explains that after he found out he was HIV positive, the police took him and put him in a detention prison in the countryside. But when they found out that he'd progressed to AIDS, they tossed him back to the streets. He shows us his certificate, plops it on the table, a photo ID with his name and HIV status. "Never come back here, they tell to me. If they catch me now, I just show them this. They won't arrest me." He seems proud of this.

Minh is dying: a shooting star, his glow weakening, falling into the darkness. Like the sex workers in Chennai and Bangkok, his dreams of beauty and love are not fantasies but strategies to survive the terror inflicted upon him by not only the streets and society but his own family. Van told me that HIV infections have increased most significantly with young men, boys even. They clean up after other users have abandoned needles, fighting over the dregs of each needle to get high.

Tuong is still preoccupied. He takes our picture and then one of Minh alone. I watch as Minh proudly offers his best pose, but in my mind I see him, naked, floating out of his clothes and up into the soggy trees, disappearing into the darkness of the rain.

Minh unconsciously favors his right side, hiding his scars and sores. As we walk, he pushes a bicycle through the drizzle and oily streets. I can't help staring at the sores on his feet; a single limp band-aid flaps off one ankle. He could use fifty more just for one leg. We give him money and buy him two disposable cameras and tell him we will see him in a few days. I want him to take pictures of whatever he wants: his friends, his family, the streets where he works, so that Tuong and I can learn more about the street life. He is disappointed, looking at the money and the disposable cameras. Earlier he'd asked for money to buy a cyclo, a bicycle-powered taxi to drive tourists around. I considered it, but knew

I'd better first ask Van. "I will see you again?" he asks, his body now sagging.

"Yes, we will see you."

Japanese tourists, European backpackers, and Americans amble about the central tourist district of Ho Chi Minh City. A girl rides on her belly on a homemade wooden dolly. She wears sandals as gloves and has her left foot tied to her thigh so that it won't drag on the street. She is severely deformed and unable to speak; she grunts for us to drop her a coin. Tuong whispers, "She is probably that way 'cause of the agent orange." Further on, three white-faced, transgender males prance by in heels; they smirk and smile, eyes aglow in make-up, with dyed hair and long nails—hummingbirds of the night.

We walk and walk until we come upon a sleek new hotel. Puffy and happy Chinese and Germans dominate the lobby, drinking and discussing business. On a stage with a white grand piano, a sign advertises "The American Buffet." We sit down and eat our way out of the sadness of the past few days, going back again and again to fill our plates. We eat so much that we decide to walk the two miles back to our hotel. It's a clear night, warm and clean after the rain. We pass crowds of young movie-goers pouring out of the cinema, lonely women selling noodles from carts, sex workers mingling by the disco clubs, couples flying by on motorbikes, garbage collectors sleeping in their empty wheelbarrows.

❋

It takes nearly an hour by motorbike to reach Van's weekly meeting with HIV-positive drug users. We cross back and forth over tributaries of the polluted Saigon River and through slums that hug its banks, until we come to a little outdoor café in a new quarter the government has set aside for a manufacturing zone.

"Bring more people," Van implores this group as the meeting begins. "Helping others helps you."

"Trends," reads the pink t-shirt of a frail woman sitting to my left. Her shriveled body is no more than skin tightly wrapped around a shell of bones. A gray pallor shrouds her sad face. Her sunken eyes and hollow cheeks make her nose long and her head too big for her frame. Her husband sits slumped next to her, a dingy white construction hat in his hands, and an expression on his face of a trapped man. Across the table, two men seethe, arms folded, eyes narrowed to slits. Another man hides under an Adidas cap. A child sits on a window ledge behind a mother with one eye. Van tells me after the meeting that these drug users go to this half-blind woman's food stall when they are sick and have no food. "She is like a saint to them," he says. "We give her a little money for their food."

As Van counsels them to keep working and take walks together, I wonder, why does he do this? "Every month they die," he tells me. "Last month there was four, twenty-five already this year."

The world of drug users and AIDS has a potent mythology in Vietnam. Drug users are known to attack the police and anyone who comes between them and their addiction, sticking needles in their arms to draw blood and then threatening to stab and infect whoever comes too close. Drugs, according to the government and UNAIDS, account for most of Vietnam's growing HIV population. Seventy percent of drug users in Ho Chi Minh City have been infected, adding to the long, sad history of opium's effect on the Vietnamese, whose mountainous poor still use opium as a way to deaden their hunger. It's not just the urban and rural poor—the government admits that at least 20 percent of those employed by the state have serious drug problems as well.

Cigarette smoke hangs in the heavy, humid air. The male drug users take every drag deep into their lungs, then fall into fits of coughing. Van introduces us and Tuong translates, whispering as he leans toward me so that I can keep what little eye contact the group offers. Most say but a few words, look off, say something else, shrug; then the next takes their turn. I gather from Tuong that someone is missing. Some in the group shake their heads. "He got caught stealing," a man reports. "Stealing a bike," Tuong whispers, when I ask what he stole. This bicycle story actually brings a few smiles to their faces. The following day, however, I learn that the man was missing not because he stole a bike, but because he was dead.

Rain clouds smudge the afternoon sun. The man in the corner mumbles out his story between coughs. He tells the group that he became so sick once that he couldn't get up off the floor, so his fellow addicts didn't know what else to do but give him more heroin. Perhaps it is the cigarette smoke or the graying afternoon, but for a moment it appears that his body has vanished, fading into his own shadow, leaving his clothes and the smoke hanging in the air. "When they gave me the drugs," Tuong translates, "I got up off the floor and could see again." The man laughs at the absurdity of it, but in his hollow cheeks his laughter sounds more like a dying man's rattle.

The husband with the construction cap now speaks as if I am the only one present, imploring me to understand, his face and body reminiscent of those tortured depictions of Jesus on the cross in Medieval churches. Tuong listens very carefully, translating what he can: "He says the government makes the HIV people and the drug users attend meetings each month, to check on them like criminals, and if they don't go they are taken to jail. He collects trash, pushing a wheelbarrow around all day. His job is all he and his wife have and it makes him feel better when he works. He doesn't know what he will do if he loses his job." While her husband speaks, I steal glances at his wife. I am drawn to her body: the deep eye sockets, the black needle stains down her arms, but mostly it is the mechanical rise and fall of her breath that upstages the drama of her husband's account of their life. Each time her chest collapses in its exhale, I wait in sympathetic terror, holding my own breath, thinking that it will be her last. But then up again comes a spurt of life, her lungs laboriously suck in more air, though they are so weak she has to massage her nostrils to draw in more oxygen. It is so painful to watch, that I find myself breathing more deeply, hoping somehow to help her. I have a macabre image of wrapping myself around her frail body and breathing into her, pumping her emaciated body back to life. She reminds me of my grandfather, dying of emphysema in a VA hospital: like a fish in the sand, his lungs working against the odds.

Van tells me after the meeting that he doesn't know how she has stayed alive as long as she has. "Some go quickly. The young go very fast. But others, like her, they go on and on; nobody knows why."

With the permission of Van and the group, Tuong circles around the table as they talk, taking photos as he translates. He sets up his shots, focusing on their faces, moving in close and then back away, using his camera not as if taking a photograph but as if offering his respect, his acknowledgement of their suffering. Photography for Tuong has become a way to express what he can't in language sometimes. "I start to take more and more when I come to America. With my photographs I don't have to worry if people understand my English. I can communicate the things I feel without speaking." Watching him, I now understand how he'd lost part of his hearing the year before, trying to photograph the dragon dance during Chicago's Chinese New Year celebration.

When drug-users have all had a chance to speak, Van turns to me and asks, "Do you want to speak now?"

Ever since sitting down in this café, I've found myself trying to hide my health by contracting my body, hunching over, crawling into the black ink scribbles in my notebook. I have to ask myself again and again: Why did you come? Why do this to them? Why show them a future they aren't allowed to have? I can feel their eyes on my skin, looking at who I really am under the façade of muscle. They can see that the American obsession with physical beauty and youth is nothing more than the fear of death.

Tuong looks at me and pleads, "Please Michael, speak slow, okay?" At least, I think, it will be his words and not mine.

How absurd it all has become, I think: America destroying Vietnam only to build it back up with tourist money. Fifteen-year-old girls from poor rice farms selling themselves to plump European fathers who'd throw their own daughters out of the house if they were caught having sex with their boyfriends. Drug users shooting heroin to stay alive.

Tuong telling dying people that this American, his teacher, tried to kill himself by having sex with another man because he was too ashamed of the sexual pleasure men gave him. Minh, the uneducated shoeshine boy, who speaks several languages and lives on the street because his father, a worker in a factory that makes Mickey Mouse dolls, will beat him because he has AIDS.

I open my mouth and try not to think, as I tell my story to these people gathered around me. At one point I hold up my notebook, showing them what I am doing and telling them it is their book, too. "Our book," I say like I am some kind of politician. But that doesn't have much effect on them until Tuong says something, something on his own about me that makes his lip quiver. What, I never find out, but after he does, they seem to lean in toward me waiting for what I have to say.

Van suggests they ask me questions. A man, who hasn't said much, asks very politely if I am sure I have HIV because it doesn't look like I am sick. Van explains that I do yoga, delicately emphasizing how I am taking care of my body, rather than mentioning I have access to anti-retroviral drugs that they don't. Intrigued by this mention of yoga, a debate breaks out among the group over just exactly what yoga is.

The next question, though throws me. "They want to know how you got it?"

I know what I have to admit—something even drug users in a traditional culture like Vietnam can find offensive—that I have contracted HIV from having sex with another man. In a way it is a test. I swallow, and the image comes to me of the drunken, drugged nights I shared with men in apartments in Chicago. As I sit here, looking down at my feet and unconsciously over at Tuong's empty pack of cigarettes, I think, what difference does it make to them how I have gotten the disease? "I had sex with men. I drank, I did drugs. I wanted to kill myself." I reel off the list, gaining more of their confidence with each confession of social transgression.

They still aren't satisfied. "What happened when you found out?" A man in the corner asks. I shift and squirm, grab the sides of my chair. I remember the office of the social worker and the indifference in the voice of the woman behind the desk: "You weren't expecting this were you?" I see myself in the shower that day I found out, wanting to pound my fist through the bathroom wall. "I was angry," I tell them, my right hand forming a clenched fist under the table. "At who?" Tuong asks, not necessarily for them but for himself.

"I was angry at the world," I tell him, my fist now rising out from under the table. I look at Van and he is nodding, as he must have nodded at words like these many times before. Then a shiver goes through me, and I can feel the power of my anger and how I have learned to chain it down with words and muscle. Out of habit, I look out at the river in the distance, imagining a way out. But in front of the suffering and the nearly dead, what is there to hide?

In Tuong's face, I now see my own: a frustrated foreigner unable to speak, like the hundreds of immigrants who have sat before me in classes, desperate not simply for the knowledge of how to put words in their proper order, but desperate to be translated out of the past into the language of the future. I look at these people sitting around me, their gray bodies sapped of the color of life, yet on their faces, to my astonishment, I see compassion.

"I don't want to die," I spit out, doing everything I can to not to break down. Tuong whispers my words and when I look up it appears that their faces have left their bodies and come within inches of my eyes. "I want to make more people understand. I don't want anyone else to have to . . . to feel the shame that I have."

Out of Tuong's body come my words. I listen to his voice and the emotions riding the waves of his diphthongal glides, and as I do, I realize that what I have said, what experiences I believe are mine and mine alone, are not really mine at all.

Then a man asks about the origins of AIDS. I try to explain the African monkey theory, but he isn't having any of it. He believes it comes from America. And no matter what Van or Tuong or I say, we can't convince him otherwise. And why would he, a man who lived through the Vietnam War, not think that AIDS had come from the same place that had dropped bombs and sprayed poison down on his people?

When the meeting is over, there is an awkward shuffling around. They walk away slowly. But something feels incomplete. I want to shake someone's hand; I want to touch someone, hug someone. I walk up behind the fragile woman with the pink t-shirt, who leans on her husband as they hobble to the road. She raises her head to look at me, but then drops it again to watch her feet so as not to fall. Without speaking, I put my arm around her shoulder. She turns and looks up, smiles and then, embarrassed, buries her head into her chest. It feels like I have placed a log on a dying wildflower.

As we climb onto our motorbikes, dark clouds sink over the streets and soon it begins to rain. Van worries that I might catch a cold and stops to buy me a cheap plastic poncho, but as we are buying it, the rain begins to pour, so we run into a tailor's shop.

The rain sweeps over the city and soon the owner's wife rises from her sewing machine and finds two small wooden stools. We sit there, Van and I, watching the rain and the children playing in the downpour. I learn that Van writes lyrics to folk songs in his spare time. He tells me about plays he has directed and puppet shows, too. "I like the puppets," he says moving his hands, mimicking a puppeteer. And he tells me how difficult it is for him to become close to these people, only to know that they will soon pass away. "Young people," he sighs. "They die too quickly. I have to take their pictures. We go to the picnic, we make the party. I think they need this so much. And then I take my camera. I take the photo with the happy faces. Because when they die, they have to have a picture for the funeral . . . for us to remember them. We tell them, 'we support the end day.' It is important for them to know that they will not die alone. I know they will die soon, so I take their photo. But sometimes I don't take them in time. Some die: no picture. A couple of weeks ago a boy die, a good boy, who was working with us as the peer counselor, but he loved the drugs too much. The night they called to tell me, I couldn't sleep. I couldn't because . . . because I don't have a picture. So I just write down everything he told me about his life. I write and I write: the secrets, the stories, all the things I remember he told me. Then, I go back to sleep."

VI

Chiang Mai Province, Thailand (July, 2001)

The morning after our day with the dying drug users and the street kids, I told Tuong I'd had enough of Vietnam.

"But what about our plan to go to Hanoi? Don't you want to go see drug users on the Chinese border? What about the village with all the people who have Agent Orange, don't you want to go interview them? And my relatives, they want to see you again." He couldn't understand what was wrong. Neither could I. Out of guilt, I found one of the few ATMs at one of the swanky new hotels in Ho Chi Minh City and withdrew a million dong. I called Van and told him that I couldn't meet with the Cambodian sex workers or the high school students he'd wanted me to speak to, and that I was flying back to Bangkok the next day, making up some excuse as to why I was leaving two weeks early. We met, and I handed over every dong I had and told him to buy Minh, the shoe shine boy, a cyclo and to use the rest for his other programs. I hardly gave him a moment to speak. When he pulled away in his antique motorbike, I sat down on the curb and wept.

As soon as they closed the doors of my plane to Bangkok, it was like that day of the eclipse in Ben Tre all over again. I was trapped, not only in a metal tube full of people but trapped in a mind that, for whatever reason, was no longer under my control. Around me, all I saw was confinement, shrinking space, people getting bigger. The plane revved its engines, picked up speed and lifted off. The only thing to do was to shield my eyes from seeing the flight attendants or the door or anything that reminded me that I was on a plane and couldn't get out. So I studied the veins and lines in my hands, hoping to keep my mind off the panic. I don't know what was more terrifying: the thought that I might hurt someone, the thought that I was losing my mind, or the shame both would bring me. Then, I closed my eyes and took several deep breaths, exhaling as slowly as I could. Finally, I could open my eyes and listen to the happy voice of the New Zealander next to me telling stories of scuba diving.

❋

This is my fifth day back in Thailand. I arrived by way of Chiang Mai, where I found myself sitting in a hotel room drinking beer and scaring myself with my suicidal fantasies while walking about taking pictures of temples and graveyards. Then, on my way to Doi Inthanon, Thailand's tallest peak and most sacred mountain, my driver pulled over in the town of Chum Thung, and told me here was an ancient temple that I must see. So I walked into the temple, lit my candles and incense, sat down and closed my eyes. Five minutes later a woman tapped me on the shoulder and asked: "You want to stay here and be a student with Phra Ajan Song Sirimangalo?"

The rules are straightforward. Meditators must follow the eight precepts and refrain from: destroying living creatures; taking what's not theirs; enjoying any kind of erotic behavior; using incorrect speech; drinking intoxicating liquors or taking drugs; eating at the wrong times (i.e. after noon); indulging in self-beautification; and lying in luxurious sleeping places. Meditators also shall not leave the temple grounds, sleep during the day, read, write, or practice other spiritual disciplines. To keep the mind focused and not tempted by the flesh, meditators must not kiss, touch, hug, hold hands, sunbathe, socialize, dance, sing, listen to music, gossip, be nude (except while bathing), or go without proper undergarments.

Two pleasures, however, are allowed: smoking and eating yogurt.

Along with the Thai novices from Bangkok and Chiang Mai, there are a handful of other *farangs* here who have pulled in, as I have, off the Eastern journey highway to add to their store of mystical experiences. We have donned the same white pajamas that all *bikkuni* wear and bow with folded hands at the heart to show respect to the monks and elders. There is a nursing student from London, who has made it a whole month, and now has a shaved head and says she wants to stay and teach English to the monks. The rest of us fall far short of her discipline. There's a French loner, who seems sick, or depressed, or both, and who never comes out of his cottage except at meals. There is an American couple from Minnesota, who leave after only three days. Then, there's an Irish guy, in his early twenties, who keeps asking me: "Is something supposed to happen? I listen to the abbot and I do what he says, you know, I do the sitting and walking, but . . . but nothing happens. Is something supposed to happen?" And there is a woman who arrived today, a Chinese woman I thought at first. But when she opened her mouth, I knew she wasn't from Taipei or Beijing: "Do they really expect us to wear this . . . this uniform?" I could even place her geographically. She was a pure, red-blooded Californian.

❋

I am sitting on a yoga mat, a folded blanket, two towels, and a pair of pants in a twelve by twelve foot cottage. My feet are numb, my back hurts, my stomach growls, and my mind, full from a lifetime of defilements, flits from thought to thought.

In a few minutes I will be let out to report to the abbot on my progress in the study of insight meditation. I will enter his sitting room, bow three times, crawl up to his feet, mumble a prayer of homage, then wait for my questions to be translated by an ant-like old woman with a bald head, who could pass for an eight-year-old girl: "He say, 'Do you have pain?' He ask you, 'Do you have thoughts?' He want to know, 'Do you see lights?'"

The abbot says the world is full of heat, turmoil, and confusion. All mental and physical phenomena are impermanent, tinged by suffering, and not of the true Self. Only purified minds can truly perform good deeds.

Thai Buddhists claim the practice of Vipassana is the single most important teaching of Lord Buddha. After my first session with the abbot, the old lady translator told me: "You practice every day, every minute, keep the mindfulness always for seven years and two things can happen: when you die, you not get reborn, or . . . you get nirvana."

❋

We line up outside the abbot's office and wait our turn to see him. We're now down to just the French man, the London nurse, the Californian, and me.

"You late," says Lon Pol, the translator. "We say meet here every day, five o'clock. Why you late every time?"

I have no answer.

"Michael, show me walking." Every day she finds something wrong with what I'm doing. One day my shirt wasn't buttoned right. Yesterday my feet were dirty. So as the monks walk by, she scrutinizes my technique. "No, no, you walk too fast." The monks bounce along, joking like frat brothers, in their saffron togas draped over one shoulder, no doubt heading out for a smoke, as a gang of them do twice a day behind my cottage. I can't blame them. Most of them seem bored, as they are here to please parents and will only stay a year, if that.

Inside the abbot's quarters, I take my turn, kneel, prostrate three times, and chant to the Buddha: *namo tassa bhagavato arahato sammasambuddhassa.*

Phra Ajan Sirimangalo, a plump jelly ball of a man with a brown, bald head sits seemingly half asleep on a kind of golden throne, surrounded by a tiered altar filled with Buddhist statuary, golden bowls, jars with scrolls of sacred texts, urns filled with lotus and marigolds. Behind him are pictures of him with Pope John Paul II and the Dalai Lama, and, as in every room in this country, sacred or profane, a portrait of Thailand's King and Queen. Lon Pol reminds him that I'm on my sixth day, meditating for half-hour intervals. Vipassana demands greater and greater levels of concentration as the student progresses in his practice. Meditation begins with the student focusing on the breath with the eyes closed. In my case, I'm asked to take my attention from my breath to a series of energetic points, starting at the bottoms of the feet and onto ankles, knees, hips, back, chest, shoulders, and the chakra centers of the body.

Back at my cottage, I take one step inside and walk back out. I can't stand another minute cramped inside this cottage, trying to will myself into believing that this was what I really wanted to do: sit for ten days confronting a remarkably predictable and banal mind. I sit out back. Beyond the temple grounds, rice fields extend far into the undulating landscape. I entertain thoughts of one of the monks finding me alone and offering me one of his cigarettes. I often have this fantasy, of breaking through their persona and finding out who they really are under their costumes.

Gazing out at the rice fields, I can see someone walking, one of the Thai novices, I think. But as she gets closer, I can tell that walk, it's the Californian, Jenny. She looks sad even from a distance and I think of going out and talking with her, but then I remember: *no socializing, no talking*. As she gets closer, she looks my way, then turns. I study her movements, her athletic body, absorbing her loneliness into mine.

❈

I'd believed at first, that the panic attacks that began in Vietnam were due to the stress of travel. The word "panic," after all, comes from the half-man, half-goat, over-sexed satyr of Greek mythology, who terrified lonely travelers along their journeys. But sitting alone these six days, observing my mind as it cycles its plots of fancy, its primal tantrums and tiresome complaints to fill the void of silence, I realize that panic always comes from within.

The instruction given by Phra Ajong via Lon Pol is well-meaning, but no more beneficial than the badly photocopied student guide, which we are not supposed to read until we leave. But I don't need another book to read about meditation or another retreat; what I need is a teacher. My two-minute sessions with Phra Ajong are useless. Sure, it's a problem of language. If I could speak to him directly in Thai, I'd test the man's wisdom and patience at every turn. But Lon Pol is so subservient, I don't bother. It was obvious from the first day that her job is to keep the *farangs* and the donations coming while not taxing Phra Ajong with our ignorance and poor manners. The Buddhists, like everybody else in this country, have learned how to profit from the desires and dreams of Western tourists. What can anyone learn about meditation or any spiritual discipline in a week or a month? I should be grateful that someplace like this exists for troubled souls like me.

For the first couple of days, I was relieved to not have to be any-where, talk to anyone, observe and record anything other than the work-ings of my own mind. I needed to rest and to get a hold of myself. I need-ed structure and the discipline of meditation practice. Since stepping onto the plane in Indianapolis three months ago, I'd hoped to find a place along my journey where I could sit down and let the past empty itself out. I knew my mind would want to play tricks. I knew it would exploit the first moment of fatigue and boredom to feed my ego with intellectual spins and riffs. I knew that I'd wander into fantasies of grandeur and lust. I was not naïve to the cunning and stubborn nature of my mind, when it was challenged by the discipline of yoga and med-itation. I was eager to dismantle the machine of thought, but I was not prepared to witness the rage that my mind held and the sadness that it protected.

As the days pass, the rebellious tantrums and wild fits of anger only intensify, making me feel strangely not only physically younger but emo-tionally younger as well. I'm scared by the ferocity of my fury. Not knowing the mechanics of the muscles or the electrical circuitry of the nervous system is one thing, but to not know why certain emotions hold the body in a constant state of fear and shame seems not only foolish but deadly.

Intellectually, I understand that anger is an instinctual response to frustration, neglect, or injustice. But for me, I've always associated this emotion with shame and the thing I fear most: lack of control. This fear came, in part, from the emotional chaos of my family, and the alcohol and depression that fueled it. I remember huddling with my sisters in the closet as the pans crashed and the cursing echoed down the hall. I vowed that whatever caused my parents such emotional explosions, I would never let myself be ruled by it.

As a child, I was content to be alone. I played quietly in my room building and imagining worlds of my own design. When I played with others, especially games with my sisters or the neighbor kids, something happened inside me that I couldn't explain. One moment I was deeply involved in playing, and the next, I could see the game board flying out of my hands, the bat whirling toward a kid's head. I would lose my tem-per, stomp home, heaving with sobs at the imperfections of the world. It got so bad that I was banned from playing games. My parents feared these explosions were signs of some developmental delay and held me back a year from entering school. But it did no good. I lived with emo-tional outbursts well into grammar school and brought home report cards with uniform perfection until my parents turned to the back and read the notes written in red ink: "Mike is an excellent student but often cannot control his temper." Somewhere in adolescence these rages disap-peared, and presumably I regained my control. But the disappearance was an illusion: I'd only learned how to swallow the rage.

Beneath the anger, as I have been discovering during these long days of meditation, exists another realm of emotional history and attachments: anger's shy twin, sadness. As anger fills space with emotion and action, sadness swallows and suppresses, using the body to contain and mask true feelings. I would like to think that this sadness stems from what I have seen and the stories I've recorded in my travels. But the people that I've been drawn to—the activists and healers, the doctors and community leaders—have used HIV and AIDS as a kind of vaccine against despair and sadness. AIDS has strengthened them spiritually, not weakened them.

Sitting with the sadness these past days, feeling it expanding and retracting with each breath, I'm reminded that there's no escape from karma. It lives in every action, every thought, every breath and drop of blood. It was I who took the poison, it was my hand that put the drinks and the drugs to my mouth, it was my body that ached to be filled by nameless men, it was my mind that plotted its demise. This isn't an explanation; it is the cycle of karma itself. Sadness begets sadness, suffering begets suffering. The sickness of self-destruction is that once attempts are made on one's life, by whatever means, then it is no longer necessary to try again, because shame will endlessly repeat the act without the body lifting a finger.

Rilke said that the melancholy that comes over us sometimes is not necessarily of our own making but grows from our sensitivity to the land itself, the weather, the stones, and the trees that have their own kind of emotional life and history. I have always believed that there was some deep sorrow in the land of my birth, Indiana, a state denuded of trees and drained of its swamps and bogs, its prairies plowed, its rivers dammed, its lakes polluted, the heart of the Midwest cut and squared for human consumption. Indeed, the land reflects the spirituality of its people. Here, in my homeland, the fear-driven men and the obedient women ripped open the cold, shit-sodden earth year upon year until they collapsed and were plowed under, leaving their children to pick up where they left off. Calvin's pinnacled churches pierced our factory-smoke sky. In this world of providence and merit, there was no compassionate Christ for the poor or sick. There was right and wrong, hard work and hell. On a black sign in a soybean field facing the highway outside my hometown was the story in six white words: "The Wages of Sin are Death."

Generation upon generation, this brown on brown, sad world of beer bottles and bricks and clods of dirt seeped into my blood. It tarnished everything I touched: my house, my dreams, and my body. It was only in those desperate naked dashes in the middle of the night and innocent embraces with a boy in our barn that I could find release.

I learned to find this sadness wherever I went and with whomever I met. I knew how to find the dark tooth in the back of their mouths, that stutter, that eye unable to tell a lie. I remember the first time I found out about how Lawrence's father had killed himself, explaining the mystery I'd turned over and over in my mind since I'd first met him. I knew some kids didn't have fathers for different reasons, but Lawrence never said why his was gone. So when I finally heard the truth from his cousin, I wanted confirmation. I figured he needed to tell me. I was his friend. "Why?" I asked that day as we rested between games of one-on-one in my backyard. "Why did he shoot himself? I mean, why would someone do such a thing? In the mouth? In the alley behind your house? Why?" Leaning up against the ash tree by the court, Lawrence refused to take his eyes off the top branches, hoping to hold his tears in his sockets, but like dripping blood they streaked down his dusty, black face.

When I began to teach writing, it was the first thing I asked students to do: write about the saddest day in your life. Dutifully, but nervously, they would. Story after story, loss after loss, I read them: the war stories, the refugee camps, the gang shootings, the Christmases in the projects. It had become my trade, the way I connected with people. It was no surprise that I'd taken my pen and notebook out to the edges of the world to hear more.

✺

Outside the temple each evening, I see the old women walking in meditation, moving like cats after prey, foot by foot, as they inch across the stone terrace. Many of the women are widows who have come to spend their last years in the company of the monks and the abbot, living in little cottages around the perimeter of the temple complex.

In the soft spill of moonlight, the temple looks even older than its five hundred years. The golden bot next to it, supposedly housing fragments of the Buddha's finger bones, looks like a spaceship coming up out of the ground. There's a breeze, and bats swoop and swirl picking off mosquitoes. Among the other Thai and Western meditators, I have little trouble concentrating on my feet. The clear night air lifts the bones and softens the muscles. I walk in meditation as if I've practiced for years. Then an owl atop one of the pines shatters the peace, and the temple dogs begin to bark, and I lose my balance.

Lon Pol sits draped in a long white shawl far away in meditation. I figure it's best to leave while she's meditating so as not to get called over. She likes to talk after meditating, telling her stories about the abbot or the Buddha. I pick up my sandals and tip-toe to the gate, but I am stopped at the steps: "Michael, you come, we talk now."

I don't want to stay. I know we'll only get into another debate, as we did the night before, when I'd tried to argue with her, hoping a traditional Theravada Buddhist would see my postmodern points about desire and the body: "Desire is *not* always bad. Desire is wisdom; it teaches us things." Tonight, I say nothing. I listen to her stories of Shakyamuni and the tinkling chimes of the temple, until the bells signal that it's time for bed.

❀

At breakfast, instead of sitting with the Thai novices and mindfully eating yesterday's leftovers from lunch, I sit beside Jenny with the *farangs* clustered around Lon Pol. We whisper a few exchanges about where we've been—the travel resume, always the first conversation topic for Americans abroad. She wants to teach English in Taiwan; she has worked with some relief organization in India, traveled some in Nepal, wants to stay in Asia, and has that idealism and rebellion that come from traveling far from home for the first time. I consider lying when she asks about me, but it's hard to lie in a place where you spend all day confronting lifetimes of deceit.

Lon Pol is lecturing us for eating too fast and talking too much. "Even when eating we should practice; we can think, 'I am chewing, chewing, chewing.'" A scrawny, rat-like kitten with a hairless tail cries under our table for food. Jenny befriends it, cradling the ugly thing and giving it some milk from her bowl. Jenny comes back to the table and Lon Pol drones on: "We lift our spoon, lifting, lifting, lifting; now we are chewing, chewing . . ." Suddenly a dog goes after the kitten, and Jenny shrieks as the kitten scampers for its life up a nearby tree.

"Please eat and leave the cat," Lon Pol commands, embarrassed that this woman under her direction has caused such a scene in front of the other Thais. But Jenny pulls the frightened kitten off the tree, brings it to her chest and runs like a girl to her cottage as Lon Pol calls, "You must take your bowl back to wash! Come back!"

After this scene, I'm too worked up to meditate, so I rip off my shirt, drop my pants, and roll out my yoga mat. After seven days, I've had enough. Madly, I jump into my asanas, moving from pose to pose with defiance, trying to concentrate but feeling so much anger coming up and out of my body I feel like screaming. With the windows shut and the morning humidity and midday heat, sweat pours from my body. After showering, I unzip my duffle bag, toss out my notebooks, unwrap the t-shirts around two bottles of stashed Heineken, and plug in my computer. I look at my bags and imagine how quickly I could be packed and on the road. But I tell myself to stay until at least the day after tomorrow. Tomorrow is my birthday, and I don't want to be alone. Instead of leaving, I decide to break another rule and hike into town.

I wait until afternoon, when everything gets quiet, sneak through the back, put on another shirt over my acolyte's outfit, and head down the main street looking for an internet café, and it's not long until I find one. An hour is gone in no time as I gleefully read, tap, click, and send until I've drained two cans of Coke, eaten three packs of cookies, and written half a dozen long letters.

Buzzed on sugar, I saunter up the road, when I can't believe my eyes: *a 7-Eleven*. I never thought a convenience store could look so good. I buy everything: candy, gum, two newspapers, film, cookies, ice cream, and several little cartons of yogurt. At the counter, I realize I've overdone it and put a few things back, remembering that I still have to make it through the gate.

Back in my room, where I've left the Heinekens in my sink full of cold water, I sit on the floor, not to meditate, but to open my bag of goodies and drink my beer. Impatiently I tear the large bag of M&Ms with my teeth and they scatter, so I crawl about the room picking up M&Ms and popping them in my mouth.

❄

At breakfast, Jenny corners me before we sit down. "Where were you yesterday? You missed the report with Phra Ajong."

"I went out."

"Out? I thought we weren't supposed to leave?"

"I had to check my email."

"Email? Where?" She grabs my arm and then drops it.

"In town. You want to go with me? I'm going again around three."

Later that afternoon, like two high school students, we skip out. She wants to stop everywhere: a bakery, a market, a store that sells paper that she wants to buy for one of the old widow ladies. At a fruit stand she buys fruit, tasting them and then putting them up to my mouth, "Try this."

"Are you going to stay the whole time?" She asks.

"I don't know. I really have to be on my way. There's some people in Chiang Mai I should try to interview."

"But you seem so into it. I saw you doing the walking meditation last night, you can really do it. I'm impressed."

"I finally learned that you have to slow down, way down."

"I hate this place. I mean I like the people, the old ladies. Have you met the dog lady? I love the temple and the little spirit houses. I walk around a lot. I can't stay in that room, it has this smell. It makes me sick." Her body is full of energy, flipping from subject to subject, curious, full of questions. We make it to the email café and spend a half hour typing away; I watch her between letters and wonder what we'd be doing if there were no computers. Then I get lost answering some letters when she taps me on the shoulder: "I'll be outside. Take your time."

We stop and eat at a little vegetarian restaurant. She talks about going north, wondering if I might be interested in going with her. "Have you been up in the triangle, with the Hill Tribes? Are you going to do research there? It's bad up there, isn't it, with the drugs?" She tries to get me to talk about my work, but I turn each question back to her. We meander slowly back toward the temple, stopping on a bridge to watch ducks and a churning, wooden, water wheel.

"You know what today is?" I ask, looking down into the water.

"No. What is it?"

"It's my birthday."

"Your birthday?" I can see she's looking at me, but I don't move. "Why didn't you say something? You know, you're a very odd person. There's something about . . . something doesn't seem right. I'm sorry. I . . . I've been thinking about you, and what you're working on. Why are you doing this?"

I hear her but listen to the water, pull myself into the scene of the ducks, like I'm one of them and not really in this body leaning on this bridge. For seven days I've been relieved of being the guy with HIV. I was just a guy traveling, writing a few stories, my turmoil confined to my cottage. Today, walking with her, I'd forgotten about all of this.

"I mean, why go to all of these countries and write about this?"

Her face demands the truth, and I know that if I don't admit it, she will ask the question anyway.

My answer comes out like a sigh: "Because I'm HIV positive, that's why."

"Oh, I thought so. I'm sorry I didn't mean to—"

"No, no, no. I should have told you."

"That's why you're so into yoga, isn't it?"

"Yeah."

I go into my spiel, using words to stabilize the emotions and turn my legs and arms to stone. Her eyes widen, her face seems to expand and eclipse the temple and everything around it. She wants to know everything: all the usual questions people want to know, think they have a right to ask once I tell them, believing that it conveys concern. I tell her whatever she wants to know.

"So it sounds like you . . . you kind of wanted to get infected, like you wanted to, like, kill yourself?"

Essentially she's right, though I'd not had anyone really put it to me like this before. Not by a woman, anyway, a woman who had entered my romantic imagination. "Yes, I guess you could say that," I say mechanically, as if we're talking about someone else.

As we get closer to the monastery, she starts to cry. "I'm sorry, I'm sorry. It's your birthday, and I'm asking you all of this. I'm so sorry."

I want to hug her, but here in the open, I know I can't. We walk side by side toward the temple. It's getting later in the afternoon. People are filling the street, going home from work, coming out to shop. Then in another burst of emotion, she offers: "I tried to kill myself once, too."

I say nothing, afraid to look at her, afraid of this endless stream of suffering that seems to reveal itself in everyone I meet. We walk on to the 7-Eleven, buy ice cream and sit outside, watching each other try to eat as it melts down our wrists. We walk slowly back into the temple grounds alone with our thoughts.

She takes me to see the dog lady, one of the old widows who gets her name from feeding the temple dogs and cats. After she quiets her barking dogs, we enter her cottage. The dog lady has silver hair and is dressed in white silk pants and a white cotton smock. In every corner of her cottage I see a cat: one on the bed, another wrapped around itself in a chair, two lying in a box on the floor, one on the windowsill, one on top of the dresser. But it's not the cats that are so surprising, it's her walls. They are covered with long sheets of paper, old calendars turned around, and other scraps of used paper, all with Pali written in large red lettering.

"What are these?" I ask.

"These are teachings of the Buddha. I put them up to make them stay in my mind," she smiles, pointing to her head.

As Jenny plays with the cats, the dog lady shows me her scrapbook, pointing out pictures of her as a nurse in Bangkok and of her husband, who died in a car accident years ago. "I have no children," she says, explaining before I can ask.

"I show you something." She gets up, waving for us to follow. Outside in a little walled-in patio, she points to an old dog lying with several kittens nestled beside it. "See, she thinks she is the mother." She looks down at the old dog, which is licking the little kittens. "It is the second time she take kittens, first time she feed them." At this, she snickers, covering her mouth with her hand, her shoulders shaking with pleasure at this oddity of nature, as if this dog's action proves the wisdom of the Buddha, when he said that even dogs and cats can attain enlightenment.

❀

I make some calls to set up a meeting with a Thai Christian minister who runs an AIDS social service agency in Chiang Mai. I tell Lon Pol that I'll be leaving the next day. I meditate that day with a calmness and focus I've not had in the eight days since I arrived. Jenny agrees to go with me, at least to Chiang Mai. We make no real plans. A woman from Chiang Mai, a wealthy hotel owner, who has been at the temple for a week, says she'll give us a ride.

I wake early. Our ride has her luxury Toyota pulled up with the trunk already open. "Where's the Chinese girl? I want to go now."

Lon Pol, aware of this woman's status and her financial support for the temple, is not happy. "She is very nice to wait for you. She take you to Chiang Mai. Where is the girl?"

"I don't know? I'll go look for her."

"No, you can't go back there, that side for the women."

The woman looks at her watch and sighs. I put my luggage in the trunk. I see Jenny walking to the dog lady's cottage. I almost don't recognize her in her tight-fitting jeans, sweater, and red lipstick. "I'm not ready. I want to say goodbye to the dog lady, I'm sorry, I couldn't sleep."

"But our ride is waiting."

"I don't care. Let her go. You can go. I'll just go later. I'm so mad at this Lon Pol. She came into my room and lectured me on how I dress— can you believe it!" And Jenny stomps off.

The woman closes her trunk and gets in her car. Lon Pol advises me to go: "She is only like a child, leave her. You must go now." I look back toward the dog lady's cottage, but then get into the car.

All the way to Chiang Mai, I regret my choice, playing back the scene in my mind, seeing Jenny standing there, her brilliant red lipstick, her anger, her voice now gone: "I'll see you—maybe in Chiang Mai, okay?"

The wealthy woman goes on a long diatribe about this and that, the economy, the lack of tourists, her problems keeping good staff, but reassuring me that I will like Chiang Mai and her four star hotel, which will only cost $110. "I give you special price." When I mention that I'm here to write about AIDS in Thailand, she goes on another lecture, blaming the epidemic on the irresponsibility of the poor and ungrateful young people, telling a story to illustrate about a friend's son who'd died of an overdose. "Terrible, terrible to do this to his mother. Just a selfish child. I don't tell her this. But that's what he was."

She goes on and on as I clench my fists, wondering how much further it is to Chiang Mai. "They are all dying," she continues, as if she were talking about livestock. "It's terrible. It seems every time I come into work, I've got to hire someone new. 'Where's bell boy?' I ask. 'Oh, he die,' they say. 'Where is cook?' 'Oh, he die too.'" In my mind I envision her on that table in the After-Death Room at the monastery in Lopburi. I see her naked old lady's body floating in formaldehyde. I consider telling her my status, but hold my tongue, just as I did the day before during my last audience with the abbot.

Lon Pol had told me that he had agreed to take some of my questions at our last meeting. I was now his official acolyte and thus had earned a few moments with him. Through Lon Pol, he answered my questions about the role of Buddhism and Thailand's clergy in helping the country respond to HIV and AIDS. He said that meditation and the way of the dharma would help all who suffer. "It makes the mind strong; it help with difficulties of pain." But AIDS, he said, "is caused by desire and people breaking the precepts [of Buddhism]. They not follow the right path, so they die."

I kept thinking this was the time to tell them. I could feel the words in the back of my throat as I listened to Lon Pol translate his pronouncements. I wanted to tell him. I wanted to give him this as my donation: *Look at me. Look at my body, my legs and arms, my face and chest. I'm AIDS. I'm HIV. Me. I'm the sex worker. I'm the drug user. I'm the homosexual. Me, right here in front of you. I am Desire.* But I didn't. I listened, dutifully, as Lon Pol told me they help sponsor some program for drug users. Then the abbot reached his hand out as though touching something hot. His face brightened, and he looked more alive than I'd seen him in ten days. "He say," Lon Pol whispered looking down to the floor, "The people, the people who let the desire take them, it is like fire. The people who have no control of their desire, they burn. If you go to them, and be with them, you will be burned too."

VII

Chiang Mai, Thailand (July, 2001)

Pastor Sanan easily spots my blond hair at a bus station where we'd arranged to meet. He takes me across Chiang Mai to a split-level house discreetly situated in a wooded lot across from a Presbyterian college. Like many AIDS-related organizations, no sign marks what this place is or does.

Pastor Sanan is self-conscious about his English and wants me to hold my questions until his assistant arrives. He is a sturdy man of about my age, wearing the same relaxed, loose-fitting silk shirt you'd find on any Thai man who is dressed for a casual affair. He hardly fits my image of a Christian pastor.

Their ministry, like the many other non-governmental organizations in the area which deal with HIV and AIDS, began ten years ago when civic and religious organizations in Thailand felt compelled to respond to the epidemic. Over the past decade, their work has evolved into something of a social-service agency. There is no self-righteousness in his voice when he describes the AIDS ministry. He pats my hand: "We serve Lord Jesus Christ with the healing, to touch the sick persons, not to forget the poor. We serve because our Lord teach us that way: to care for the least among us."

A couple of other staff members join us, including his assistant, who is fluent in English. Her name is Julailak Khampeera, but she asks to be called Pon. She wears khaki pants and a man's golf shirt, her hair short and boyish. They confer about what to do with me, then Pon writes some things on a legal pad.

"Tomorrow, I pick you up at seven o'clock," Pon says, showing me my schedule. "We come here for morning meeting and prayer, then we go to outreach communities. Tuesday, we visit New Life Friends Centre, meet with AIDS group and activist, Samran." She looks over at Sanan, who nods his approval. "Wednesday, you go to visit Phra Jahn, Buddhist monk who work with AIDS patients. He is at his retreat center, outside of Chiang Mai. I call for you. Thursday we meet with Phra Phongthep, Buddhist monk who has AIDS hospice. Today, you meet the doctor, he is coming soon. He see our clients. You can talk with them if they give permission. I wish I could take you to visit some more people, but I have other work to do." Pon looks up from her notebook. "This okay for you?"

I hardly know what to say. I expected some suggestions, phone numbers, directions, but not a five day tour with a translator and transportation. "Thank you, that's great. I'll be ready."

Pon and Sanan together explain their programs, one of which Pon calls "Clear Sky." "When AIDS hit, the sick were rejected from society, so we try to change the attitudes of people—people in our own church." Serving twenty to thirty people a week, they advise their clients on treatment, diet, and alternative care: Thai massage, meditation, and yoga. "We try to empower the people," Pastor Sanan says, "to show them they have choices, that there is a network of people who can help them, that they have the rights."

He confesses that he has learned from those who have had to face death: "Before I afraid so much of death, but working with these people with AIDS, I don't have the fear anymore. They are like everyone, they want the dignity, they want to die with the power." Then he adds something that seems amazing to me after the conservative responses I've heard from Buddhists, Hindus, and Christians in America: "If we ask people to change their behavior to prevent the AIDS, why can't society change, too?"

Dr. Sangrog Pradupkeow, a short man with a confident air, explains that things are much better in the North than ten years ago. People are living longer because there are more services and better health care. Yet, he laments, "Despite all the work, we have much more we need to do."

I'm impressed that he comes to volunteer every week. How easily he works with the patients, touching and listening with concern, like the doctors in Chennai. A few are taking the retroviral treatments via special programs at Chiang Mai's hospital. He asks them about diet and the traditional treatments they're using; he gives advice for skin problems and checks for symptoms. Between clients, he tells me a story of the time he had to remove a kidney in an emergency. He makes a fist with his right hand. "This big, the cyst was, that we had to remove. I told the head nurse, we need some ice. So my nurse told somebody to go buy some ice, twenty-five *bhat* of ice," he laughs. "We took the kidney out, packed it in the ice, and put it back. Ha! Would have cost hundred thousand dollars in America. We did it for fifty cents!"

"Why do you do this work for the ministry?" I ask.

"I do it because it's my duty," he says sobering up, waving to the next patient.

The clients are poor and mostly in their thirties and forties. A man wearing a Nike hat, shielding a thin, serious face tells me that he is sad when he sees others with AIDS. For himself, he says, "I feel strong," making fists with his hands. But I wonder how strong a man can be whose friends have all died.

When I ask about the V-1 cure, he tells me sniffling that, yes, he has tried it, shrugging like it's not such a big deal. He now uses a traditional medication and believes it's working. He doesn't know what it's called. It's something he found in his village. He cooks it for an hour and drinks it. When I ask him if there's a chance to take the newer antiretroviral drugs, he says: "I hear about them, new ones each year. But I don't think I'll ever be able to get them." He knows they could help him. There is a pause. Pon knows he wants to say something else. The man becomes nervous, not sure what he should say. "The cure," he says pressing his hands down onto the table, "is not something that should be kept in the bank like money. It should be given to everyone, whether they have the money or not."

In his eyes and voice, I recognize that intelligence I've seen before in the faces of people with HIV. It's a wisdom about life, knowledge about this disease that an expert can never detect or discover from where he stands. Even though this man believes he will get better in the future, he sees the epidemic getting worse: "I wish I could go back and avoid it, go back to the time when I was healthy. I miss the past," he says looking out the window, as if the past is a place he can still find his way back to. Then his sister arrives to take him home. After he leaves, Pon tells me that his sister is as sick as he is.

I talk next with three women. They are small, poor, terribly self-conscious and nervous, but one jumps to answer my questions, telling me she is part of a group called Friends For Life, an organization that Pon reminds me I will see in a few days. "Groups help, talking to family and friends help," she tells me. Another woman shakes her head, she has no group. They talk about their maladies, about headaches and diarrhea, about spots on their skin, rolling up their pants and pointing them out to me. Then they turn to food, debating which ones are best to eat. "Meat," says one. "The good vegetables and the fruit," says another. "No," a third chimes in, "fish is best."

The talkative lady says she's fifty years old, her birthday just was the other day. She has had the virus for six years. I tell her that I've had it for five and that I, too, just had my birthday. It turns out we have the same birthday. Self-conscious about her bad teeth, she tries to smile without showing them, but her emotion can't be contained.

Pon drives me to my hotel in her mini pick-up truck. She tells me about her husband who is a youth pastor and studying for his divinity degree. I debate whether to reveal that I, too, once studied theology and wanted to be a minister, something I rarely admit, but figure it can only help me make a better impression. "You? You studied theology?"

I laugh. "You don't believe me?"

She pulls the truck into the hotel drive. "Yes, I believe. I see you tomorrow, Michael."

I am drained from a day of interviewing. Pon drew me a map of where to find a swimming pool and that's right where I head after doing my yoga practice.

Later, back at my hotel, typing my notes, the phone rings. I look at it, confused, wondering who could possibly be calling me. Then, I think, Jenny? I grab it. "Hello?"

A small voice I don't recognize answers: "Is everything okay?"

I can't figure out who it is.

"Did you find the swimming pool?" It's Pon. "I hope it's okay that I called you, but I worry if everything is okay? Your room, okay? I come tomorrow at seven-thirty, okay?"

After I hang up, I lie on my bed like a stone. Her call, meant to reassure me, has the opposite effect. I think of Jenny, somewhere in town, and wonder again why I'd not decided to travel with her. The room, so quaint and warm before, now becomes a mirror of my loneliness: the one bath towel, the empty shelves and dressers, the wide empty bed. My breath shortens. The panic is back.

I get up, but I have nowhere to go. I've read all my books. I decide to take a shower. It doesn't help. I consider going out: on the way back from the pool I had seen several clubs. Chiang Mai, while not Bangkok or Pattaya, has its share of bars that cater to the restless and hungry. Instead I drink another beer and watch TV.

That night I have a nightmare of the man in the Nike cap. In the dream his face decays before my eyes as I interview him. As if in time-lapse photography, his skin breaks into boils, rots, and then falls off, leaving only his eyes in his skull. Not blinking or flinching, his eyes remain fixed on mine, as he tells me about all the people he has watched die before him.

❄

On my second day with the Christians, Pon greets me with a bag of pastries and a cup of coffee poured from her thermos: "Today, we make the home visits and stop to see the HIV-positive people who live in a community house outside Chiang Mai."

At the ministry, though, the day begins with worship. The AIDS ministry is sponsored by the Church of Christ of Thailand, a small conservative sect of the Methodist tradition, which has several small congregations in Chiang Mai. Pastor Sanan is glad to see me, knowing I didn't have to join them. The staff meet in the conference room in the basement. Hymnals are passed around and Pon pulls a Bible from the shelf, sits down next to me, and slides it over. "It's in English," she whispers.

When, I wonder, was I last part of a Christian religious service? I've been to weddings and funerals of course. But it must be over fifteen years—ironically, with a small group of Christian activists, like this one, that I joined while in divinity school. Everyone in that ecumenical group worked in some way in activism, with battered women, in street ministries, with immigrants as I did, or with the poor as did the nuns whose house on the South Side we used for our meeting place each Friday night. It was our own community-based church, following the liberation theology model spawned by Gustavo Gutierrez, Ernesto Cardinal, and other Latin American priests and activists.

Pastor Sanan and the staff stand. We sing an old hymn I remember. Though they sing it in Thai, I hear in their voices the familiar rousing march and rhythm of so much church music that I grew up with. I try to hum along out of respect. Pon, hearing that I know the tune, thrusts her hymnal in front of me, though of course I can't read a word of it.

Then there is the lectionary. Pon flips through my Bible to a passage in Isaiah. As they take turns offering their interpretations, I float back to those Fridays on 47th Street in Chicago, sitting in a circle with the black ladies from next door, the nuns and ministers, activists and students, as we passed around a loaf of bread. As the Thai Protestants wrestle with the wisdom of Isaiah, I glance up at the familiar face of Jesus on the wall: that tilting head, those empathetic eyes, that tan (but not too tan) skin. It's the same handsome Anglo-Saxon Jesus that was mounted on the wall of every Sunday school class I ever attended. Save for the long hair, it's the image American Protestants have sent around the world: clean, holy, youthful, strong, and white. To see it here, in a country steeped in traditional Theravada Buddhism, with a King and Queen who are seen as nearly divine, seems absurd. But then, looking at the faces of these people before me, clapping and singing with their open hearts as they prepare for another day of devoted service to the poor and sick of northern Thailand, who is more absurd: I—who have come from a Buddhist monastery taking on the garb and discipline of monks—or them? The service ends in a prayer. We bow our heads. I look up at their closed eyes, their intense faces, hear my name evoked by Pastor Sanan, and quickly drop my eyes.

✻

Eva, a high school student from Sweden who is a volunteer for the summer, joins Pon and me as we head into the countryside to meet with the HIV-positive clients the ministry serves. The first stop is a house next to an auto repair shop on the outskirts of a little town next to a large flooded rice field. A frail, young woman in a plaid shirt waves at us from her porch. As I step out, she steps back, her happy face now full of fear. Pon reads her concern and introduces me as someone living with HIV. We sit on the woman's porch, talking and drinking iced tea. Earlier Pon had told me that this woman, perhaps no more than thirty, had lost two children and a husband in the last two years to AIDS. "She was very sick and wanted to die, but we got her into a special program so that she could get the new drugs."

Her skin looks pasty, but her eyes register a hunger for life. Embarrassed but happy, she whispers to Pon that she has gained another two pounds. She has problems with her skin, rubbing her arms and pointing to her neck, asking me what I recommend. I suggest a cream I used once, and Pon writes it down.

Knowing I might help her with the drug side effects, Pon asks her to show me the medication she's using. I recognize it. "Drink a lot of water," I tell her. Then I turn to Pon. "Have her eat starchy food—it will lessen the effects of nausea." I turn back to the woman, "It's okay, the bad feelings go away after awhile." Then I show her some yoga poses. She sits beside me on the floor and I put her feet up on the wall. Eva and Pon try them, too. "Do this one, if you can't sleep, or have emotional problems."

A man walks up the steps, stumbles by us and collapses on a couch inside. Pon shrugs, whispering that he is her friend who stays with her sometimes. He comes back out, asking Pon if we can help him with his eyes. He is emaciated, his eyes watery and vacant. I wonder if he sleeps with her. The healthy with the healthy. The sick with the sick.

The diesel fumes and the mechanics next door pounding and revving engines force me out to take a walk. Behind her house, two boys and a girl, up to their thighs in mud, drive a team of water buffalo through a flooded field of rice. Next to a barbed wire fence, a spirit house rests on a wooden stand. In this red and green doll-house temple, a stairway leads to two tiny porcelain monks standing before a bowl of fresh rice balls, a cup of water, and cuts from a red bougainvillea. The woman sees me walk over and waves. It's here that she feeds the dead, which the Thai believe will wander, haunting the living, if they are not cared for and given offerings every day. I've seen many of these spirit houses, but for the first time I understand why they are so important.

We drive another ten miles through farm land, down a narrow, overgrown lane and past a few cottages. Pon stops in front of a cement-block house. Two women stand in a dirt yard talking with a thin woman sitting on a porch eating a bowl of noodles. Pon gets out of the truck and approaches the woman, rubs her shoulders and arms, fixes her threadbare shirt. She seems in good spirits, answering questions between bites. Eva and I sit on the steps. One of the ladies in the yard is the sick woman's mother. As Pon strokes the sick woman's hair, the woman's mother and Pon speak as people do of the sick, referring to them in the third person as if they weren't there.

The sick woman's eldest son arrives on a motorbike. Our attention shifts to this vital young man, who parks his bike and bounds up the steps to be next to his mother. He's beautiful and reminds me of a young man I met at the baths in Bangkok. As he rubs his mother's shoulders, I feel such loneliness that I turn my eyes to the ground in embarrassment and yearning. Pon tells me that she lost her husband recently, and her two teenage sons and mother now take care of her. "He quit school to go to work to make money for them," she whispers.

The woman looks at her son as if she knows her life will soon be carried inside his. She begins to cry as she speaks of how proud she is of him. The son, embarrassed, turns his head from us. As she weeps, I watch him, a lotus bud about to burst and flower, a body that speaks only of the future. Her sobs silence the barking dogs. Then for the first time she looks at me and asks Pon to tell me that she and her husband had bought this house just before they'd become sick. She points to the posts and the door and the roof, the embodiments of the future they believed they would have together.

Pon takes away the tears with questions about the present, asking her about her recent visit to the doctor and the new medications. The woman mumbles, blowing her nose. Pon gives her a hug and tells her she'll be back next week, waving goodbye and signaling to Eva and me that it's time to head to our next stop.

❀

The next day, Pon takes me to another a community support group called New Life Friends Centre. The organization is located in a residential neighborhood in Chiang Mai. When we enter, seven or eight of the members are sitting on a mat, eating. Paper butterflies hang from the ceiling. Filing cabinets, bookcases, and desks fit between couches and chairs. It's a community center and office all rolled into one.

The people in the room all look young and healthy except for a woman who has sores on her legs. The brochure states that most are single, have some education, and are employed in manual or service jobs. Their president, Samran Takan, looks both slightly older and better off. Slender and well-groomed, he sports a stylish haircut and wears a silk shirt and jeans. In a profile of him by the national daily framed on the wall, I read the story of how a taxi driver saved him when, after his diagnosis, he'd taken a taxi to a park intending to hang himself. The taxi driver noticed the rope and his forlorn demeanor and talked Samran out of killing himself.

Samran reminds me of the AIDS activist I met in Chennai, the president of India's Network Positive, Ashok Pillai, a well-educated man who also had a flair for leadership and self-promotion. Both are featured prominently on posters and brochures, describing their organizations.

AIDS activism is as political as any other movement, and activists eventually must become more political as their movements grow, as someone like South Africa's Zackie Achmat attests. Achmat has something akin to celebrity status in South Africa, recognized wherever he goes. His decision not to take the antiretroviral treatment was both a defiant stance of solidarity with the thousands who have no access to medications and a smart PR move to keep himself and TAC (Treatment Action Campaign) in the news.[1]

Referring to the troubled period in his life, Samran admits that he was so sick that he had no other place to go than the AIDS clinic in Lopburi. "My family had no money to help me. I was prepared to die," he tells Pon, "but then I got better."

"I've been there. What was it like being a patient at Lopburi?"

He acts like he doesn't understand. I look to Pon, and her body language tells me that he doesn't want to talk about it. "Sit down and eat," she tells me.

Noticing plastic packets holding HIV drugs in an educational display, I turn to the subject of medications. The members of New Life receive free medications by participating in experimental trials offered by NGOs and Chiang Mai University. This is why Pon encourages her clients to join groups like New Life Friends Centre. When I ask Samran what will happen when this research grant ends, he smiles sarcastically: "Find another experiment."

Without these doctors and their research, these people would not have treatment, as none can afford the expense of the cocktail treatment, notwithstanding the government's recent cut in the price. If Thailand bought the cheaper generics that companies like Cipla in India and others in South Africa and Brazil now sell, many more people could be treated. But because 25 percent of Thailand's exports are to the U.S., the Thai government is hesitant to break their one-sided trade pact with the U.S. for poor people living with HIV.[2]

What they want to know, of course, is what drugs I take, how well they work, and what they cost me. I'm not sure how to explain that I not only have access to the latest and most powerful combination therapy, but can now take "holidays" (periods of six months to a year not taking the drugs), knowing that I can return at any time. But Pon tries to explain. Their response is an awkward silence.

After I give my blood cell count and viral level, one by one they state theirs. However, it's too expensive for them to have their viral count taken, so they only know their CD4 counts.[3] I ask about insurance. Most Thais have to pay for their own insurance, Samran says. The government can only afford a very minimal safety net, offering some public health programs and drug discounts, but not nearly enough.

From the time Pon introduced me to the group, one woman has made me uneasy. One moment she mocks my sincerity, rolling her eyes, and then the next she's flashing seductive smiles. Yet she has not said a word until now. She turns first to Pon and then to me with a confrontational voice. Pon tries to soften her questions: "She wants to know, 'Why are you here? Don't you have your own groups, in Chicago?'" The room quiets, and everybody's eyes turn toward me.

"Yes."

She fires back, "Have you asked them these questions you've asked us?"

She smiles at my discomfort. "Well, not really, because I don't belong to any of them."

"Why, not?"

"I did once, but . . . but they depressed me, so I quit."

When Pon reluctantly translates, they all laugh at my explanation. Pon, however, finds my admission anything but funny.

I try to switch subjects, but they want to know about vaccines and why Americans are so interested in coming here to experiment on them but can't make their drugs available. I try to express my agreement, but Pon, who is exhausted, can't make my confusing explanation of how difficult it is to make a vaccine sound like anything but an evasion.

The woman with the sly, seductive smile barks back something in Thai.

"What did she say?" I whisper to Pon.

"Rats. She say, they are like the rats in the experiment."

In the midst of this awkwardness, the building shakes and our conversation is silenced. I look out the window and two F-16s disappear over the mountains. I point up: "This is part of the problem." Samran agrees. The day before, I read that Thailand's military will purchase four more fighter jets from the U.S. "They're coming from the border," Samran explains, referring to Thailand's on-again off-again movement of troops to keep Myanmar's unpredictable army in check.

Pon has been up since five. She bends over, stretching and moving about to keep herself awake and to signal to me that she's ready to go. I'm so flustered at the turn of the conversation that I forgot that I wanted to offer to teach a yoga class for them. I make an effort to plug yoga anyway. "See what Pon is doing?" I say, walking over to her and forcing her head down when she naturally lifts her head to translate. "Stay there," I whisper to her. "See this is good for Pon. This is yoga; this is what I do to keep healthy. You know yoga, right?"

Confused, they wait for Pon to explain. "Let's do what Pon did. Bend over and bend your knees, relax your neck and shoulders, shake your head and hands."

Samran mimics me and they all follow him, bending over and shaking their heads. He rises and asks Pon something. She frowns. "He says he wants you to teach them yoga. But I can't stay, Michael, I have to go. Maybe tomorrow."

"I'm going to that Buddhist monk who treats AIDS patients tomorrow, and then the other monk, what's his name? Then I go back to Bangkok." Pon gives them my schedule. They confer, all talking at once.

"When you leave—Saturday?" Pon asks.

"Yes."

"They say you can do it Friday, in the morning, before you see Phra Phongthep. Someone will be here to translate. Can you do it?"

"Sure, okay, Friday morning."

"You come?" Samran asks in his English, putting his hand on my shoulder. "Friday, okay? We pick you up."

❋

Pon has been eager to introduce me to the monk who runs an AIDS hospice. However, as we drive through the outskirts of the city, she offers a warning, "We have trouble before. He has a hard head. Only do things his way, you know? But a good man, very intelligent. You will see."

Her caveat doesn't surprise me—a stubborn, opinionated Buddhist monk? After Phra Ajan Song at Chum Thung and the bizarre day I spent the day before interviewing the so-called "rocking" monk, Phra Jahn, I'm prepared for anything. Indeed, the "rocking" monk will be hard to top. All afternoon on a mountain retreat outside of Chiang Mai, I rocked and spat into a paper cup as I took his meditative cure along with a room full of devoted followers, while this monk warned us of ozone holes, UFOs, globalization, Western consumerism, and America's secret plan to take over the world. After he learned that I was seropositive, he begged me to stay, too, and work with him and his entourage (many of whom he claims have been cleansed of the HIV virus). "Please help and work with us, make website, make people know of the powers of 'rocking meditation.'"

Friends For Life Centre, not to be confused with New Life Friends Centre (where I taught yoga that morning), lies in a wooded grove, down a dirt road, on the outskirts of Chiang Mai. We walk through a raked garden of fire-orange flowering bougainvillea and white lilies, stepping on flagstones that lead us past little signs tacked onto tree trunks with passages from the Dhammapada: "Many talk like philosophers and live like fools." Ahead, through the garden, is a set of rudimentary wooden buildings attached to a small, elegantly designed building made of glass, grandly named The Wisdom and Peace Library. When we enter, a monk, tall by Thai standards, comes shuffling out of an office in sandals with a computer print-out in his hand. Phra Phongthep Dhammagaruku has a boyish face with fine lips and large round-framed glasses. I forget and stick out my hand. It hangs there unclasped. Pon is nervous, knowing she's going to have to translate for two strong-minded men.

"Sit down, sit down," Phra Phongthep directs us like we've come for business. "We talk right here, okay?" We sit at a long table full of books and papers. He begins in English with Pon's help, but soon his face registers frustration as he struggles to express himself. "I can understand but I cannot speak." So with Pon's help and his emphasis on certain words, he relates stories about his childhood that led him into the monastery and then into AIDS advocacy. "I love to study the teachings of the great Buddhist scholars, the social activists, and communist thinkers. But when I first became a monk I think I can leave the world to meditate and study, but the problems of the world are all around us, even in the monastery."

When I ask him to tell me how he began the hospice, he describes how he found a thin man lying outside his shelter in the monastery. "I knew he must have AIDS, so I try to find a place for him and collect money to take him to the AIDS clinic at Lopburi." This experience left a deep impression. After much thought and talking with doctors, many of whom warned him against it, he decided that he must work with the growing numbers of those infected and dying in his community. His abbot, however, would not allow him to work on his project while in the monastery fearing it would keep people away from the temple.

The mission of Friends For Life is not only to care for the twelve patients they have, but to educate others on the use of dharma and meditation as a means to alleviate suffering. In fact, unlike at Lopburi, people cannot just drop off their family members and hope that they will be cared for until their death. Phra Phongthep emphatically states that those family members must agree to actively participate in the care of their loved one, or else they won't be admitted.

I have to smile as I hear Pon, the Christian, translate Phra Phongthep's speeches about how AIDS is the direct result of society losing sight of the Buddha's teachings. Indeed, he is a man of many strong opinions, and not just against social ills such as sex work and drug use, but consumerism and greed, which, for him, are the true causes of the spread of AIDS in Thailand. His criticism doesn't stop with popular culture and materialism; he also chastises those traditionalists who don't believe monks should engage in political and social matters.

A phone rings, and he is called away. In the library behind us, there is a long wooden display case in the middle of the room. "What's in here?" I ask Pon, pointing at the case. Walking in, I am not surprised to find a skeleton in the case under glass, with this warning on a card beside its skull: "I was one day like you, but one day you will be like me."

"Why do they *do* this?" I whine in disgust.

"That's what many temples do, Michael, they use the skeletons to teach." Coming back in the room, Phra Phongthep smiles at our discovery.

"Ask him why they do this," I order Pon, my anger rising. "I want to know, as someone with HIV. Do they do this because they want to scare people?" I speak so quickly she doesn't quite understand, or perhaps she's afraid to offend him. So I grab her as if to scare her, pantomiming: "Do they want to scare someone? Is that what this is all about?"

"Yes," he says in English. "To make fear, make people afraid. So they change before death. Dead too late."

"Yes," I shoot back, "but this is a person's body; it's not right to use it."

"No." Pon explains, her voice now rising, "He says she wanted her body used for this."

Then he lifts his finger in the air, as if wanting me to stop my thinking. He goes back to his office and comes back with a piece of paper. Conferring with Pon, he asks, "English teacher, right; you can help me?" Pon says he has something for me to translate from a grant that he is writing. He hands me a sheet of paper written in Pali, but in a column next to it reads in English: "CLINGING, OPENING, CLINGING, GRASPING, OPENING, GIVING, GRASPING, SUFFERING, GIVING, PEACE."

"It's a prayer or meditation," Pon says, pointing to the heading, *Kam Bae Meditation*.

"I can't read it, but I can try to help."

With Pon's help, he describes the meditation. He makes a fist and shows it to me. I nod. Then he opens it. "Opening, right?"

"Yes."

"Clinging?" he asks, pulling in his fingers tight.

"That's right," I say making a fist and releasing it as he is doing.

"It is simple, yes? For dying people, simple meditation. For people—" He struggles for a word and turns to Pon who completes his thought: "It's for the dying people who have no strength."

"Yes, yes," he says, looking at me, hoping I'm getting it. "'Bae' mean 'opening.' This help them. Practice for the dying people, you see?"

Phra Phongthep invites us to lunch and a tour around the hospice. We sit at a table under a wooden roof between the two wings. Five residents join us. One of them is the woman I interviewed at the AIDS ministry who was embarrassed about her teeth. She is glad to see Pon, but she drops her head when I greet her in Thai. A resident brings out a pan of rice, and the cook sets a simple dish of fish and vegetables on a rustic wooden table. The woman leads us in a short prayer: "We thank the earth, we thank the farmers, we thank the cooks so that we can live."

The monks, three of them, eat in a closed-in porch, separate from us. One is thin and looks sad. I assume he's the one Phra Phongthep mentioned who was seropositive. Those who are too sick to come to the group meals are fed by the residents. Those at our table politely pass me the rice and the ladle for the food. The residents move slowly, bent over their food, withdrawn. As we eat, a light rain begins to fall.

After lunch, Phra Phongthep shows us the wards for men and women. Three residents from lunch are back in their rooms, sitting alone, like animals in a zoo, conscious that we are looking at them but seemingly resigned to where they are. We drift by them like ghosts from another world. One man sleeps. Another, too weak to move, stares as if waiting for someone. Off by himself, a man lies in a bed under mosquito netting. "We keep him separate. He has tuberculosis," Phra Phongthep tells us.

He takes us out into a garden. The mosquitoes are terrible, but I am glad to be out of the wards and into the sunlight. There are fruit trees and a little pond. He giggles like a boy, telling us that there are fish in the pond but no one can catch them. Then he picks some red berries from a tree and places them in our hands. "Eat."

Before we leave, I ask him for a picture, something I have done everywhere. Pon takes my camera and directs us to stand before the Library of Peace and Wisdom. He stands straight, proud and firm, a man whose beliefs have become embodied in his work. I take the camera and ask for their photograph now: the Christian and the Buddhist. "Oh, no," he says, shaking his whole upper body, moving back.

"Why not?"

Pon laughs nervously at another of my American cultural miscues. "He say that someone might use it to blackmail him."

But I will not take no for an answer. Bashfully, he walks over to Pon, and they stand stiffly for the picture.

As we walk to Pon's truck, he puts his arm around my shoulder and with his other hand clasps my biceps. Together, strolling through the garden, his touch reminds me of the sensations that I still feel from the bodies I touched that morning teaching yoga. As he releases me and we bow, it occurs to me that perhaps more than ideas or words, we are led in this life from touch to touch, body to body, until our physical form is worn away.

Driving back, Pon and I talk about Phra Phongthep as a way to talk to each other. "He liked you," she says, "he talked different around you than before with me."

"He likes you, too," I say, noticing her sudden nervousness. "I can tell he admires you, because you are doing difficult work. You don't talk, you act; you do things."

We try to find more things to say, then silence closes around us as she drives me to my hotel one last time. Over the past five days a bond has developed between us. We surprised each other with how quickly we could speak about those things that mattered. We talked, of course, about HIV and AIDS and Thailand's attempts to educate and inform its people. Pon wasn't afraid to ask about how I'd contracted the virus. She wanted to talk about homosexuality and bisexuality; she wanted to talk about yoga and how it had helped me spiritually and psychologically, and how it might help others.

We also had passionate talks about Christian theology and the teachings of Jesus, and how they informed her ethical and political beliefs. She was hungry for conversation, eager to match wits and debate. "My dream is to go to school, too, and study theology," she told me. I could see how she longed to go to school like her husband and have books and papers to write. For that reason and others, she could not understand how I could have left seminary and such an opportunity. "Why did you do that?" she asked me once parked in front of restaurant where we'd eaten. "When I hear you talk, I think, you would have been a good minister. Why?"

Another time, she stopped me in mid-sentence as I was waxing on about my interpretation of the Book of Job: "Can I ask you something? What do you believe in? I mean not your ideas and all of that, but your faith, what is your faith?" Every day we approached this Kierkegaardian cliff and edged toward the realm that always makes me squirm. To her it didn't gel that I could talk so passionately about ideas that were sacred to her and not be able to say that I believed in the crucified Christ. When I tried to philosophize my way toward some acceptable answer, she didn't buy it. "No, no, I don't want theology and words; I want to know what *you* believe."

I want to leave her with some answer to those questions that she has had the guts to ask me during our time together, because I sense in Pon that she isn't asking, as so many Christians do, out of a need to convince herself of her beliefs. No, Pon's interest in my work and life is motivated by something far beyond herself. She has asked out of what I can only call love. But as we arrive in silence at the AIDS ministry, my mouth is dry and my mind empty. I am a blank; I am full. I have traveled thousands of miles across south Asia and have no answers for her or for myself. All I know is that it no longer does any good to speak out of self-preservation or to fill the space of silence. I can only say goodbye.

VIII

Indianapolis, Indiana (September, 2001)

I am stretching on my parents' family room floor in Indianapolis. My father sits nearby reading his newspaper. I'm exhausted. Yesterday I drove seven hundred miles, returning from a road trip to Colorado to see an old friend. She'd invited me to come out and relax after my trip to Asia. We hiked and climbed, swam in cold mountain lakes, and lay naked in the sun. She insisted I drink all the beer in her refrigerator and not read or write a word about AIDS. She took me into the foothills of the Rockies to meet her father, an eighty-year-old rancher whose body looked like the apple trees he'd planted fifty years ago next to his barn, gnarled and humbled by the weather. He told me he'd rescued a calf earlier before we'd arrived, pulled it out of a cow's uterus. "Saved it, by God!" Watching him watch football on TV, I thought maybe I ought to stay on his ranch and become a cowboy, live with old dogs, dedicate myself to the care of animals, and leave the human world to its own designs.

At my friend's apartment one day while she was at work, the man who lives upstairs noticed me doing yoga on the lawn. "Hey, what's that, yoga?" he called out, leaning over the railing of his porch. He was Filipino, a waiter, home on his day off. He watched me, while I became self-conscious, smiling in that way gay men smile when they know you're afraid to admit that you are as much aware of them as they are of you. He asked questions, trying to get me to reveal what he already suspected. I told him about where I'd been traveling. Curious but confused, he pried further: "Why go *there*?" So I told him.

As it turned out, he'd just quit working at the Denver AIDS Hotline. "It's getting bad again. These boys, these young ones, they just don't learn. But I'm tired of it, you know?" I looked up, the sun in my eyes blocking him from view, wondering why, of all the houses in Denver, this man was living upstairs from one of my former girlfriends?

"Why don't you come upstairs? Do you get high? What else have you got to do—you're on vacation, right?"

I declined, reluctantly, did some more back bends, and went to an empty coffee shop down the street, where I worked on an essay for a magazine which was supposed to be about a trip I took with my father to revisit the minor league parks he'd played in during his baseball career but ended up being about the conversations we tried to have about my health and homosexuality.

Warm sunlight pours in through the family room windows bathing both me and my father as we go through our morning rituals. He reads the sports page. I go through a modest series of yoga poses. He is relieved to have me under his roof, surprising me and himself. I've caught him putting his hands on me as he wobbles about the house, pretending to steady himself, but really, I think, he just wants to touch me, to make sure I'm still there.

He gets up now and goes to the kitchen, bringing me a cup of coffee, then stands at the window looking proudly at the glimmering sunlight on the old swimming pool in our backyard, which was why he bought the house when we moved here thirty years ago when I was fifteen.

"You go swimming yet?" he asks, watching me do a shoulder stand, knowing how much I love to swim. *The Today Show* plays in the background. As I do another pose, Katie Couric interviews Ted Kennedy about some benefit in honor of Jackie Onassis. In down dog, I can see Couric between my legs: her tight black boots and pleated skirt, her bouncy hair falling over her eyes. Then her happy face goes blank. Real news comes over her ear phone: "Apparently, we've just heard that there's been a small plane accidentally hit one of the World Trade Towers. I think we've got a camera . . ." I come to my knees. Ted Kennedy disappears. There is smoke rising from a corner of one of the World Trade Towers. My first thought is about the Filipino man who told me why he'd moved to Denver: "Remember that bomb at the World Trade Center? Ninety-five? Remember? I was there. I was working there! I went home with ashes, ashes all over me. I quit my job that day and moved here the next week. New York—who needs it?"

I turn to my father still behind his newspaper and a voice comes out of me that I don't recognize: "That's not an accident."

"What?" My father peers over his paper.

"Look, dad."

We stare at the TV all morning, chair next to chair, talking to each other without our eyes leaving the screen. More than once, the thought comes to me that the world might finally be coming to an end. But then, looking at my father's sagging body under his t-shirt, I'm comforted, at least I will die with my father and not alone.

Chicago, Illinois (September, 2001)

In Chicago, my home where, after nearly twenty years, I have no apartment, I park my old Ford Escort. The seats are full, back and front, with clothes, some books, and my bike, the few things I did not sell before I left for Asia. People walk like they are wounded, like the AIDS-stricken Thais standing in line that day at the police headquarters in

Bangkok waiting to be saved by the V-1 Immunator. At the bank, people stare at one another as if to say something, then turn away, embarrassed, take their money and shuffle to their cars. Nobody uses their horns. A strange politeness rules the city. I have returned to attend a symposium I helped organize on the economic and social problems facing Africa. The attendance is light: half of the African speakers are stranded in Canada because of the terrorist attack, including activists I'd met at the AIDS conference, Eunice Odongo of Kenya's WOFAK and Dr. Gbodossou of PROMETRA from Senegal.

Harvard economist Jeffrey Sachs fills the screen in the ballroom of the Chicago Hyatt. He tells us all a new set of dramatic facts to illustrate the rich world's indifference to Africa's AIDS-inflicted decline. He offers an analogy: if the rich nations, with a GNP of $25 trillion, could spend one tenth of one percent of that wealth to help Africa climb out of its health-care disaster, "one penny out of ten dollars," then millions of lives might be saved. Next, up to the podium steps Charles Wiwa, the nephew of the martyred environmental activist Ken Saro-Wiwa, who was murdered for questioning the colluding forces of Shell Oil and the Nigerian government in their destruction of land belonging to poor Ogoni farmers in Nigeria's southern delta. As we sit with our hands folded in our ironed shirts and matching outfits, Wiwa paints a picture of African activism: a crowd of poor Ogoni women marching up to the barbed wire gates of Shell's compound that sits on their ancestral homeland. The women are naked. (An ancient ritual to express utter disrespect.) They chant, condemning those who've come to poison their land and the waters of the delta where they have fished and farmed for generations.

We break for coffee and pastries, after which a Ghanaian minister, who was seated next to me, offers a prayer before his talk, as do all of the Africans before they speak, aware of the emotional tension in the audience. His words resonate across the room, shaking the water glasses, as he moves to his final trope: "On this day of tragedy, we must see that AIDS is an act of terrorism, too." His talk is laced with religious sentiment and unapologetic spiritual references to Jesus and the Holy Spirit, as he describes how poor women in his community, who have lost their husbands to AIDS, have created a new community where they care for one another's children and provide for those who are ill.

Finally, Madame Museveni, the wife of the President of Uganda, regally floats into the ballroom with her retinue. We clap when she tells us of Uganda's remarkable success in reversing their numbers of infected and in instituting programs to promote prevention. Of course she doesn't tell us that her husband has declared himself president for life, decided condoms are evil, and that she has begun to support national tests on young women to see if they are virgins.[1] We eat our chicken and cheesecake and congratulate ourselves for putting on such an important conference. Before we adjourn, the committee proudly announces that there will be a website to keep information flowing across the continents.

I leave in a hurry to attend a yoga workshop, hoping that twisting and deep breathing in a room of ninety, spandex-clad torsos will take my mind off the embarrassing conference and those planes that keep crashing into the World Trade Towers every time I close my eyes. For four hours, people cry and whimper between poses and glances at the Sears Tower in the distance. But we're caught by the fierce gaze of Ana Forrest, the guru of Santa Monica, who at one point growls at a despairing woman who can't seem to get it together: "Let go of it! You've got to learn that you can't change anything but yourself!" After a day of talk about debt relief and 15 million orphans, tuberculosis, and Nigerian women storming the gates of Shell Oil, I'm trying to let go of it, while balancing on one foot with my thigh over my shoulder in the bird of paradise pose. But it's not working. I'm falling, and falling, and falling again.

I'm not thinking of changing the world, I'm really not. I'm not thinking of New Yorkers flying to their fiery deaths, or the women in Chennai who are being thrown out of their homes, or the children on the streets of Saigon high on cheap heroin. I'm thinking of the Ghanaian pastor and his big-barreled body blasting out the wisdom of the Holy Spirit from the podium: "On this day of darkness, we pray for you America— America the great land! For we know, we know! Christ is on the cross! And there will be a salvation!"

❖

Per Erez sits at an outdoor café in Andersonville, a North Side, Chicago, neighborhood that is a mélange of lesbians, middle-age gay men, old Swedes, Middle Eastern businessmen, and upwardly mobile whites from across the Midwest. I'm staying down the street, sleeping on a couch at a friend's condo. Like Per, he is yoga teacher, too.

Per's spider-like body shines as does his characteristically serene face framed in his short thin locks. We'd met a few years before, when he'd contacted me after reading an article in a local New Age magazine. It featured me on the cover as "yoga teacher of the month," lauding my "heroic life, battling HIV" and teaching yoga at an AIDS clinic. "You don't know me, but I know you," Per began our phone conversation that day. Per was the real yogi living the "heroic life." He'd been seropositive for twelve years and taught yoga for a living (not just twice a week like me). He'd also been teaching people with HIV well before I'd even been infected. It was Per, in fact, who'd encouraged me to go to South Africa and offer the yoga workshop, a workshop we'd first put together here in

Chicago. Per never questioned why I needed to sell my things, leave my job, and try to rediscover what I'd experienced in South Africa by traveling to Asia.

When I bring up the terrorist attacks, he's the first person who responds with a shrug. And why wouldn't he?—the son of a Costa Rican mother who fled her homeland and a black father who worked most of his life in a coal mine, and the brother of a woman addicted to crack cocaine? Indeed, why would a gay man, who has lived his whole life on the outside of outside—why not sigh and shrug at inexplicable suffering that much of the world confronts every day? When I tell him of the things I saw in India and Thailand, he makes the connection without a second thought, "Sounds a lot like this place used to be." Then he pauses, and corrects himself: "Like it still is."

Per came to Chicago, like so many other gay men from small towns in the Midwest, naïve but eager to find a sense of community. As a man of color, however, he's never really felt at home on either the South Side, where he first lived, or on the North Side, where he lives now. He told me once, "I always felt safer being a gay man on the North Side and a black/Latino man on the South Side." He worked at different jobs, trying to acculturate himself to the ways of the urban world as a young gay man finding his way in, but in his second year in the city, he was raped and infected by a gay white man he thought he could trust.

As he listens to me rattle on about my travels, I recall the painful way he looked as he described for me those first months after he'd learned of his diagnosis. "For months," he said, "I walked around numb, anesthetized, barely able to get through my day, going to work on the North Side and coming home to the South Side. I knew I was infected. I knew something was wrong." Then a friend told him about TPAN (Test Positive Aware Network), a community-based organization primarily run by an HIV-positive staff and volunteers that provides services for people with HIV. Here he joined one of the many peer-led support groups. "We were all in our twenties. Each week we just talked about whatever was on our minds. It became my community. People knew your name and really cared. This meant a lot to me then. I mean, these people called you when you were sick, they checked in on you." This was in the late eighties when there were no effective treatments. "People were dying all the time. You came in to the office there on Bellmont and you'd see this black board with white letters spelling out the names of those who'd died that week."

It is at TPAN that Per, like so many other activists I've met, found self-healing by becoming a part of a community and activism. Soon after he joined, he became a volunteer in one of their prevention programs. On the weekends, he passed out condoms and canvassed the bars and bath houses for donations for TPAN, but in reality, he was there as a reminder to those gay and bisexual men in denial of the growing epidemic. Per's choice to plant himself in the middle of the gay social scene and announce his status was not easy. Friends who had once greeted him and wanted to date now turned their backs, afraid even to talk to him. Eventually, he took on the position of outreach coordinator, developing safe-sex programs and taking them wherever gay and bisexual men congregated. It was also at TPAN that he began to study yoga with a teacher who recognized from his enthusiasm that he should become a teacher himself.

Per's interest in alternative therapies and yoga intensified when he became sick after taking the first combination treatment. Like many doctors at the time, Per's pushed him to take the cocktail treatment when little was known of its potential side-effects or toxicity. "I wasn't sick, my numbers [T cell count] were good, but they thought I should take it. Soon after, I became sick." The thoughtlessness of the process made him distrustful of any further treatments and reinforced his belief that he needed to become active in maintaining his own health. In 1990 he went to the Kapalu Yoga Training Center in Western Massachusetts and found his calling. "I soaked it up. I needed something like yoga to calm me—to cut away the anxieties about my health."

I'd let his pragmatic wisdom, spiritual activism, and good health distract me from the painful realities he and other people of color must still confront, in a country more like those I visited than Americans would like to believe. Per's story and life remind me of those heartbreaking yet transformative passages in James Baldwin, where he describes with poetic accuracy the coming together of race and sexuality and how it shaped the spiritual crisis of his youth that would define his life and inspire his literary genesis:

> [T]he anguish that filled me cannot be described. It moved in me like one of those floods that devastate countries, tearing everything down, tearing children from their parents and lovers from each other, and making everything an unrecognizable waste . . . it was though I were yelling up to Heaven and Heaven would not hear me. . . . Yes, it does indeed mean something—something unspeakable—to be born, in a white country, an Anglo-Teutonic, anti-sexual country, black.[2]

※

It's been nearly six months since I last saw my doctor. Illinois Masonic Hospital, closest to Chicago's highest concentrations of gay men, was one of the first hospitals in the country to set up clinics solely for those with HIV. It was in this clinic, too, that I was asked to teach my first yoga class for people with HIV. My doctor, Malte Schutz, son of a German physician, is, like many of the best HIV specialists in the country, gay and almost religiously dedicated to his practice and research. On my first visit in 1996, after going through Chicago's Public Health clinics, I came to him, terrified and sick. I will never forget the way he treated me that day, spending what seemed to me over an hour to answer all my questions and educate me on what was going on in my body. It wasn't the talk of medications that I remember being so important, it was the hope I heard in his voice. Emerging from his office, I believed for the first time since I'd been diagnosed that I was going to be okay.

Since the eighties, when Dr. Schutz had begun his practice, he'd cared for hundreds of patients, watching many of them die, as he contributed to the science and the development of new treatments for HIV. In our fixation with science heroes and medical celebrities, we tend to forget that the story of AIDS epidemiology and treatment is like the story of all medicine: a collective tale written by thousands of physicians, scientists, nurses, caregivers, and patients, who have all contributed to the growing body of knowledge around this disease.

On this visit, as usual, he is on top of everything, asking all the pertinent questions, and most important of all, confirming what I'd hoped—that despite not taking the meds and traveling through the third world, my counts were good. I ask him to give me names of some doctors whom I might interview for my project. He thinks for a minute: "Have you thought of going to Cook County Jail? I know a doctor there: Kirby Cunningham." In two minutes he has the doctor on the line, handing me the phone as I sit on the examining table.

At Illinois Masonic, with its rolling file cabinets, efficient nurses and staff, computerized thermometers, and elaborate charts diagramming my medical history, the contrast from where I have been is stark. All in all, I'm in and out of there in less than forty-five minutes, and that's with stopping to pick up my meds at the pharmacy on the floor below.

But the treatment I receive is not available to all of the 11,000 plus men and women who live with HIV in Chicago.

❀

From the North Side, where my clinic is located, to the South Side of Chicago, it's only a few miles, but the cultural and economic distance can be as great as it is from Asia or Africa. Ever since African-Americans moved north in the two great internal migrations of the 20th century, Chicago has found subtle and not-so-subtle ways to segregate its white and black citizens. Nothing typifies this more than the bulwark of housing projects that flank the Dan Ryan Expressway (which itself was built to separate the black South Side communities from other white neighborhoods). At bus and El stops in the Loop at five o'clock you see the divide: those going south are black, those going north are white.

South from the Loop stands the nation's largest public-housing project and the longest stretch of projects in the world: the infamous State Way Gardens and Robert Taylor Homes—twenty-eight identical, sixteen-story apartment towers. The projects were supposedly erected to ease the desperate need for housing in the sixties, but in reality they made a great deal of money for Mayor Richard J. Daley's friends and managed to keep some of the poorest blacks in the city corralled in a corridor between State Street and the Dan Ryan Expressway. At their peak in the early nineties, some 200,000 people lived in Chicago's public housing projects. Nearly the entire population within the projects is black, more than half are children, and a staggering number are single mothers.[3] But it's not just poor blacks who live in this so-called "black belt"; it's middle-income blacks as well. Forty-two percent of Chicago's population is black and over 90 percent of that number is concentrated on the South and West Sides. When people compare Chicago with an apartheid-era South African city, the difference in segregation is not as great as one might hope. Of the 1.7 million blacks who live in Illinois, 1.4 million are in Chicago, and over a million live either in the "black belt" or on the West Side.

As a boy, I remember passing these monstrous, gray towers on visits with my family to the city. Looking out our station-wagon windows, I stared at the upper windows of the projects, noticing the fence-like grating over the stairwells and hallways, the flapping curtains, and below, the children playing in dirt lots and goal-less basketball courts. Whether it was here in Chicago or behind our house where I grew up with neighbors who had dirt floors, seeing the poor and how they lived always terrified me. The Depression had left a deep impression on my parents and grandparents. Though no one talked about it, my grandfather's suicide in the thirties had a lot to do with the shame and fear of poverty. My parents, forever the teachers, would pull our car over while on vacation on some winding Appalachian road or driving through Indian reservations in Arizona and point out how badly people had to live, while my sisters and I cowered in the backseats. Though these roadside lessons were meant to illustrate the injustice of poverty, unconsciously they also imprinted upon us this fear and shame.

I make my way south to meet with Howard Spiller, who I met first at the HIV Planning Council, a collection of the city's HIV activists, service providers, and organizations. Spiller lives on the far South Side in a small house with his sister in the middle-class neighborhood of Morgan Park. It takes him some time to get to the door and a little more time to remember who I am. A few years ago, Spiller suffered a stroke due to the onset of full-blown AIDS, and he walks and talks with some difficulty. Yet within his sturdy, stocky frame and intense face there is a man very much in motion. He gets his coat and we are off to visit his neighborhood clinic, located in a small strip mall down the street from his house.

The Luck Care Clinic, Spiller says, is supported by both the city's Public Health Department and the South Side's Roseland Community Hospital. It was founded by Dr. Sherry Luck, a progressive black woman who devoted her medical career to providing health care to her community, opening the clinic in 1994 as the first clinic on the South Side to serve people living with HIV and their families. Luck Care turns no one away. It provides pastoral care, group therapy, and substance-abuse counseling. The clinic also offers referrals and helps clients find housing and locate food pantries. In other words, it's a social service agency as well. Four or five black men sit in a waiting room as we enter this small, homey clinic. Spiller walks about as if he works there, stopping in each cubicle to say hello to the staff and introduce me: "This is Michael, he's been around the world writing about AIDS, and he wants to put us in his book." Spiller is an advocate in the truest sense, as he moves between people like him, who are dependent on the city's social services, and to those in power who can take these services away.

The men waiting are close in age to me or younger, yet they look worn, unnaturally aged, shrunken. Nevertheless, they greet me with openness and warmth, their eyes and bodies reaching up and out to make me feel that, even in this hallway of a strip mall, this is their home and I'm welcome in it. Perhaps their warmth is because I have come as Spiller's guest. Or, I wonder if they sense in me the flood of memories I am having of India and Thailand as I wander through the clinic, memories from the far side of the world that have strangely led me to people in my own city I would never have met. Spiller tells me how crucial clinics like Luck Care are for those in the black community with HIV, people who for economic and cultural reasons don't want to travel to the larger service providers downtown or on the North Side. I'd heard much the same from a journalist and friend of mine, Leroy Whitfield (also a black AIDS activist). Whitfield once reminded me of the age-old suspicion blacks have understandably fostered toward predominately white-run health care facilities. The suspicion, he believes, comes not only from sky-rocketing health care costs, which often prevent people from going to a doctor, but also from the historic disregard for the rights of black patients. Clinics that care for lower income people often depend on grant monies that are tied to scientific studies of one sort or another. Many blacks are suspicious of such studies: the memory of the Tuskegee syphilis experiments continue to haunt them.[4] This suspicion and distrust might explain a recent survey taken that indicated that over 40 percent of African-Americans believe that AIDS is a secret plot by white scientists to kill them.[5] This same belief persists across Africa as well.

Spiller introduces me to a case-worker whose job is to track down the men who come into this office for care and don't return for follow-up visits or for their meds. Many of the men have no permanent address, due to family problems, loss of jobs, incarceration, or drug use. This woman's work is crucial, not only for these men, but for the protection of others.

Spiller tells me more about his life as I drive him downtown for another Task Force meeting that evening. He wants to loan me a video to show how sick he was when his mother and sister came to Washington, D.C. to take him back to Chicago.

"Look at it, it's me in the hospital. Go ahead take it. We made it to use in my case against the doctor."

As I pull my car to the curb along State Street, he turns and asks, "Are you married?" Which really means: Do you have a boyfriend?

"Uh, no. No, I'm not."

"You aren't?" He squints like it hurts to hear this. Then he gives me a hug and reminds me to give him back the video tape. I watch him, hobbling down the street with his briefcase, his shoulder into the winds whipping off the downtown buildings.

Later that night, house-sitting at a friend's condo, I pop in Spiller's video. I hear women's voices but there's no picture. Loud rumblings follow, clicks, and finally blurred images appear: A ceiling, a tiled floor, a hospital bed. Then out of the confusion, a man's face comes into focus. Propped up by two pillows, it's Spiller. His eyes are unfocused. One side of his mouth droops to the side. A warm female voice speaks: "Baby, we're here, now. How you feeling?" The camera closes in. Spiller tries to speak, but only half his mouth moves. Tears fall. A hand wipes his wet face. I turn it off.

❈

Not sure what my future holds anymore in this city, I move back and forth between friends, family, and stints at art colonies. My car, stuffed full of my things, seems the only place I feel at home. Two images haunt me from my travels in Asia, or really one, because one is the reverse of the other. In Asia, people lived their lives not so much for themselves but for those who surrounded them: their families, their friends, their lovers, their co-workers, their community groups. When I entered the go-go clubs of Bangkok, the female sex workers seemed to care for each other in a sisterly way, their hands fixing one another's clothes and hair, their exhausted bodies holding up one another's spirits. I have the same image of the peer educators at Sahodaran in Chennai, fidgeting and fussing with one another's shirt collars, hands in one another's pockets, staring into one another's faces like mirrors. I also met ghosts: bodies thinned and emptied of spirit, bodies detached and disappearing, banished and shamed away, like animals, who know they must leave the pack to die alone to save the living from the stench of their putrefaction.

Traveling, as always, has made me distrustful of everyone back home. Instinct drives me on. I plan for another trip to West Africa and continue to look for activists to interview. I write and I swim. I meditate and I do my practice. I spend time with Tuong. We go eat at Vietnamese restaurants in his neighborhood, where he asks me again and again what we're going to do to help Pham Van in Saigon. "I want to go back there. Do a documentary, you come with me. We can make a film to help Mr. Van and the street kids?" Then one day he calls and tells me he needs to talk to me.

"I got bad news. I got a call from my brother. My nephew. You remember him who had the drug problems? Guess what? He got HIV now."

Tuong sits slumped in the booth at the restaurant. The waitress brings us tea. Tuong sighs, apologizing: "I know you don't want to hear about it. I think maybe not to tell you but—my parents want to send him the drugs. Can we get them? I've got the money, my parents will pay for them."

"Tuong . . . Tuong, they're like seven hundred dollars a month."

"Seven hundred?!"

"That's just for one of the three I take. I mean, with insurance I don't pay that amount, but that's how much . . . but, it doesn't matter. You can't get them anyway."

"But maybe, you can get some extra and—"

"No, I can't. You have to have a doctor prescribe them. You need to get him here, Tuong. Can't he come for a visit and then stay?"

"Oh no, Michael. They'll never let him come here, not now."

In silence, we drink our tea and watch the Vietnamese bustling about on Argyle Street, working feverishly as if everything they have could be taken from them at any moment. After that, we spend more time together, talking about what to do, going over it again and again until Tuong doesn't want to talk about it anymore.

Of course my family in Indiana are supportive, especially my sisters, who wish I'd just stay with them so that I won't be so alone with all "these sad stories." They are loyal and protective and would come pick me up like I'm one of their own teenage sons if I'd just call. But I don't. They seem like they have enough problems. My parents, as they have been for much of my adult life, remain confused and worried.

Most of my friends seem uncertain, some even afraid about what to say to me. Some surprise me, and read my body and see perhaps better than I how I have been affected. They take me out to eat or to go listen to music. They offer their homes, send me books and newspaper clippings, support me without making me think I'm being supported.

One such friend, Erin, a former yoga student of mine and massage therapist, one day offered to give me a massage. After she'd worked on me for over three hours, I barely could get off the table. As I sat with her afterwards, she asked, "What happened to you over there?"

"You don't want to know."

"Yes, I do," she said, her diminutive body erect, her powerful little hands fluttering. "You have to let people help you. You can't do this by yourself, you know. "

After that, Erin became my ally. Unlike other women I'd dated or wanted to date, she accepted my bisexuality and dealt with my HIV status with little fear. She'd had her "dark days" as well, with drugs and punk bands and death. At twenty-four, her husband had asked her to commit suicide with him. When she refused, he shot himself with her gun. She was the only one who understood what I meant when I talked about ghosts. "You've got to keep going toward the light," she'd tell me. "Keep walking toward the light."

❁

As I travel south from Chicago's loop on Lake Shore Drive, Lake Michigan gleams an emerald blue in the late-afternoon sun. Along the lake stand the great temples of the American Midwest—the halls of Science and Art, the showrooms of commerce and technology, the arenas of sport and heroes. But in the shadow of these icons lies another city. Further south, behind the flowers and ornamental trees, stretch neighborhoods where the sounds of the Delta fused with the cold realities of this northern city to create rhythms and voices that reflect the tortured spirit of all those who've come to Chicago dreaming of a life it could never offer.

I am headed south to Jackson Park, one of the city's largest parks skirting the lakefront. Here on this pleasant October afternoon, behind the Museum of Science and Industry, I am meeting two AIDS activists. David Ley, a square-jawed, handsome man with wavy salt and pepper hair, sits in my car as we wait in the parking lot. A psychotherapist by training, Ley specializes in working with gay men who live, as he does, with HIV. "I call our community 'worried, well people,'" he half-jokingly tells me. David has watched the epidemic take away his friends and, from time to time, overwhelm his own health; yet he perseveres against the bitterness by buoying up his patients, his clients, and his friends. From his work in issues around AIDS and gay men's health, he has become an advocate for community-based programs that serve a growing population of people living with HIV.

We are here to meet with a friend of his, Dave Jimenez, a sociologist and activist, who has worked for years with the Latino gay and bisexual community as well as with several other marginalized, at-risk populations, including the one he wants to show me this afternoon. Jimenez pulls into the parking lot in an old BMW and parks next to us. After chatting a while about his work, he takes David and me into the park. Jimenez blends street advocacy with his research in ethnographic sociology at the University of Illinois at Chicago. Currently, he is working on a survey where researchers and advocates are trying to understand the social networks of young gay and bisexual men to see how diseases such as HIV and other STDs may spread.[6] Jimenez also has done important work in trying to show how the stigma of HIV deters people from getting tested and treated for another serious health problem in poorer communities—tuberculosis.

We wander through the parking lot past a group of black men in their forties and fifties, who have come to socialize and meet other gay and bisexual men in the park. Strolling over a small bridge, we pass four or five other younger men in their twenties and thirties. They are dressed in the familiar urban style of sports jerseys, baggy pants, and gold chains. They are outgoing, if not flirtatious, sliding in and out of the rhythm of their high energy conversation to say hello. We walk by a single young man engrossed in a book, two men with shaved heads entering each other's numbers into their cell phones, and a single man who looks perhaps in his seventies. Ahead, sitting on the back of a park bench, two twenty-somethings toke on a twist of marijuana. The wooded island is overgrown with fallen trees left from storms, which provides camouflage for the men who want to meet other men for sex. One man slips out from behind a thicket next to the lagoon and another man follows. How different is this park from those riversides and beaches in Chennai, I wonder. As in Chennai, men often meet here to have sex but also to exchange sex for money or drugs: a reminder that much of the epidemic in the black and Latino communities, where over a third of gay and bisexual men are reportedly infected, revolves around the dangerous mix of drugs and alcohol with sex.

Parks have always been a place for gay and bisexual men to meet clandestinely. But for non-straight men in the black community, who feel uncomfortable frequenting predominately white gay bars on the North Side and often don't want to spend the money or time trucking to the other side of town, these parks are more accessible and less exposed. Of course, it's not just black gay and bisexual men who need to meet in the quiet corners and back seats of vans in Chicago's parks, it's an entire city of working-class people who don't have the privacy in their cramped homes and apartments to meet with their lovers, particularly young people who have few places but their cars to be intimate. "Maybe there are other factors, too, we don't know about," Jimenez, the ethnographer, suggests, smiling with his cherubic face. "Maybe people like to have sex in these kinds of situations."

Walking toward the museum, we come to another remnant of the Columbian Exposition, the Japanese Garden with its trickling falls, manicured trees, bridges, stone lanterns, and tea house. Sitting on a platform of the tea house, Dave and David talk about the state of AIDS prevention in Chicago, wondering where it's going and how it's changed over the last few years. Both are worried about the low priority the Bush administration has given to public health and AIDS prevention, which they see as going hand in hand. They've seen how the stinginess of the government and the poor distribution of available funds have inordinately hurt those most in need of health care—the working poor. They are also concerned about the growing AIDS business, the bureaucracy, the overlapping of programs and the competition for funds. "It's hard to know who's doing what anymore," David says wistfully. "Small is still beautiful. Bureaucracy always kills the spirit of people trying to do innovative things on the ground. Everybody is so worried about funding and numbers they barely have time to let programs work."

We walk on in the soft afternoon light. I can't help recalling that first time I discovered this park during my divinity school days. Eager to escape my books and myself, I was drawn to the unusual diversity of birds that flocked there. That day, too, I saw who else came to this little birder's paradise, or one part of me did. It was as if I were living in two bodies, seeing the world with two sets of eyes, focusing on a vireo with its bouncing tail, and then staring as intently at the young man watching me from a nearby bench.

In the parking lot, Jimenez recognizes one of the case managers who works at AIDS Task Force, a program sponsored by the Public Health Department. Jimenez introduces us to Willy Leaks. He's here because he knows he can find some of his clients. He is relaxed. It's Friday for him, too. "This is their place. They feel more at home here than in their own homes," he says. Jimenez asks him how long people have been coming here to cruise. "Oh, people have been coming here for years. These bus drivers, see?" He points to a couple of parked buses waiting for tour groups from the museum. "They would have to hang around in their buses. Then it became known as a gay hangout. This is going way back. So black and white men have been coming here for a long time."

More men have arrived. A guy has brought out his cooler, another has turned up his car stereo. "It's party time!" a lanky guy in a Bull's t-shirt booms, his arm waving us over. But we have to be on our way to our next stop—Jordan House, a residential home for recovering addicts, the mentally ill, men recently out of prison, and people living with HIV and AIDS. Before we do, we stop and eat at Morry's Deli. At the counter, ordering sandwiches, I recognize a man but can't place him. As David describes how he became involved with Jordan House, the tall man at the counter notices me.

"Hey, I remember you. You played ball at the Y, didn't you?"

"Yeah, that's right, I knew you looked familiar."

"You still play there?"

"Nah, I was too old *then* to play."

He laughs. "Good to see ya, man."

Watching him leave, I lose myself in a reverie of those days when I played ball at the Halsted Street Y, before I sidelined myself, fearful I might get a scrape or cut and infect someone. The Y was also where I met lovers, including Eric, a black photographer who held me together after my diagnosis and refused to let me abandon my body's other passions.

❁

It is a sunny winter day, warm even, as I drive through Chicago's West Side to get to 26th and California, the euphemism for Chicago's criminal justice system. The criminal court building is said to process more cases than any other court in the world, and next to it looms Cook County Jail, one of the largest jails in the U.S. Spreading out over nearly one-hundred acres, eleven multi-story blocks of cells house over 10,000 inmates, most of whom are young, poor, and black or Latino. Most are here because they were caught for drug-related crimes—getting them, using them, selling them, stealing or killing for them. Over 100,000 inmates a year pass through Cook County on their way to court, back on to the street, or to one of Illinois's correctional facilities. Nearly 2 million men and women are incarcerated in America's jails and prisons, thanks to the stiffening of sentences related to drug possession and trafficking in the eighties. Some 40 percent of that staggering number are black. Considering how many are on probation or parole, the number of men and women under custody or surveillance in the U.S. reaches close to 6 million. In most European countries the number of incarcerated citizens is eight times lower.[7]

Steel spirals of razor fencing reflect blinding sunlight, as I enter through a side door of Cermak Health Center, which is a part of Cook County Jail. There I am to meet Dr. James Kirby Cunningham, a veteran physician who has been serving Chicago's marginalized communities infected with HIV for going on two decades. For the past three years, Cunningham has been coming to the jail twice a week in a new program designed to address what most prisons have neglected, the precipitous rise in HIV infection rates for men and now for women. Estimates put the numbers of infected at Cook County somewhere between 4 and 5 percent.

I pass through a series of locked gates, and a doctor's assistant, who is also a priest, introduces himself and leads me down an elevator and through a tunnel into what feels more like a bomb shelter than a hospital. Here, among hulking prison guards, the priest introduces me to Cunningham as he emerges from a little cubicle. Dressed in hiking boots, khakis, and a rumpled shirt with rolled up sleeves, Cunningham asks in a warm Texas drawl if it's okay if he can talk to me between seeing his patients. "They run me ragged around here." This is no joke, as he has to hike through the maze of Cook County's tunnels that link the eleven buildings to make his rounds.

At nine a.m. sharp, I can hear some commotion in the large holding area outside his cubicle and in comes his first patient. Cunningham explains to the inmate that I'm here to write about the jail. The thirty-something Latino man shrugs, barely noticing me. He holds his jaw, telling the doctor that he's got a toothache. He also complains that his methadone treatment is too high. They go over his numbers. His T cells are high. He doesn't seem concerned much about his HIV infection. What he wants from the doctor is to see if he can get off his floor. "They're just a bunch of gang-bangers. I want to get out of there." He also wants a painkiller. But Cunningham pointedly tells him he doesn't have any. The man is in for armed robbery. Cunningham suggests that when he gets out, he should consider a treatment program.

The next man who enters reminds me of the infected men I saw in my travels in Asia: ghostly and thin, his shoulders hunch even though he is a tall man of only about thirty. A new inmate, he is in for possession. He'd been off his meds for a year, but now he's taking medication again. Cunningham tells me that many of the men only get treatment when they are incarcerated. His viral load is high, but coming down now that he is back on medication. Cunningham pleads with him to keep taking meds, "Why weren't you taking them? Why didn't you come to see us at Core?" (The Core Center is a state-of-the-art HIV/AIDS service center in Chicago where Cunningham sees former inmates once a week.) Cunningham asks him a series of questions, bluntly and quickly: "Do you drink? Do you take drugs? Have you had sex with men?"

Like all the prisoners, the man wears a shabby yellow-brown uniform with missing buttons and frayed cuffs. "I be tired all the time. I am trying to stay away from drugs but I smoke weed, see, because it helps me with my appetite," he tells Cunningham, before turning to me, noticing that I'm writing down what he has said. "I can't sleep. I've lost eighteen pounds. Can't feel anything in my feet. I'd be glad if you wrote about me, then maybe it would help somebody."

"You can't expect me to rescue you. You've got to take care of yourself," Cunningham pleads. Like so many physicians and health-care professionals who work with the incarcerated, half of his job is that of therapist, parent, and job counselor. I'm impressed as he goes from ethnicity to ethnicity, adjusting his rhetoric each time. He must sift through layers of truth to find the right words to keep these men directed toward a healthier future. Yet, he is aware that he is often the only one who listens to problems he can't really do much about it. They want off floors, they want more blankets, they want blocks that have warm showers. One young man, in his early twenties, spends his whole time during the visit pacing, leaning over Cunningham's shoulder as he writes, pleading, whining, desperate for attention. It's painful to watch a young man with so much energy, so much need. "I'm gonna die up there doc. You gotta get me out of there. There's no heat, no hot water. A person with HIV can't stand this stuff."

"What are you in for?" the doctor asks.

"Possession and burglary. Six to thirty years. I wind up back to drugs. You love me Doctor Cunningham. You gotta help me. You gotta." He pulls up his shirt, "I got a bullet in me, see?" He turns to show me. A scar pinches and discolors a section of skin on his back. "I can't be treated like this."

Cunningham says he'll try to help, but reminds him to see the health educator on his ward.

"Who's that? What educator? I never seen that guy."

Cunningham writes him a slip for an extra mattress and pillows and a lower bunk. When the young man leaves, Cunningham sighs: "It's a never-ending cycle in here. They don't have anything out there." The real work, he says, is to get the government to decriminalize drug use and change the sentencing laws. Or at least, the city or state should provide more than the minuscule number of treatment programs to the thousands of men and women who are clearly suffering from drug addiction. Cook County's Criminal Justice system apparently has only enough money to offer fifty convicted drug offenders the standard detox program. Fifty!

From Cunningham's vantage point, stiffer sentencing has done nothing to deter drug use or its sale. If anything, it has made thousands of young men wards of the state and more embittered, hardened criminals, who return to neighborhoods where they cause themselves and those around them more harm. And in the case of those men with HIV, the harm to others is literally poisoning families and whole communities.

I'm inspired by Cunningham's work and see the systematic nature of the problem from his perspective inside the prison. Yet, Cook County is one of the few jails in the state or the country which has even hired a well-trained, knowledgeable HIV physician to coordinate and run a program. Elsewhere, it's much worse. In Alabama, for example, Amnesty International has reported serious violations of the human rights of prisoners with HIV, who are regularly denied adequate health care and treatment. In other states the story is the same. Officials either don't believe prisoners deserve the treatment or the states simply don't have the money to spend on an expendable constituency. I look at Cunningham counseling, doing paper work, evaluating physical and mental health, doing the jobs of four of five people at once, a seventy-year-old man who could be enjoying himself on some golf course in Arizona. But here he is in the dungeon of America's prison system trying to keep a population of desperate men alive and a disease from spreading.

The enormity and complexity of the job he has taken on makes me think of Dr. Yepthorani and Dr. Madhivavan at YRG Clinic in Chennai, Dr. Pradupkeow in Chiang Mai, doctors I met in Chicago and Vietnam and South Africa, individuals who refuse to be deterred by the odds and mountainous problems. Like these doctors, Cunningham works with what he has.

An African-American man comes in with handcuffs, though they are loosened for his visit. He looks healthier than the others, more spirited, greeting me with bright, sensitive eyes. He seems forthright and confident, and no wonder, he's getting out in two days.

Cunningham's main concern is that he get into a month-long rehab program run by Catholic Charities. "Let me call for you, you should do this, this will be good for you, help you out."

"I want to doc, but I want to see my daughter. That's all I want, I want to see my baby."

He looks at me and smiles while Cunningham puts the call in to this program to see if they have space. "I got a daughter. She is eight years old. Doc . . . Doctor Cunningham, I need to see her first, make sure I can see her first."

We talk a bit. I tell him I'm positive too and writing about things here and around the world. "You look good though man. You look REAL good. You gotta be exercising or something? I don't like these pills, they make me sick. Do you have problems?"

Cunningham gets off the phone and tells him he can see his daughter but that he has to stay there for a month. "They will arrange to pick you up when you get out, okay? They have a van."

"Doc, these meds are kind of making me sick. I think I'm taking too much."

Cunningham goes over to his files to check on what meds the prisoner has been taking. The inmate turns to me: "I don't even know if I'm positive; this one doctor said I was and then another said I wasn't, but they got me on them anyway." He shrugs.

"Well, you've no viral load and good T cells, but let me check something." Cunningham leaves the room to look at some other files outside the cubicle.

I don't know why, but the man comes right out and tells me his lover died two months ago. "I think about him every day," he says, looking down at his handcuffed hands.

"Where did you meet?"

"In my neighborhood. We had a good thing. And then, he got sick."

He asks me if I have a lover. And I say yes, thinking about Erin, who I slept with the night before. I know he thinks I'm referring to a man, but I don't correct his impression. He seems able to read me anyway, able to see my whole complex sexual history. In him, too, I see a masculinity rare among men, rarer among inmates, one that is free from bravado and hype, and not afraid to show vulnerability. "After he died, a month later, I lost my job. I was a cook. And the boss, I liked that guy, too; I was working good for him, but he has to test everyone for drugs and I didn't pass. So I got fired. Then I started to sell some stuff I got from a friend. I mean it was just weed."

Cunningham comes back in with another file. "Good news. You're right, you're not positive." The inmate shakes his head and smiles. I can't believe my ears. Apparently this kind of misdiagnosis happens all the time, according to Cunningham. The news doesn't seem to have much effect on the prisoner though. One less thing to worry about in a host of other difficult circumstances he must face when he gets out. He stands. Cunningham reminds him about the rehab arrangements. I want to somehow celebrate for him. But all I can do is offer to shake his hand when he goes, but since he can't do that with handcuffs, I pat him on the back as he walks out.

He turns back to me: "Good luck."

"Yeah, you too, man."

Cunningham shows me a list of misdiagnosed patients to stress how common it is. He explains that as they move from facility to facility, doctor to doctor, files get lost. "We just can't keep track of everything." Sometimes, he says, men assume they are positive because a girlfriend or boyfriend has tested positive or died. Some know that those who are HIV positive get better treatment, so they accept a diagnosis. Others are so depressed and warped by addiction that it doesn't matter to them. Cunningham is trying to develop a smoother system so that these misdiagnoses are kept at a minimum, and drug regimens can be maintained. But it's just one of the many problems he faces with impossibly limited funds and staffing.

Another problem is the resistance inmates have to HIV testing. When they are admitted, they are tested for syphilis and other STDs but not for HIV. In fact, a fourth of the city's new cases of STDs are discovered in entry physicals of new prisoners at Cook County Jail. Citing these statistics, many law-makers and prisons officials in Illinois believe mandatory testing will assist public health officials in prevention as well as provide timely treatment for those infected. However rational this may seem from the outside expert, the fear of rape and the stigma of HIV is so great that it can have devastating psychological effects on inmates, particularly on young first-time offenders. Rape and sexual assault is a very serious problem in America's penal system.[8] Unquestionably, prisons and jails need to have the resources and funds to establish programs that make it easier for those at-risk for HIV to seek testing and receive counseling and treatment.[9] When prison officials at Cook County admit that as many as 4,000 HIV infected men and women may pass through the jail every year without getting tested, it doesn't take a epidemiologist to figure out just how critical it is to spend the money necessary to provide prevention and treatment programs for the incarcerated.

Cunningham's office hours are over. He leads me back upstairs, but not before we pass through a tunnel that opens into a waiting area. *The Jerry Springer Show* blares from a TV high in a corner, echoing down the tunnels. Men on one side of the hall, women down the other, separated by big-bellied guards. I avoid looking at the prisoners, telling myself I want to respect their anonymity. The writer in me, however, tells me that I must face them. Sad and forgotten, they look like abandoned children, lost and confused, their dispirited bodies docile yet hungry for whatever care and affection they can find from those around them.

❋

I first learned about Rae Lewis-Thornton two years ago. I was on my way to teach a class and spotted those familiar letters—HIV and AIDS—on a poster. Under a blurry photocopied black woman's face, I learned that Lewis-Thornton had been on *Nightline*, featured in *Jet* and *Ebony*, and on the *Oprah Winfrey Show*. AIDS, as I would discover, was her calling card, or rather—her calling. Reading further, I discovered that this virus we shared had propelled her onto the national lecture circuit.

I had returned from South Africa only a few months before. The acronym that I had once avoided now drew me to anyone who uttered it. Part of me wanted to hear Lewis-Thornton talk and to introduce myself. This was what I had learned in South Africa: connect, support, act. But, reading her resumé, I could only feel envy. I wanted to be in the Golden Eagles Room telling my "dramatic story of transformation and healing." Sure, I thought, talking to her in my head, you can come back to your old school and give a talk on AIDS; you're a professional black woman—you're the story the media wants to tell. The students can handle you. You're not gay or bisexual. You don't have problems with addiction.

I never went to Lewis-Thornton's talk. But when I began looking for people to interview, I remembered that day and my childish envy, and decided to give her a call.

"You're late," Lewis-Thornton sighs loudly, looking at her watch, when I arrive for our lunch meeting.

She is dressed in an expensive black business suit with a stylish coiffure and heels. She's big-shouldered, tall, almost muscular. Like me, she's devoted to a serious regimen of exercise and fitness training. After a few strained pleasantries and a reminder that she's got only an hour, she comes to the point: "I don't know you and don't know where you're coming from, but let me tell you, I'm a straight-up-Jesus Christ-died-for-your-sins-and-was-raised-up-and-is-coming-back Christian woman. And I don't hide nothing!"

As she introduces herself, I glance over at the next table to catch a woman's mouth so wide open I can see lettuce in the back of her throat. Remembering that she's a seminarian, preparing for the ministry in the Baptist church, I'm unsure what to say. But she's not done: "God wrote me into history. I understand my mission. All my experiences have led me to this work. Ask me anything."

After a while of nodding and writing notes, I realize this confrontational style is how she operates. "I wear my religion on my sleeve. I can't help it, Mike. I feel like I don't have any time to waste."

"I understand completely," I finally break through, catching her between bites. "I studied to be a minister, too, and I'm on a mission just like you. Why do you think I asked you to come meet me?" I confess to her about seeing her poster at Northeastern and its effect on me, but don't let her respond, spilling out my story as fast as I can: from getting tested on the South Side to South Africa to South India all in one breath.

"Okay, then," she says, sticking out her hand for me shake. "Mike, we're talking on the same page."

She eats in a rush as she runs through the highlights of her own story, her hands flying, her jaw jutting out, changing expressions with each episode. She's so theatrical, I get caught up in her performance and forget to write.

Lewis-Thornton learned that she was first infected when she donated blood for victims of a train wreck in Virginia in 1985. Ironically, she'd organized this blood drive because donations had dropped severely due to people's fear of contracting AIDS from needles. Two weeks later the Red Cross gave her a call.

Her eyes open wide and her cadence kicks in. "Me? HIV? I didn't use drugs. I dated only respectable, educated men. How could I get it?" But then her theatrical style softens as she recounts telling her boyfriend, a young minister. "I needed some comfort then. I called my boyfriend and told him to come over. When I told him, I got another shock; he cursed and called me a whore, then took his things and slammed the door on my face. I never saw him again."

Lewis-Thornton has faced adversity all her life, both her parents suffering from alcohol and drug addiction. (Her father was killed by the time she was three, and she didn't see her birth mother until she was eighteen.) She says she responded to her infection like all the hardships she'd faced in her life: "I threw myself, like always, into my work." For seven years, she kept her status to herself, working hard in various political campaigns (Jesse Jackson's Presidential campaign and Carol Mosley-Braun's Senate bid), finishing college, gaining a master's in political science, all at a bristling pace, achieving the highest honors. Then her health declined and her doctor informed her she'd now progressed to full-blown AIDS.

It was around this time that a high school teacher asked Lewis-Thornton to come speak to some of her classes on AIDS. "I'd never done any public speaking; I didn't know what I'd say." Soon she was booking speaking engagements across the country. "I learned to make it so that people can touch me, come up to me," she says with confidence. "I let them ask me anything; I like to work in the Q&A, you know, that's where they reveal what's really going on in their lives. I can feel what people need. My life is about helping people heal, helping them take care of themselves. I believe in ministering to people where they are. I'm interested in bringing souls to Christ's love."

I'm torn as I listen to her self-confidence and passion, as she mixes her Sunday-sermon rhetoric with street vernacular: "People need to deal with their shit." Part of me admires her deep conviction that she is being led by God, but I wince when she scoffs at those "with these new age beliefs" and wish she'd come down from her pulpit and just eat her lunch. I have to tell myself that I'm just the journalist here, recording her story. She doesn't have to like me or hear me out.

However, when I ask her about the role of the black church in response to HIV/AIDS, she doesn't mince words. "The black church has to learn to separate the sin from the sinner. We can take the sinner not the sin." She laments the culture of fear that pervades not only the black church but also black culture. "Black culture is killing us! This 'don't ask don't tell' is not conducive to healing." She recalls an African proverb that she uses in her talks: "He who conceals his disease cannot be cured." She fears that some members of the black church hierarchy are afraid to speak out because they themselves have things to hide about their sexual life.

"Bisexuality is rampant in the black community. Half the men in our choirs are gay. Everybody knows that!" She booms with exasperation, confirming everything I've been told by gay and bisexual black friends and lovers. Yet she acknowledges that there is a growing number of AIDS ministries created by black churches. The week before, I'd attended Trinity United Church on the South Side, one of the largest and most powerful black churches in the city. Their AIDS ministry not only serves those in their congregation, but has begun to train other black congregations in developing similar programs.

When I ask this born-again political veteran about the politics of AIDS, I brace myself uncertain where she will land. She lauds what agencies are trying to do and is aware of how little money there is for AIDS in Chicago, but wonders if the black community could do better themselves rather than working through agencies that still are controlled by what she calls the "old-gay-boy network." "We understand our community better than the gay community does. Let us have the money directly."

"Dollars follow the numbers," she says, "and we got the numbers now." She is right. African-Americans account for 54 percent of all HIV/AIDS cases in Chicago. Nationally, the infection rates are rising faster than ever among young black gay and bisexual men.[10] And for black women, AIDS is now the leading cause of death for African-American women between the ages of twenty-five to forty-four. To put it into better perspective, African-Americans now have the same rate as that of Thailand's: 2 percent.

Feeling more comfortable, she asks me about the medications that I'm taking and how I'm handling the side effects. "I'm doing okay, I swim and do yoga, but I can't seem to keep on any weight."

She scoffs, "You look great." Her pride wavering, she points to her double chin and thick neck. Like many people living with HIV she suffers from lipodystrophy, a condition whereby HIV medications affect metabolism, causing fats in the body to be distributed unevenly. "I exercise religiously; it's the only way I can control this condition somewhat. The weight comes and goes." She's angry that doctors and pharmaceuticals know no more about it than they do: "They could do something if they wanted to, but they don't care."

Out of nowhere, she evokes the name of Emmett Till, martyr of the Civil Rights movement, who was murdered in the South for allegedly whistling at a white woman in 1955. Her voice rising in emotion, she recounts the story of how Till's mother refused to hide his bloated and beaten body so that the world could feel her outrage at the injustice. "You know, Mike, to be here, in this age and time of AIDS, I wouldn't have it any other way."

"Divinity School is not easy, either. How are you holding up?"

For the first time, the preacher in her quiets. "I'm exhausted with the reading and the intellectual bullshit. I just can't take it sometimes."

I chuckle, recalling similar feelings about divinity school. Her real worry is that her outspoken style and straight talk about sexuality and AIDS may keep her from being ordained.

"I still get sick and cry before I speak at churches," she confides. "But God is there in my restlessness, Mike. He's there too."

When I tell her I've been to Cook County Jail and wonder what she thinks about the problems there, her spirit ignites. Apoplectic, she accuses the state and federal government of willful neglect in ignoring the health care needs of inmates. "They know these men are just going to spread the virus back into the black community." She's so upset that, for a moment, I think she might just get up on her chair and begin to preach to the whole restaurant. Instead, she stands and opens her arms. "Mike, I got to go. Give me a hug."

❁

I meet separately with two of the most dedicated AIDS activists in the city, Jim Pickett, a freelance consultant for AIDS service organizations, and Charles Clifton, the director of Test Positive Aware Network. For several years, I've noticed the columns they have written and have admired their outspoken advocacy for the rights of HIV-positive people in the city. They are eager to talk with me, offering ideas, suggesting people whom I should meet. Like other gay HIV-positive activists, they see the entire HIV community, particularly gay and bisexual men, as part of their flock. So I shouldn't have been surprised when they both suggest I get more involved in their programs.

The following week, I find myself standing by the side of a highway north of Chicago across the road from the heavily-guarded gates of the corporate headquarters of Abbot Laboratories. In my hand, I hold my poster: "No profits over people." It is the same sign protesters carried through the streets of Durban that afternoon before the AIDS conference.

We're trying to call attention to Abbot's decision to suddenly raise by 400 percent the price of one of it's HIV medications, Kaletra, a drug I'd popped into my mouth an hour before on the bus ride out. Abbot apparently thought that it could slip through a price hike for one of the most important drugs in the cocktail without anyone noticing. But thanks to Pickett, Clifton, and ATAC (AIDS Treatment Activist Coalition), about fifty of us show up to ask why Abbot, which continues to show healthy profits like almost all major pharmaceuticals, needs to suck a little bit more blood from those struggling to stay alive. Along with the AIDS activists, we are joined by a handful of medical students concerned about the ethical practices of Big Pharma, and a collection of seniors from AARP, outraged by Abbot's pricing practices that leave them broke and busing to Canada.

While pacing and chanting, I start chatting to a woman by the name of Ida Blyther-Smith. She, too, is HIV positive. Ida tells me she's a former nurse and founder of a shelter and half-way house for ex-offenders and people living with HIV on the far South Side. "I'm an activist. Everything and anything that has to do with AIDS—I'm there. City Hall, Springfield, Washington, D.C." Brushing back her reddish hair, Ida tells me she's written a book. "It's not published, but people ought to read it. You've heard about the 'down low'? Well, I know all about it. My late husband fooled me for years, but I took him back and cared for him until he passed last year. People said I was crazy, but they don't know anything. He was my husband, what was I supposed to do? Leave him on the street to die?"

An old lady in a Lexus sticks out her tongue as her husband whisks them by. Ida doesn't notice, just like she'd ignored the police cars and the excited police dogs, when she'd bolted across the road to press her case to the wealthy in their limos and luxury SUVs. She doesn't argue either when two sheriffs escort her back to our cordoned soapbox.

As we are leaving, I pound on her bus window and put my hand to my ear, indicating I'll give her a call. Driving south back through some of the wealthiest communities in the U.S., Lake Forest, Wilmette, Kenilworth, I keep thinking about Ida, marching out there onto the highway to stick her sign into the windshields of stockholders. Watching her reminded me of the African sculpture I used to look at on my lunch hour when I worked at the Field Museum. She had the same fierce stance, feet planted and apart, eyes bulging and alert, that same spirit ready to jump right out of her skin.

❉

The elevator opens onto the second floor of the City of Chicago's Health Department. Row after row, cubicle after cubicle, desk after desk, computer connected to computer, phones ringing in all directions. A glance at the size of an office like this reminds me that there's more than HIV that concern those in the field of public health. In fact, this city, which reversed the flow of the Chicago River in order to conquer its dysentery, has always had monumental problems maintaining the health of its polyglot composite of peoples. It's a city that never seems to learn from one disaster to the next—building too many wooden houses too close together resulting in the fire of 1870, creating a public housing nightmare, mishandling the heat wave of 1995, when over 700 people died.[11] "It gets hot in the summer, deal with it," was our mayor's famous retort to the media. Indeed, HIV/AIDS is not the city's biggest problem. Chicago leads the nation in syphilis, murder, and deaths attributed to heroin, and suffers from an epidemic of type 2 diabetes and respiratory ailments.[12] Like everywhere else, Chicago's public health problems begin with its chronic poverty. And, in the City of Big Shoulders, 20 percent of the population lives below the poverty line, nearly 650,000 people.

I am here to meet Fikurte Wagaw, the coordinator of the city's HIV and AIDS program. She is a petite, energetic woman with an intense but informal air, whose parents emigrated from Ethiopia when she was a child. Primarily, her office balances the needs of those most affected: men and women of color, gay, bisexual and transgender men, injecting drug users, sex workers, the incarcerated, and a growing number of teenagers. "The dynamics of disease are different from community to community," she tells me, "and so are the dynamics of sexuality within each one." She talks about how difficult it is to create an ad campaign that's appropriate and effective, but doesn't offend some group. It's her job, too, to disperse the funds and make sure everybody is getting a fair shake. Not an easy task.

I admit to her that it was through the city's public health infrastructure that I was tested (at an STD clinic on the near South Side) and subsequently saw my first doctor (at a clinic in a Puerto Rican neighborhood on the West Side). She nods, fully aware of the shame and stigma that pulls people away from their own neighborhoods and doctors to get tested and treated.

Wagaw concedes frustration with the bureaucracy of public health: with its duplicating layers of government policy, funds, and mandates. In the end, she asks, who is responsible? Who, ultimately, pays the bills and the price for inaction? The federal government? The state? The local government?

It's touchy. "There's a lot of turf wars," she admits. There is also some deep resentment and a lack of trust, particularly in the black community, which often sees the city as an enemy rather than an ally. She tells me of a recent meeting initiated by predominately white AIDS organizations. The idea was to invite African-American clergy to become more involved in prevention programs and help them disseminate more information.

"Hardly any of the ministers showed up. They don't like to always come to the North Side." Though she doesn't state it, I know she means: it's more than a problem of geography and traffic.

That afternoon Wagaw has invited a visiting social worker from Ethiopia. She has set up a meeting for him with her staff. So we pile into a tiny conference room around a table of cold cuts and cookies. Three staffers are former Peace Corps volunteers and another three are HIV positive. The Ethiopian describes his work with orphans on the streets of Addis Ababa. He speaks of the growing numbers who roam the streets: "Sisters and brothers cling to each other; gangs form to find food and survive; some turn to crime and sex work." The room is silent when he finishes, not because these people haven't seen or dealt with the neglected and forgotten of American society, but because of the enormity of the work this man has taken on. The contrast is dramatic: the budget of Chicago's public health program surpasses what the nation of Ethiopia spends on a population twenty times as large.[13]

The Ethiopian is here at the invitation of several black churches, where he will be giving talks to raise money for his programs. "Whatever I can do, I know it will help." His faith strikes a chord with us in the room, reminding us that, for much of the world, social work and health care is not just a good job on the way to a better one in the AIDS business, but a calling to serve one's country and people.

In the corner of a coffee shop in Lakeview, Chicago's most populous lakefront neighborhood, Mary Lewis sits, pen in hand, her tortoise-shell glasses match her smart orange and black sweater. On the table before her lie files and a guide on how to write an effective book proposal. Her eyes are sad, her face gaunt, her thin legs hidden in black stretch pants. Yet, there is a directness to her gaze that tells me I'm in the right place.

On the phone, a few days before, she'd agreed to talk to me about the memoir she was writing, which dealt, in part, with her life with HIV. Lewis had worked as a freelancer and editor for years, and I'd hoped that she might offer me a bit of advice on the business of writing about AIDS. However, when she explained to me how she had to give herself daily shots of interluken (a very powerful HIV drug, given as a last resort), I cut the conversation short. "Let's just get together. When would be a good time?"

Nervously, I sit down, eager to impress upon her my seriousness by mentioning some of the places I've traveled and my ideas about writing a memoir myself. But she stops me in the middle of my favorite anecdote: "Why do you want to do this? I mean, why do you want to tell someone this story? You have to have a clear reason, a purpose to do this. I'm not sure you know what that is."

At first, I read her directness as envy, but when I can't come out with a clear response except some stuttering cliché about helping people see the human face of AIDS, I realize it's not envy, it's experience.

Lewis grew up in Chicago on the South Side. Her father worked as a fireman, her mother was a teacher. "I'd always known I wanted to be a writer," she says, recalling how a librarian in her neighborhood gave her Bronzeville Boys and Girls by Gwendolyn Brooks. "It was the first time I read a book with black kids as characters." Children's literature led into her career as a writer: first working at a New York TV station doing children's programming, then as Junior Editor at Ebony, followed by several more years in publishing until she was asked to do a book on black teenage girls.

As with many black women, her infection came as a complete surprise. "I didn't have much awareness about AIDS," she says frowning. "Sure, I enjoyed myself and lived somewhat freely, but I dated professional men." Her voice is measured, her words chosen with precision as she recalls those days before she was infected. I can feel there is more than the writer at work here. It is as if the words keep her emotions anchored to the facts rather than the painful journey her body has traveled since then. As she tells me of those years before her infection, I imagine her as the attractive young woman working in the hustle and verve of print media, rubbing shoulders with journalists and the black professional elite, like ABC news anchor Max Robinson, whom she met and dated for a time.

I recall an image of Robinson delivering the news and then of an even stronger image of his photo behind the face of another newscaster, announcing his death along with the words: "He died as a result of complications due to . . ." Arthur Ashe got the good sportsman's award, Magic Johnson got the hero's praise, but Robinson, the first black anchor on national TV, got buried in the back pages, because his death revealed the truth that was not fit to print, that he was a man "on the down low"—a bisexual black man.

"I was busy getting ready for my book launch when I heard that Max was ill," Lewis says as if it were yesterday. Then her sister pointed out Robinson's obituary; she became worried and decided to get tested. She was stunned when she learned the results, though he'd confided in her about his bisexuality. "It bothered him but it didn't bother me. I liked being with him." She speaks fondly of their conversations about his interest in art and writing. She is not bitter, but philosophical: "Men like this are sacrificing their lives to a lie. I know they want to keep it a secret to protect their family. But eventually something happens."

Not having symptoms, Lewis buried herself into her work to keep from thinking about it. "I didn't want to let go of my career; it was my life. I had a condo and a car, a comfortable lifestyle. I worked seventy to eighty hours a week. I wasn't taking care of myself, but I didn't want to let people see who I really was. I feared I'd lose my work. This was in the late eighties. People were doing crazy things in response to AIDS. I needed to keep the façade."

Lewis got a chance to go to Seattle for a job and thought this would be a productive change. For a while things went well there, and she began to feel that clarity and purpose to her life that often accompanies confronting illness and mortality. "I knew it was time to speak the truth about my life," she says, referring to a long letter she wrote to her family during those first weeks in Seattle asking them to acknowledge the history of sexual abuse in their midst. Then, a few months later, she became ill with parasitic ailment she'd caught from her roommate's cat. With Seattle's long winter setting in, far from home and friends, her family in shock over her letter, Lewis found herself alone in a hospital.

Six weeks later, thinned to the bone and broke from hospital bills, Lewis had recovered enough to go home. But what home? She couldn't return to her apartment because of the cat, so she slept on a friend's couch until she realized she had to move back to Chicago. In Chicago, her friends put her up and she turned to Cook County Hospital for treatment. Like many of America's public city hospitals, Cook County has dealt with the epidemic from the very beginning. At the time, there were few women seeking treatment, but Doctor Marge Cohen, a pioneer in developing treatment for women, gave Lewis a renewed sense of confidence. And with AZT, she began to feel better and returned to freelance work. Still, she had little money and knew she'd worn out the hospitality of her friends. She applied for Social Security, hoping to qualify for disability under a new law that included people living with HIV and AIDS, but she had too many assets (like a car) and made too much money with her freelance work. She turned to one of Chicago's leading advocacy and social service centers for people living with HIV, Howard Brown Health Center. Without these programs and her therapist from Catholic Relief Services, she admits she would never have made it.

Lewis had not really thought about writing about her life as someone with HIV. But friends encouraged her to put her story into a memoir, including the equally painful subject of sexual abuse in her family. During this time too, she took a freelance job on The Faces of AIDS project, a book that gave a picture of the diversity of those living with HIV in the Midwest. AIDS organizations backing the project, recognizing that they had, in Lewis, a woman who could articulate the realities of living with HIV, asked her to speak at various media events for the book and other forums. She became a reluctant activist: "It made me uncomfortable. I didn't like the role of me, a black woman, being a poster child and spokesperson for white-run organizations. I didn't need the HIV- professional role," she says with a note of exasperation and perhaps a tinge of bitterness.

With the advent of the cocktail treatment, her health improved. She worked harder on her memoir. A lawyer at the AIDS Legal Assistance Foundation helped her reapply for Social Security, and Lewis got it, as well as a reimbursement for much of the money she had to pay for hospitalization back in Seattle. With this support, she could move out of subsidized housing and find a safer and more comfortable apartment.

"I really felt I'd gotten my life back," she tells me. "I worked on my memoir and other freelance jobs. I'd even gotten a part-time job at a bookstore to get out and be with people again." But her health troubles never seemed to go away. The cocktail drugs along with medications to counteract a hormonal imbalance wreaked havoc on her body, affecting her in ways no one could explain. Her weight went up, her breasts enlarged, and then her weight dropped. It was a nightmare. Her body, both inside and out, warped in ways that left her unrecognizable even to herself. From one of her chapters in her memoir, this is how she described it:

> "That's me?!" A half-sob, half-wail keens from my mouth while I gawk at a naked, misshapen, mirrored form. Swerving from towel to reflected image, I shake my head, wishing I was in a funhouse or that I was ignorant. But this is my bathroom, and my eyes are laser beams that have ripped open the pattern that was keeping me from seeing and not seeing my body. . . . Astonished, embarrassed, repelled, I'm trapped in the wreckage of truth. . . . Be nice to me, I beg the mirror.[14]

Then, even as she was making progress on her memoir, more trouble arrived: Social Security determined that she was no longer eligible and wanted to audit her, claiming she owed them thousands of dollars. "I shouldn't have taken on that part-time job at the bookstore. It raised a red flag." She had to collect and copy hundreds of papers, find a lawyer, and fight to keep her disability. "I felt my floor had fallen out from under me. I felt more frightened than when I had first been diagnosed. I dreaded the thought of losing my apartment." And if this wasn't enough, her doctors then told her that she was showing resistance to the cocktail treatment and asked her to begin a powerful new treatment with debilitating side effects.

As I listen to Lewis's story, I can't help wondering: Will this be me, next year, two, three years from now? Will I have her strength to fight every battle? To stick needles in my arm twice a day? To fight the government for my health, for my right to live? To have the courage to keep looking at myself in the mirror and accepting my body for what it is and what it needs? Will I have the courage to keep on writing?

Despite her travails and weakened body, her teeth and lips have a fierce beauty and power. She is not silent in her suffering. She speaks, she bites, she persuades. The writer in Lewis holds on: "If I can only write an hour a day, that's okay." Her discipline and faith in herself have become her source of strength. Like many of the activists I've met in Asia and South Africa, Lewis has learned to use suffering, both hers and others'. When she gives me advice on how to structure my memoir, she tells me that in writing hers she found that she was many different people. This was what she wanted to reflect in her memoir: the interrelated stories of the people, experiences, and selves that make up a life. Remarkably, she admits that "it's HIV which forced me into one being."

She tells me how writing has helped her, not so much to heal but to go deeper into her life, layer by layer, revision by revision. "The more I wrote, the more revisions I made, the more I realized it was helping me live with this disease." Writing about HIV, however, did not give her the answers; to her surprise, it gave her more questions. Yet she sees that turning the landscape of her inner life into art has given her a power that she didn't believe she possessed. "Writing forces you to make things tangible. It forces you to give voice to something that needs to be said."

"It's like you have been scarified. You know, the ritual Africans use? Marking their faces? You're scarred, marked as a member of a group. It's like that. A rite of passage. Like a naming ceremony. You must bear the pain to have your identity, to become who you are."

IX

Chicago, USA (February, 2002)

In a brilliant white damask gown, Baaba Maal, Senegal's world music superstar, gently guides an elderly blind man onto the stage to a stool and places a microphone in his hands. Two musicians follow, a drummer and a man with a flute. Maal's indigo face radiates as he greets us. But the crowd here on Chicago's North Side is confused: Where is the rest of his band? On this cold February night, we have come to be swept up into the spirit of Senegal's Afro beat. We have come to dance. But times have changed. In a paranoid, post 9-11 America, African Muslims who drum and dance could be a threat, so they remain in Dakar and Paris without visas.

Since Maal can't perform with his usual band and troupe of mesmerizing dancers, he chooses to sing traditional praise songs. The crowd listens politely, unaware that as Maal's voice spirals upward, singing now in Wolof instead of his native tongue Pulaar, he is praising the all-merciful Allah. I try to pull out the few Wolof words that I can still remember. But this old sentimental habit depresses me, as I can barely recover a few words from a language I once could speak even in my dreams.

For nearly twenty years, the music of Senegal and West Africa has allowed me to hold on to this world where I hiked, as a Peace Corps volunteer, between Wolof and Mandinka villages trying to help poor peanut farmers and their families. With a CD of Youssou N'dour, I could use the mythic sounds of the talking drums and the driving beat of the electric guitar to make me believe that I was still connected, still concerned, still conscious of that world. But now that I am about to return to Senegal for the first time, I realize how far I have drifted from it.

The blind man's face shines from within, and as he sings, his head rocks from side to side, giving the impression that his body has become his voice. I close my eyes, and I'm back in my thatch hut listening to the African night and the chanting of young men as they sit around a fire singing in honor of the Prophet's birth.

Dakar, Senegal (March 2002)

I arrive in Dakar as I left nineteen years ago: on a thick, sultry night, the air like a mouth swallowing me as soon as step off the plane. Crowds jam the gate, waiting for relatives who boarded as janitors from Atlanta or cab drivers from New York but exit as family heroes clad in Nike wear and flush with gifts.

I have no time to float off into nostalgia as I'm quickly surrounded by four young men, whom the Wolof call "saay saay" (fast-talking con men). I try to refuse their false offers of help in my bad French and mix of English and what little Wolof I've relearned from my old Peace Corps handbook on my flight. But it's no use, they are too dramatic and slick. I'm saved by my host and interpreter just as I'm ready to get into a fistfight.

Abdou-Karim Sylla, a jovial, stocky, thirty-something Wolof in jeans and a Temple University sweatshirt, pays off the punks, and we head into the night to find a hotel. I have arrived on the eve of Senegal's biggest holiday, Tabaski, or Eid al-Kebir, as the rest of the Muslim world calls it. Fortunately, Abdou-Karim finds the last hotel room available in Dakar and drops me off.

I'm exhausted, but with the booming Senegalese music from the bar below I have no choice but to hit the ground running. As I enter the bar, Youssou N'dour is wailing away from a video projected on the wall behind me. Elongated shadows of a dancing couple cross the screen. Men sit at the bar. Couples huddle around candles on corner tables. I'm, by far, the least well-dressed in the place. Western suits, tailored pants and shirts for the men; tight-fitting jeans or dresses with slits up the sides for the women.

I order a beer so I can practice my Wolof and try to distinguish myself from who I really am—a tourist. The cold tang of Senegalese beer makes me feel instinctively the presence of my old Peace Corps colleagues with whom I must have drunk a thousand of these very same green bottles of Flag.

Discovering I know some Wolof, the bartender flirts, asking questions, wondering if I'm staying here at the hotel. More couples make an entrance, more women decked out in heels and gauzy tops. Another of the waitresses smiles at me as she dances with a customer. It's a holiday, people are in a good mood. Or is it just another night in Dakar—a city full of young women from all over West Africa, looking for a way out of poverty, hoping a relative or a "friend" can find them a job cooking or cleaning or doing something that over 25,000 other women do in Dakar to survive, sex work.

Without looking for it, I have entered into the story that I have come to tell, a story that began here twenty years ago for me, as I sat in that thatch hut listening to the BBC, learning of a mysterious, new disease with an acronym to make it easier to remember, as if that would ever be one of its problems.

❋

The story of Senegal's "lutte contre le SIDA" (the battle against AIDS), as it is called here, is one that everyone wants to tell, as it stands in stark contrast to what has happened elsewhere in Africa. Here, in this country of 9 million people, the rate of HIV infection has remained relatively flat; in fact, it has fallen off to where it now affects only 1.4 percent of the adult population. A success story, or so we are led to believe.

As the story is told, instead of ignoring the alarming predictions of the World Health Organization and the United Nations back in the mideighties, Senegal took these predictions seriously. Senegalese doctors not only helped discover the first cases in the country but also the second strand of the virus—HIV 2. So there was pride involved from the outset, and support from Harvard's School of Public Health. The Senegalese government acted quickly to consolidate several health-related agencies and put them under a single office known as the AIDS Board, with a cabinet level director who reported to the president. This coordination of government offices and NGOs also extended to powerful Islamic brotherhoods and organizations. Though Senegal is not a theocracy, government leaders have always understood that their success depends on the support of the powerful religious leaders who control not only a great deal of wealth in the country, but command enormous respect among the population, particularly peasant farmers. From the beginning of the pandemic, imams and the rural marabouts (clerics) did not oppose the prevention methods of the government and NGOs. Islam may be more influential in containing HIV than many outside the Islamic world care to admit or explore. One important factor in holding down infection rates in Islamic countries such as Senegal is the relatively low consumption of alcohol, which has proven to be a serious contributing factor in other, non-Muslim, African countries. In Senegal, although there are certainly men who drink, there is still a powerful taboo against the use of alcohol, particularly in public. The Islamic practice of male circumcision, which many public health officials believe can markedly reduce heterosexual transmission, may also contribute to Senegal's success.

Another critical factor in Senegal's low infection rate is the health care the state provides for those women who legally register as sex workers in the major cities. Following the socialist policies of France, Senegal legalized prostitution in the sixties. In Dakar, all sex workers must register at government-run public health clinics or be arrested. With support from international agencies, HIV testing has been added to the basic health care services these women receive when they register. However, there are thousands of women who refuse or are too ashamed to register and remain outside this system, and their number is growing, according to organizations that work with sex workers.

Geography also plays an important role in helping slow the spread of the virus into Senegal from its neighbors. The country is surrounded by the Atlantic Ocean and the sparsely-populated Sahelian savannah and desert, which act as natural protective barriers from the heavily-infected areas in West Africa. This relative isolation is beginning to change, however, as Senegal is becoming home to more and more refugees from civil wars in Sierra Leone, Liberia, and Côte D'Ivoire. Dakar is also now overtaking Abidjan as the commercial center of West Africa and thus has become the destination for so many of the region's young people. Moreover, as more Senegalese look abroad for work, they bring cultural influences and diseases home with them. Globalization, as everywhere, is a two-edged sword, and the increased movement of people in and out of Senegal may come with a cost.

※

On my first morning in Senegal, Abdou-Karim comes to pick me up so that I can spend this holy day devoted to feasting with his relatives. Half-asleep, I try to absorb a city that I can hardly remember, as it passes me by in a kind of jetlag dream: convenience stores, ATMs, women in jeans with cell phones, young men in hip-hop dress, and silver SUVs negotiating traffic. Despite these advances and worldly influences, my heart warms when I spot the images that, for me, are still Dakar: the towering minaret of La Grande Mosque, the cobalt blue and mustard car rapides stuffed with passengers, and the dramatic seascape along the Corniche.

Abdou-Karim lives in a middle-class neighborhood, though he and his wife have little money and must share a cramped compound with his older sister and her children.

When I enter, Abdou-Karim's wife and sister, who are busy preparing for the day of food, offer the traditional greetings, asking about my family and their health. They are glad to see me, knowing I bring work for Abdou-Karim, who must rely on occasional translating or guiding visiting scholars. His children, dressed in their best clothes, shyly come up and shake my hand, murmuring their greetings and giggling in surprise when out of the back of my mind come the traditional responses. One of Abdou-Karim's sons sets a chair under a mango tree so I can watch the ritual sacrifice that the day centers around.

Abdou-Karim and his nephew grab a screaming sheep, wrestle it to the ground, and slice open its neck. A crowd of neighboring children jumps back to avoid the spurts of blood until Abdou-Karim directs the steaming red jets into a hole in the cement patio of their courtyard. As he cuts through the sheep's neck, whispering prayers under his breath, I recall the first time I saw this ceremony in my village. A cluster of elders stood around a similar hole in the middle of the chief's compound, whispering prayers over the sacrificial sheep. The solemnity of the chief's large family, all in rapt attention as the blood poured out of the sheep's gurgling neck, mesmerized me more than the actual ritual slaughter. In silence, they waited for the completion of the ritual, as if time itself had come to a halt and only through this sacrificial act that it could be restarted. Tabaski is the day to honor the faith of Ibrahim or Abraham, the patriarch of Judaism, Christianity, and Islam. The Kaaba, the tomb at the center of the holiest shrine in Islam in Mecca, is where Muslims believe Ibrahim is buried. In honor of Ibrahim's act of faith in offering his own son, the Senegalese offer lamb to the poor, their neighbors, and their extended families.

In my village, I recall bowl after bowl of lamb was sent to the families that lived off the charity of the village chief, families that often ate only once a day.[1] Soon three thin, barefoot boys show up at Abdou-Karim's compound door and present their rusty tomato-paste cans to collect offerings of food. One boy wears only a threadbare man's suit coat that comes to his knees; he holds it shut with one hand for fear it will open and reveal his nakedness. Other street children follow. So, here in a country with an average per capita income of $426 per annum, the people practice their faith by giving away food. I ask Abdou-Karim how much a sheep costs, and he tells me proudly that he got his for a good price at 40,000 CFA, nearly $60.

❋

When I learned that I'd been assigned by the Peace Corps to work in Senegal, I had no idea I was going to a Muslim country. I didn't even know where the country was located and knew next to nothing about Islam. In the weeks before I left, I fantasized about living in a remote village where people practiced ancient rituals and held elaborate festivals with masked dancers evoking the spirits of the dead. Like almost every kid in America, I'd grown up with images of Africa supplied by Tarzan movies and the National Geographic. How disappointed I was when I landed in a conservative Islamic village of Wolofs and Mandinka, who had abandoned the rituals and ceremonies of their animistic ancestors long ago.[2]

Today we are headed to the Grande Mosque to meet with a cleric who heads L'Institute Islamique, a center for Islamic studies and culture. But we are having a hard time finding a taxi, as each doubles his price as soon as they see me, which infuriates Abdou-Karim. Finally, we find one. I climb in and see a familiar face staring back at me on the dashboard— Osama Bin Laden. This isn't the first time: I have seen his face on buses, taxis, and t-shirts. Abdou-Karim says you can buy his tapes in the markets. I glance at the taxi driver in his turban. He's oblivious of me, but the anger in me is still there from the attacks of seven months ago, and part of me wants to point to the photo and ask the driver, who's that?

Our taxi passes through the neighborhood of Medina, a mix of sprawling open markets, small shops, and what seems like an endless number of makeshift fix-it shops, where men covered in grease attempt to salvage parts of trucks and cars that would have been junked long ago in the West. In the middle of this maze of poverty rises Dakar's tallest structure, La Grande Mosque with its towering minaret.

The mosque is off limits to me, but with Abdou-Karim's help I have secured an interview with El Hadj Demba Thiaw. Thiaw is a cleric close-ly associated with the powerful Mbacke family, heirs to Cheik Amadou Bamba, a 19th century martyr and mystic and the founder of Senegal's Sufi sect and Islamic brotherhood, the Mourides. The image of Amadou Bamba, a face wrapped in a white head scarf, can be seen everywhere, painted by hand on the sides of little shops, on taxis and buses, and the walls of homes.[3]

Even though I have an appointment, Abdou-Karim must talk his way through two sets of guards before we are allowed through the wrought iron gate. Inside, the din and dirt of the city are gone. Through cupola-shaped arches, I walk into the courtyard and peer up into the serene symmetry of classic Islamic architecture, balcony upon balcony, cupola upon cupola, the green and white tile work extending upward as if in some Moorish mosque of 16th century Spain.

El Hadj Demba Thiaw—lean, goateed, fortyish—invites us into his windowless office. He is dressed in a flowing, green gown that perfectly matches the classic Islamic emerald green tile in the courtyard. He has just returned from Mecca and looks tired.

The courtyard's open elegance gives way to the drab, institutional office of metal tables and bookshelves covered with dust. Thick books with elaborate Arabic script are stacked about the room and give it an aura of scholarship rather than bureaucracy.

From the start, things don't go well. I fumble through my first ques-tion in French, wondering about Islam's connection to AIDS. However, he misunderstands me, thinking I'm blaming Islam for the spread of AIDS. Abdou-Karim nervously corrects me. What I meant to ask was did he think Islamic beliefs and laws were stemming the spread of the dis-ease or was it causing some people to fear getting tested out of retribu-tion and shame. Thiaw turns to Abdou-Karim, admonishing him, sur-prised that he would let me ask such an obviously ignorant question. "Islam is pure," he says. "It is the people who stray from the Prophet's teachings." Through the Prophet, Allah gave man law and order so as to enable him to live peacefully and righteously rather than in chaos, he lec-tures. The law, as I remember now from my single course on Islam in divinity school, is the only way to keep humans from destroying them-selves. AIDS can be stopped cold if people simply follow the dictates of the Prophet's teachings, he tells us matter-of-factly. It is as simple as that, and those who fail to do so must pay for their evil acts. His strict moralism sounds all too familiar, reminding me not only of conservative Christians but of the response I got from the Buddhist abbot of Chum Thung in Northern Thailand.

"But what about women?" I want to know, reminding him that many women are contracting the virus from husbands who know that they may be putting their wives or partners at risk. "Women cannot refuse their husbands, isn't that right?"

"Women are to serve the husband," he states. "This is the natural order."

"But, sometimes the man beats his wife and makes her have sex, even if she refuses."

"This is wrong. No man should hurt his wife. She is a creature of God."

I keep pushing: "But these men who drive taxis and trucks, aren't they the ones passing the virus?"

"Men should not have sex if they are infected," he says. "They should refrain."

"Use condoms?"

"Yes."

He leans back in his chair stroking his goatee. "Those who are sick are to follow the teachings of Islam," he tells me: "They should not harm others, even if that means exile from the family or community. This is the righteous act."

I remember other Muslims explaining the importance of health to a believer. The pilgrimage to Mecca can't be undertaken if the body is enfeebled or sick. Fasting during Ramadan is also discouraged if one is in poor health. Personal responsibility and discipline are at the heart of a believer's faith. To be a good Muslim, action is required, deeds must be performed, and sacrifices made.

Yet, when I think about women I've met who have been thrown into the streets because they're unprotected by political and cultural "laws," I can't appreciate his theological argument for sacrifice. It's an easy position to take if you are a man with authority and power.

It all seems so perfectly clear to him, which annoys some part of me that has always rebelled against this type of religious absolutism. Yet I realize that his beliefs are not subject simply to cultural or political explanations. They are metaphysical laws that define every act, every object, every thought in this man's life. They are all a part of his faith in this towering theological edifice built on a book of laws. Looking at him, surrounded by his dusty Arabic texts, I have to accept this as his response to the world, which is no less subject to doubt than my beliefs or any other belief system.

Nevertheless, in my broken French I continue to try. "But what about other Muslim countries, Côte d'Ivoire? Mali?" (Mali has a population that has a higher percentage of Muslims than Senegal and an HIV rate of 4 percent and rising.) "And what about Nigeria?"

"Senegal is different, truer to Islam, the only country never to have a coup d'etat. We are stable, tolerant." This was true but the switch was interesting: National pride had taken precedence over Islamic legalism. The Wolofs are well known for their unapologetic sense of superiority over other West-African ethnicities. True to form, El Hadj Thiaw sums up each culture with a quick dismissal: The Malians aren't well educated. The Nigerians have too many non-Muslims, etc.

Despite Abdou-Karim's clarifications, the cleric's impatience grows. Rounding out the interview, I ask him if he has any questions for me. He unleashes: "Why come here and ask us about AIDS? We are a poor country." He becomes animated, his face angry, spreading his arms to point to the men outside who sleep in their greasy clothes on cardboard mats in the corrugated metal garages that line the streets around the mosque. "Why come here, when it is you who brought this disease, and you who, if you wanted, could solve it?"

"Why can't a group of scientists get together," he continues, "from France and England, from Japan and the U.S.? They could work on it. They could use all that they know, all the money you have, and you would have a cure, believe me, in a short time. If they wanted to do this, they would." Then he pauses, looks away and mutters, "But they don't want to."

For the second time, I have met with a Muslim scholar who has turned the conversation about AIDS into one about America. The day before, we'd talked to an Islamic scholar at the University of Dakar, Professor Mbacke, who at the end of my interview turned to me and said: "It's not AIDS that we are so much worried about, my friend, it's the culture you Americans are spreading to our children which makes us afraid, which makes us fear that they will not keep our beliefs and religious traditions. To be honest with you, as a father, I see my children watching the TV, and I think, I don't even know who they are anymore."

As Abdou-Karim and I head back to his home through the diesel fumes and dust, past the polio victims begging at stoplights, the Jaguars with UN plates, and billboards spouting happy slogans and black faces drinking milk, I marvel at how humans can withstand so much contradiction without losing faith in themselves and their traditions. In my mind, I keep turning it over: An Islamic cleric lectures me for an hour on the importance of divine law to guide society only to argue in the end that medical science can save Africa from AIDS; the same medical science, which, without the wisdom and foresight of Islamic scholars, would have vanished during the Middle Ages because of the fears and religious beliefs of Europeans.

❋

I'd heard that there were two former Peace Corps volunteers who ran a NGO called ACI (African Consultants International) which works with community-based organizations on HIV/AIDS throughout the continent. Where I'm staying near the University of Dakar, I can throw a stone in any direction and hit some international organization which deals with HIV. Dakar is home to approximately 150 organizations that work in some capacity with HIV/AIDS, not to mention UNAIDS, UNESCO, USAID, and the EU. For a country with approximately 90,000 people living with HIV, that's a pretty good ratio. The day before, Abdou-Karim and I went to an organization heavily supported by USAID that did nothing more than coordinate other NGOs to keep them from duplicating efforts.

I get lost and end up at ACI's other office where they house their cross-cultural education program aimed at American universities, offering students language classes and experiences living with Senegalese families. This augments ACI's funding, keeping them from having to rely too heavily on international grants.

My timing is just right for lunch. I try to feign polite disinterest, opting to sit alone and study some educational materials. The Senegalese staff, acquainted with this silly American trait, laugh in my face and tell me to go wash my hands. I sit down at the communal bowl and eat the national dish, *ceeb u jen*, fresh fish stuffed with tasty spices and served with rice and big chunks of vegetables. More good-natured teasing at my expense follows when I end up being the last to leave the bowl.

ACI serves as a resource center, providing and translating materials for community organizations and keeping them trained and aware of the most current information on HIV/AIDS. The days of dry demonstrations and picture-graph pamphlets I knew in the Peace Corps are over. ACI not only makes it easy for community organizations to use videos, they are now in the business of production as well. Their assistant director, Ibrahima Bob, tells me about one such video project called Scenarios. This video is a collection of short films written by students throughout West Africa that ACI helped to sponsor, along with other NGOs and the Lutheran World Service. The stories are told in a range of styles, from cartoons to comedy to serious drama, all smartly incorporating educational themes on HIV. They feature hip-hop stars from Dakar and well known actors from each country, and are directed by some of West Africa's most talented young filmmakers. ACI is on to something.

Next I talk with Louise Dia who works with co-founders Lillian Baer and Gary Engleberg on developing trainings for everyone from Senegal's National Assembly to journalists to sex workers. I ask her how she thinks things are going. I'm surprised to hear an ominous tone. "People in the rural areas and here in the poor neighborhoods of Dakar are simply not getting the message." She has the worn, glassy-eyed look I've seen in other countries among AIDS advocates. She sighs and takes me to see Engleberg.

He sits before his Macintosh surrounded by files and a large whiteboard calendar indicating when he is on the road facilitating ACI's trainings. He'd just returned from Mali. Soft-spoken, bear-like, intense, Engleberg seems to understand that I'm not there as another freelance writer. Before I can reel off my list of questions, he turns the tables, leans in and asks, "Why did you come here?" I find myself telling him my story. In minutes he has a list of organizations I should visit, people to meet, even an angle for an article.

The Peace Corps has its unstated hierarchies: there are those who sign up but never complete their two-year service; those who hate it but stay the course; those who love it and never stop telling their stories about it (the category I fall into); those who have their eyes on some kind of political career and stick around and get a job with USAID; then there are the ones who fall in love with the culture and either stay on or come home with a spouse. And then there are the Englebergs, who leave for the Peace Corps, as he did in 1965, and are so completely transformed by their work and experiences that they never return.

Engleberg's suggestions on who to see and where to go are precisely what ACI does for the scores of community-based organizations that they serve throughout Senegal. Having worked in development across Africa, Engleberg tells me, "I became a student of what worked and what didn't." What works for ACI is to identify selected organizations already actively involved in AIDS advocacy and support them via additional training, resources, and educational materials. "We have trained five case-workers who are familiar with a certain region and they serve what we call 'Poles of Excellence' or community organizations which have become somewhat self-sufficient." Engleberg believes that by helping to sustain the work and autonomy of already established community organizations, they will organically become resources for other community groups. Studies show that this approach seems to be working.

"We have an organic view of both the virus and how we as humans respond to it," Engleberg explains. "The virus reproduces very quickly; it's very smart, and so we have to keep ahead of it. We have to be just as smart, and so our job is to find natural antiviral elements in society [religious and community organizations, the arts, traditional beliefs] and reinforce them, stimulate them."

"AIDS, as an epidemic, is challenging methods of development," he tells me with the passion you hear more from artists or religious leaders than administrators. "We can't exclude anyone. We must go on the road with them. You have to go where people are, work from there."

Excited, I bombard him with questions: "What about the funding? How do you keep this going? How do you keep them connected? How do they get these resources you have here?"

"We don't provide funding, no trips to Dakar. They can come here and we can help them look for possible sources, show them how to apply for funding, give them the tools and resources to expand what they are doing. Look," he stops abruptly, "I've got a meeting. Why don't you come over to my house and have dinner?"

Later I meet him at his modest little compound that looks like a bohemian artist's studio of the early seventies, with African musical instruments, ancient batiks, and other pieces of art from West Africa. As I look at a Dogon mask resting proudly on top of a bookshelf, I imagine what my life might have been like if I had never returned to the States. Like other AIDS advocates I've met, Engleberg has learned to get the most out of his encounters with journalists. He reminds me of the Chumpon Apisuk, for whom development and activism are creative expressions that involve inspiring people to work together.

Just as we are ready to sit down to eat, a young man by the name of Osman Camara shows up. Unbeknownst to me, Engleberg has invited this young Sierra Leonian refugee, who wants to become a journalist. Earnest and wide-eyed, Camara has brought stories he wants me to read and is so eager to meet me he barely eats. His stare makes me uncomfortable, and when he finally opens his mouth, he speaks as if I am not there. "I have a dream last night, Mr. Gary. I dream of meeting someone, someone who has come to help me. And here he is." Then he turns to me and announces with complete faith. "You are my dream, Mr. Michael."

After Osman leaves, Engleberg fills me in on the Sierra Leonian refugees that he has been helping. "They were living on the streets, sleeping in the markets, unknown to each other. Katherine (Fraser), the ambassador's wife—she's the one who really got the ball rolling—decided to find an apartment for them. But quickly it became too crowded. So we established what we call the Baker Collier House. There's about twenty-five of them there. Osman is one of the more fragile ones. He's lost pretty much his whole family, as many of them have. He was tortured—humiliated, sexually, I think. He escaped out of the jungle with two other young men and made it to Guinea. When he couldn't find his mother or brothers in the refugee camps there, he somehow found his way here. It would mean a lot if you talked to him. Baker Collier is not far from your hotel."

"Sure, sure," I say.

After leaving Engleberg's house, I decide to walk to Abdou-Karim's compound. I can't get the round face and sincere eyes of this young man from Sierra Leone out of my head. I want to walk. I want to remember where I am. I've been so busy interviewing people that I've barely been able to let it sink in that I'm actually back in Senegal. I keep thinking if something happens—if I get sick and don't make the trip back to Darou Mouniaguene, I'll never forgive myself. I relish every shop I pass, every sound and smell, every person who catches my eye. I stop to buy some mangoes for Abdou-Karim's family. But the sound of the Wolof coming from my own mouth pleases me so much that I buy four or five different kinds of fruit, two newspapers, gum, and some candies. Across the street, school girls in green jumpers and starched white blouses march down the sandy street; further down, four men with shovels toss dirt up to a second floor, working and chanting in unison; a burst of cackling laughter makes me turn my head toward a hair salon full of women; I watch boys playing soccer near an outdoor mosque where men are just finishing their prayers. It is as if I have stepped out of a cave and back into the waking world, where each face, each sensation collapses time and makes me believe, for a moment, that some part of me never left this land and its people.

❋

Abdou-Karim and I travel into the center of the city. Dakar still has the feel of a colonial enclave, more Mediterranean than African, with its tree-lined streets, wrought iron grates, pale-colored stucco facades, and tile roofs. But as we reach the Place de l'Independence, which once held the exuberance of Senegal's future with its modern hotels and banks encircling a plaza of palms and trimmed grass and shrubbery, I see that its promise has faded; now sidewalks are buckling and the garden plaza of twenty years ago has browned and turned to weeds.

I need to change some cash and so Abdou-Karim takes me to a side street off the plaza, where he disappears inside a small wholesale shop which sells Thai rice and other foodstuffs. The markets in Dakar seem to spill out into every street, with informal and formal vending taking place on every corner. I can't walk a block in the central part of this city without being asked repeatedly to buy something. Of course, this was always the case in Dakar when I visited it twenty years ago. Clearly the urban Senegalese show no lack of initiative. People find ways to sell whatever they can. Women cook, sew, do hair, grow tropical plants. Men find work abroad and send what they can home. One day I see Abdou-Karim's wife making peanut-butter sandwiches for the school kids who play across the street at recess. An urban Africa of hopeless throngs of depressed and downtrodden folk is not what you find here. Yet, I sense a desperation that I don't remember.

I wait for Abdou-Karim. The heat of the day has subsided, hundreds of seagulls sweep and circle above the city as daylight slides out to sea. I always liked this time of day when the heat and struggle recedes and people clustered in their compounds to eat and drink tea. I'm thinking about what Abdou-Karim's wife might have for us to eat later, when I spot a tallish man approaching with a satchel over his shoulder, wearing a floppy cap black guys in my high school wore back in the seventies. He appears to be heading straight for me. And why not, a foreigner standing on a corner, looking content in my tie-dye shirt and sunglasses resting on golden hair? Even though he's really too far for me to see clearly, I feel that there is something wrong with him. I turn away and glance back inside the shop, hoping to spot Abdou-Karim. Glancing back at the street, I see the man's face. There's a pink splotch where his nose should be, and as he gets closer, the pinkish skin becomes a growth covering part of his nose and checks. Freckles and scars dot his face and neck. His eyes are fixed on mine as he steps up onto the sidewalk. Images of deformed faces and bodies scream in my mind in a composite chord of terror: the spastic children with MS at the camp in Kentucky where I worked one summer in college, the Vietnam Vets without arms and legs sitting in their wheelchair on the porch of the VA in my hometown, the dying and the dead at the monastery in Lopburi. I'd forgotten that here there would be no boundary, no protection from the fingerless fists begging for coins, the blind and the malformed, the sick and malnourished. Here there was no escape. They'd been waiting all day for someone just like me.

But ever the intrepid traveler, I'm determined not to show my fear. I will myself to stare back unaffected. He boldly greets me, and I try to respond in Wolof and French. He smiles. His gaze bores into my conscience. I squint to abstract his ugliness. But it takes too much effort. My legs begin to buckle and I have to concentrate to stand.

"Avez vous d'argent, pour faire . . ."

I respond in Wolof, "Amul xalas." I have no money.

He is taken aback by my quick response in his language. For a moment he appears to have given up. I look back again for Abdou-Karim. To my surprise, the man smiles, revealing a single tooth in his mouth, as he reels off a Wolof proverb.

I nod even though I can't remember what it means.

He knows I'm lying. "Comprenez-vous?"

I hesitate because some part of me understands. But my Wolof brain can only remember feelings associated with words, rarely the meanings. So I lie again. "Oui, je comprends."

He looks up in the air at the sea gulls, circling it seems more furiously, and he smiles once more and then blends back into the street.

Once he releases me from the sight of his face, the translation comes to me: "For those whom Allah favors, he asks much."

Abdou-Karim returns. "Let's go," he says, looking around like we've just scored, handing me a wad of bills as big as my fist.

❀

The next evening I take a taxi to find the community of Sierra Leonian refugees at Baker Collier House. Along the coastal road, fishing boats remind me that Dakar is still a city dependent on those fisherman who were here long before the French. Long, wooden boats cram the beach. Painted in bright reds, yellows, blues, and greens, these abstract designs symbolically honor their family names and the religious benefactors to whom they entrust their safe passage and prosperity. The taxi drops me off in Fann, a neighborhood that has become a haven for Dakar's growing West-African immigrant population. Baker Collier House looks as if it was built in the colonial period, when nearly 60,000 French emigrés huddled in Dakar and along the coast, prospering from the peanuts and trade from the interior of its vast colony.

"Hello, sir! Good evening!" Four young men startle me with their English as I reach the gate. All are dressed in various attempts at mimicking hip-hop style: their t-shirts, baggy knee-length shorts, and jeans come from Dakar's huge second-hand clothing markets.

"We've been waiting for you Mr. Michael." Osman greets me and proudly takes me on a tour of the compound, introducing me to each "brother," as he calls the twenty-some young men who live there. As we walk around, I notice what looks like a chart of some kind etched in chalk on a twenty-foot cement wall that separates them from their neighbors. At the top of the chart it reads "Refugee Problems" and underneath are subheadings: Language, Shelter, Employment, Integration, Health, and Trauma. Blue, pink, and white lines of chalk flow down the wall, forking and forking again, ending in the boys' initials.

"What's that?" I ask.

"That comes from a workshop Mr. Gary and some people did for us. It shows us the things we all need to do to survive."

A chalk board on a wide veranda that sweeps around the front of the two-story cement and stucco house spells out the week's duties and schedule: "Arizona boys clean up; California boys cooking; Meeting with Mr. Gary on Tuesday, 2:00 sharp."

Showing me the computer room, Osman tells me, "We will start our computer-training business here. We have our own website and I have written many of the articles on it." Three young men sit before an old computer and play what looks like a game of solitaire. They stand and shyly offer their hands. In the courtyard, a couple of guys are lifting weights—rebar stuck into cement casts made from the ubiquitous tomato-paste cans. Inside, we meet a couple of the refugees who are at work on antique sewing machines—one of their income-generating projects, along with making and selling ice cream.

"Mr. Michael, here, look here. This is where our president's office is."

Osman knocks on a door with a sign that reads, "The White House." A mature young man with a beaming face emerges and introduces himself as Peter Korama. Peter proudly tells me that before the civil war he had been studying to be a pastor, "When the rebels captured me, sir, I was at the School of Deliverance and Demonology of the Church of God in Christ in Freetown." Since there are both Muslims and Christians living in Baker Collier, I ask him if there any problems. "No sir, no problems. Some of us pray on Friday, others on Sunday. We are all brothers here."

On the door of the room next to the "White House" is, what else?— "The Washington Post." "Here is where the phone is," Osman points out. "It's where I will send my stories to the newspapers when I write them, once I get some jobs to report on the terrible things that have happened to the people in my county."

Osman takes me into one of the bedrooms where the young men stay. The "Arizona Boys" stay upstairs in a tight room where two queen-sized foam mattresses with mosquito netting cover nearly the entire floor. Downstairs under the kitchen is "California," where five or six "brothers" stay who have formed a rap group, called innocently "The Friendgees." The American idolatry puzzles me until Osman shows me a wall in a common room covered in photos. Almost all are Americans. Peace Corps volunteers, embassy personal, Engelberg, and other benefactors, including Kathrine Fraser whom Osman refers to as "Mother." As Osman describes the photos, many of which he took himself, he speaks in a tone that borders on worship.

"What's this, Osman?" I point at a series of photographs of the refugees in various poses as if they are acting. In one photo two men with sticks point at the head of another with hands behind his back as if tied. "We are acting out how the rebels treated us. See, they are pushing us down; here they are beating us, tying us up, and cutting off our hands." As he describes them, his eyes show no emotion.

We have to go outside and around the house to the back to get to his room. "This is Mexico, here," he tells me opening the door. "See, we are next to the U.S.A." Like the other rooms, it is covered with foam mattresses, and some shelves line the walls for their few belongings. He shows me a single stack of books and tablets, a pair of shoes, and out of his stack of clothes he pulls a pair of pants. "See these, Mr. Michael?" He holds up a tan pair of pants with rips at the knees. "They are the pants I wore when I was captured by the rebels. I wore them for all the time I was in the jungle. I told myself, Mr. Michael, I would not take them off until I made it safe. When I came here, one of the boys, he gives me one of his pair of pants."

He clutches these pants as he tells me in a monotone voice the story that haunts millions of West Africans from Liberia to Côte d'Ivoire to Sierra Leone. He describes the day he watched his father being dragged into the village at the beginning of Sierra Leone's civil war: "I was very scared, a young boy, Mr. Michael, I cried and ran away." Often embarrassed, his voice trails off into a whisper but then rises again with anger, believing that the telling will bring vindication. He takes me through his capture and then offers jumbled images of life in the camp: "We eat maybe some green mangoes, some little animals we can catch in the forest around us. They hang us in the trees, they put pepper on us, when we are naked, on our private parts. They cut off the hands and feet of some of us to make us scared. They fired the guns next to our ears." Mosquitoes are devouring me, ringing in my ears and chomping on my neck and ankles. When I push him to describe more, he can only repeat this line: "They treat us like animals, Mr. Michael. Animals."

When they made their escape, one of his party died in the jungle. They made it to Guinea and then on to the capital, Conakry, where they were put into refugee camps. There, he searched for his brothers and mother. "Day after day I'm looking for my mother or my brothers, I ask and ask, but I can't find them, Mr. Michael. I'm afraid I will get sick there. I'm so weak. So many people are sick, so I must leave." Pleading with me to understand, he looks up at me but seems to be gazing far beyond my eyes, out into the night, where he must still believe his mother and siblings exist.

As he recounts his long march to Dakar—how he stole onto bush taxis and hitched rides with truckers through three countries, some six hundred miles over jungle roads—he clings to the pants and to his words, like they are the only things he has left. "I want people to know what they did to me and my country, that's why I want to be a journalist, Mr. Michael, you can help me, can't you?"

❋

The next day I'm back at Baker Collier. Osman has organized a meeting so that I can interview his housemates. I order the typical Senegalese urban breakfast: French bread, butter and jam, and sweetened coffee with milk. Though not a stalk of wheat is grown in Senegal, French bread has been a staple in urban areas since the colonial period. Like rice, Senegal's other main staple, wheat must be imported, thus making Senegal, a country of farmers, dependent on the world market to feed its people.

We sit in a circle. I give Osman my mini-tape recorder. As I begin to ask questions, he takes over, rephrasing my English and moving around the room to record responses. The men are, of course, well aware of the gravity of AIDS coming from Sierra Leone, where rates are climbing as high as 6 percent due to the civil war. They talk about the places in Freetown where women work in basements near the docks called the "long steps," laughing about why its called this, apparently because it takes many steps to descend down into these brothels.

The men devour the bread and politely answer some of my questions, but they are uncomfortable, and a couple leave after eating. Korama, the pastor, who seems to be the spokesmen for the house, tries to fill me in: "Mr. Gary gives us the condoms. But sometimes we have to buy them." The head of the rap group now chimes in, "But they are too expensive." (Sometimes as much as fifty cents a piece.) "You can get them for almost free at clinics, but people don't go there . . ." Then he stops mid-sentence, realizing what he has to admit. "When you—when you want them, you go to the most closest place." They all begin to talk at once, explaining that they end up going to the pharmacy because it's too embarrassing to go to the shops nearby. Of course the pharmacy is where they cost the most. "There are cheaper ones, but they aren't very good," they tell me. "But they shouldn't be so expensive, Mr. Michael, should they, if they want people to use them?"

When I ask what people know about HIV, they chuckle.

"Mr. Michael," Korama responds, "many of these people in the countryside, if you ask them what they know about SIDA, they look at you as if you're coming from Jupiter." All laugh except for Osman. "Some say it's only a trick, a rumor by white people to scare us." Excited, others agree. I ask if they have ever seen anyone with AIDS. None has. "Only on TV," Korama says. I can hear a note of exasperation in their voices, as if to say: Why are you so interested in this? Why are you so sure that it is causing us so many problems, you who don't even live here? I consider going ahead and telling them my status, as I'd intended to all along. But looking at them and Osman, I decide to wait.

Suddenly they are full of questions for me. "Where did it come from? Who discovered it? Why is it not so bad here and worse in the other countries? Who got it first? How can one person get it and somebody else not get it?" Point by point, I try to offer my best answers.

"But now there is medicine, right? I've read about this," one young man asks who'd been quiet up until now.

"Yes," I say, "but not everyone can get it or afford it." Perhaps now, I think. Explain medicines; explain that I take them, and I am doing fine. I look at Osman who is snapping picture after picture with the disposable camera I gave him. But this seems more important: "Osman, easy on the pictures, save a few." But the questions keep coming: "Can you get it from kissing? What about mosquitoes?"

Osman, now out of film, picks up the tape recorder and sticks it in my face.

"Mr. Michael, one of the boys is asking now about mosquitoes. Would you tell us, can we get the SIDA from the bites of mosquitoes?"

They listen, their faces full of worry. I push back the mic. "No, you can't get it from mosquitoes."

"But they carry blood from one person to another?"

"Believe me, you can't get it from mosquitoes." I almost shout. I can see the puzzled looks on their faces. I know I should tell them. But instead, I turn the tables, making them admit what I know will embarrass them. "Have any of you been tested?" They silently shake their heads no, dropping their eyes to the floor.

"What do they look like, these people, Mr. Michael?" the tall rapper asks sincerely. "Have you seen any?"

Osman sticks the tape recorder back into my face.

"Yes," I say, choking on pride as I watch the chance to tell them slip away. Trying to redeem myself, I respond, but only in the third person. "Many people, yes, I know many. They can take drugs now, and . . . and, they are healthy as long as they take the medicines."

One by one, they get up to go, shaking my hand and thanking me for the breakfast. Where they go when they have no jobs, I don't know. To the UN Commission on Refugees to check for news of their families? To the British Embassy, where they are allowed to read the newspapers and use the internet? Osman collects the tapes and labels them for me. "We did very well, Mr. Michael. We need to work together. This is what I want. I will help you."

He's so hungry, his eyes so open that I can't speak. He walks me out to the main road. I give him another disposable camera and tell him to take more pictures and record more stories. "I'll be back," I say.

"I will do all of this for you, Mr. Michael. I will work my best."

I flinch at his earnest face as he takes down in his notebook what I tell him. "Do you want me to interview the rap group? It would be interesting for the listeners to hear their stories. Don't you think so, Mr. Michael?"

"Yes, yes do that—that would be a good idea," I say, looking down the road for one of those yellow and black taxis to come to my rescue.

❋

Over the next several days, Abdou-Karim and I travel across Dakar to follow up on the list of organizations, doctors, and agencies Engleberg has given me. We visit clinics, NGOs that work with women and sex workers, an Islamic school and health-education program, a French sociologist and former priest, and a Senegalese health educator who trains Peace Corps volunteers. Abdou-Karim sets up the visits, takes me there, and struggles to translate as I switch from English to French to Wolof, depending on fatigue and vocabulary. But to my good fortune, Abdou-Karim speaks for me with a voice that becomes more relaxed and confident each day. Despite the difficult and embarrassing subject matter, he has become devoted to our work and to me. Since I told him of my status that first evening when I visited his family, he has asked, out of respect, for no further explanations. Senegalese are a very formal people and exceedingly modest. Matters of health and sex are private affairs. But one day, he admits that he'd had to do a lot of explaining to his friends in describing what he was doing working with me. "They are like many others," he says in a tone of voice that I'd not heard him use, "they have many fears and questions. I see what the problem is now, better," he says smiling. "People are afraid, but if you talk to them about it, then they don't have the fears so much, and don't have the wrong ideas." Abdou-Karim has hit on exactly the problem and solution. It's a theme that has repeated itself wherever I have traveled. It's not only information people need, but, more importantly, the opportunity to ask questions and discuss sexuality and its relationship to health. As they relax into the subject, they steadily overcome their isolation and fear.

Abdou-Karim has confided in me about his temptations to have affairs. "It's too dangerous," he admits nervously with an innocence I'd not seen in him before. Yet, for many Senegalese men, affairs and "girlfriends" are common. Conveniently, they can say that they are testing out new potential second wives, though many men in cities cannot afford a second wife.

One Saturday, I take Abdou-Karim and his family to the beach. Xady, Abdou-Karim's wife, can't go. I forget that women are rarely allowed to leave the house—that it's up to them to care for the children, to clean the clothes, to cook and keep the household running. Xady, as is customary for a Senegalese wife, must look after me as well, as I am a guest. Conscientiously, she takes whatever laundry I have, asks politely if there are any dishes I'd like to have prepared, and buys things for me at the market. Whether Abdou-Karim has told her of my status I don't know, but more than once she has suggested that I should rest more and take it easy.

Abdou-Karim and I, along with his nephew and youngest son, hit a beach north of Dakar. It's fun to play around with the kids and swim and get away from this work. But the issues surrounding this virus are never far away. The growing tourist industry has brought with it the informal market of the sex trade. So I'm not surprised to see groups of eager young Senegalese men scouting the beaches for potential encounters with both women and men.[4] According to Engleberg, in the slums outside of this and other tourist enclaves, the rates of infection are small but growing.

❈

I've been in Senegal for nearly two weeks, and though we've met with doctors, clerics, academics, advocates, and community leaders, I've yet to meet a single person who admits to being HIV positive. Engleberg told me that in Senegal there are only a few HIV activists and a couple of organizations for those who identify as HIV positive. This is partly due to Senegal's relatively small infected population, but the more likely explanation is that it's too risky for people with HIV to gather openly.

Abdou-Karim finally makes contact with someone willing to talk. Finding the man's house, with only a name and a number, amidst the urban sprawl of Dakar is not an easy task, but by calling and asking as we go, Abdou-Karim eventually guides us to a little shop on a sandy street where we are met by Amadou Diarra Gueye, a member of a small HIV-positive group.

Gueye leads us across the street to a modest house. Inside, the rooms are empty, save for a few pillows and cardboard boxes in the main room where they have their meetings. The kitchen is empty as well. "Assez-vous," he offers, pointing to chairs by a window, where, I gather, he spends much of his day.

Gueye has the telltale signs of so many people with HIV—a body collapsing in on itself, a hollow face, and that distant, depressive look in his eyes. As we begin to talk, however, he becomes more animated, if not a bit frustrated with my French. Understandably so: he is a French-educated former lecturer of literature. It's all I can do to nod and ask my list of questions. I can barely follow his swift, embittered responses as his hands flutter and his thin fingers fumble to keep cigarettes lit.

Abdou-Karim has become so adept at knowing what I'm trying to say that I expect him to interrupt my mangled French. He sits in silence, and, for the first time, I see that he is uncomfortable. I forget that other than me, he has never met anyone with HIV. Gueye tells us that he can't return home and has nowhere to stay, so he stays here, cooks for himself, and spends most of his days alone. His wife, who he has infected, refuses to let him see his children. I listen to him describe his banishment, mumbling that he has become like "les homosexueles et les prostitutese." He turns away, exhaling the smoke from deep inside his anger. "It's like living in a prison," he says. In his voice I hear what I fear—that I too will be swallowed by that opportunistic infection called bitterness.

On the wall hangs a single photograph of a group of people with Prime Minister Tony Blair. Blair is smiling, along with several other Senegalese officials. In the corner is Mr. Gueye, smiling as well. "Yes, Blair sat in the chair that you are sitting in," he says pointing with his cigarette. He shrugs, aware of what it really is—"les politiques." Blair came to help them open the center. He looks at the photograph and shakes his head. Not only do I feel the cruelty in this purely political act, but I wonder at the insensitivity of publicizing what was going on in this house, making it that much more difficult for the HIV community to feel comfortable using it.

Under his chair is a jar half-full of an oily-looking fluid. He tells me that, along with Crixivan (a medicine I know quite well), he also takes an herbal concoction given to him by a traditional healer. It has separated into an oily mixture on top and yellowish-brown mixture below. He picks it up, shakes it, and then opens the lid for me to see and smell. It looks and smells awful, but he claims this mixture of herbs, water, and the resin from citrus seeds is helping him.

The front gate slams and I hear someone walking through the house. Hoping to meet another group member, I turn and can't believe my eyes. It's him—the man with the deformed face who had asked me for money the week before. We recognize each other immediately but say nothing as we shake hands. Without teeth, he is difficult to understand. Gueye tells him who I am, why I'm here, and my status. He stares at me and then breaks into a confession, telling me in frenzy about his health and life, until he is ordered by Gueye to shut-up and leave the room to get something. Gueye, being educated and of a higher class, treats the sick man with disdain, a common reality in Senegal, where people adhere to traditional caste distinctions related to family name, profession and ethnicity. The poor man slinks off. I'm not sorry to see him go. His face, so cancerous with Kaposi's sarcoma, turns my stomach. When the sick man returns, he tells me that he lives mostly on the street, but he volunteers passing out condoms in clandestine bars for an agency that works with female sex workers, an organization that Abdou-Karim and I had visited just the day before.

The man with the scarred face shows me some prescription for a medication, explaining that even though he can now get the cocktail drugs, it costs him over six dollars. I give Abdou-Karim some money and he crosses the street to buy some packets of cookies and bottles of Fanta. They devour the cookies in minutes, obviously starving. Gueye lights another cigarette and shows me a grant proposal for some income-generating project to sell fish in the neighborhood.

Another man enters, thirty or so, obviously from a higher class, wearing glasses and tailored pants. He and Gueye begin to argue, but I can't understand over what exactly. Abdou-Karim is so silent that I nearly forget that he is there. I glance at the grant. They want start-up capital to buy a cart and fish to start a small business. But they can't find funding. "It's just so we can start, make some money for ourselves—for us here," Gueye nearly screams, clenching his jaw and throwing his hands up in the air. I look at the numbers, again. The whole thing is not more than three or four hundred dollars. I wonder out loud in my bad French, why none of the many organizations in Senegal devoted to HIV/AIDS can't help them with an income-generating project, but only throw more fuel on the fire: "Yes, yes, you see? Computers, chauffeurs, telephones, but nothing for us!"

"Oh, yes!" the man with the glasses shouts. "They were all interested in us when Blair was coming: stopping by, helping us clean and paint, giving us some things," pointing to the pillows on the floor.

I feel helpless as they break out again into an argument about something else. I turn to Abdou-Karim, who is ready to go, but I suggest he take a few photos of us. The men brush off their pants and straighten their shirts and jackets; the man with the deformed face arranges his cap to hide himself as best as he can. We put our hands on one another's shoulders. There's finally some laughter, even from the embittered Gueye. Their bodies rise, their chests lift, their eyes reveal the image they still have of themselves as proud men.

Kaolack, Senegal (April, 2002)

There is only one main road out of Dakar, which eventually splits: one branch leads east toward the city of Thies and then north to Saint Louis and Mauritania, the other leads south toward Kaolack, which is where we are headed. There, the road splits again, heading southeast toward Mali or southwest toward The Gambia and to Darou Mouniaguene, my Peace Corps village.

It's Friday, and we crawl through the outskirts of Dakar into the city of Pikine,[5] an expanding sprawl of poverty that stretches down the coast and east along the highway, with a few modern residential buildings hinting at a tiny middle class. We pass nursery after nursery of tropical plants and flowering trees nestled between foul-smelling factories. Packed car rapides and diesel-polluting trucks pull on and off the highway. The fumes are sickening, and several of the passengers in our seven-seat Peugeot taxi are prepared with scarves that they wear over their mouths when they aren't talking on their cell phones.

Abdou-Karim and I had came out this way earlier in the week to meet a doctor who serves a poor community that includes sex workers and AIDS orphans. No taxis would drive through this sandy slum, so we slogged through on foot, noticing something rather new in Senegal: gang slogans on the cement houses.[6] In another twenty years, if trends continue, nearly a third of Senegal's population (which will double from 10 million to 20 million) will live crammed in this coastal region around Dakar. The exodus from the rural areas is unstoppable, thousands arriving each month, hoping to stay with a relative and eke out a living in the informal economy within their neighborhoods. How a nation survives the shift from a country of farmers to one in which most citizens live huddled in urban areas without enough jobs, proper sanitation, or access to clean water is a question that haunts much of the developing world.

Traffic is stopped by a woman lying in the road, surrounded by a crowd. "Dee na (She's dead)," the Senegalese in the front seat pronounce. Abdou-Karim explains that she was trying to cross but didn't make it—"Happens all the time." On both sides of the road, we pass hundreds of people carting or carrying their goods, walking home, or waiting for the over-crowded mini-buses that pull on and off the road, indiscriminately picking up passengers.

In Rufisque, once a separate city from Dakar but now connected by sprawl, a small bridge crosses a canal of stagnant water and sewage. But the bridge has another use today: shoes line each side of the road, pair after pair, creating a shoe market of the latest leftovers from the first world. Finally we turn away from the coast and head into the savannah long ago deforested, save for an occasional acacia or a stand of elephantine baobab, which ghoulishly guard old villages along the highway. I'd forgotten how strangely beautiful the baobabs can be, particularly against the backdrop of an evening sky, their spare limbs reaching out of chubby trunks like drawings made by children. Looking out my window at the dull, brown savannah repeating itself mile after mile, punctuated now and again by a lone woman carrying a stack of sticks on her head, I'm reminded of the melancholy power of this monotonous landscape.

Again and again, I'd heard how poorly maintained the road was between Dakar and Kaolack. But people said that back in eighties, too, especially the citified Dakarois, who always hyperbolized the primitive hinterlands. As the sun sets, I'm beginning to understand what they were talking about. Huge potholes force our driver to zigzag across lanes. It's a small miracle we don't hit any on-coming cars doing the same. We pass the charred skeletons of trucks and taxis abandoned in the sand, and as night falls, my respect for our driver grows. I'm mystified how he can remember or divine where the next pothole will appear. Just when I think we'd made it through the worst of it, the road becomes so impassable that it's necessary to drive off into the savannah for long stretches. I can't imagine what this road must be like in the rainy season. This is the national highway. What happened? According to Abdou-Karim, it's the same thing that plagues many African government projects—corruption and bad management.

When, six hours later, we finally get within the city lights of Kaolack, (it used to take a little more than three), we blow a tire. Even though the highways have deteriorated, Senegalese taxi drivers still possess that mechanical magic, and we are back on the road in ten minutes.

❋

Having arrived at night, the next morning I'm eager to get a glimpse of the city where I once spent many a weekend and holiday with my Peace Corps colleagues. But as we roll out of our hotel on the banks of the Saloum River, I barely recognize anything but the Catholic Church and the huge market in the city center. It appears as if the city has suffered through a war, which I suppose, economically, it has. In 1996, France discontinued its support of the CFA franc thereby forcing Senegal's currency to lose over half of its value, drastically undermining the nation's economy. If that wasn't enough of a shock, Senegal had to adhere to the strict measures imposed by the International Monetary Fund and the World Bank, including the lifting of the meager peanut subsidy given to its farmers for their crop.

Buildings that had once stored or sold goods now stand abandoned. The modern tourist hotel where we used to hang out and swim is boarded up. On street corners, pigs pilfer through piles of trash. The few streets that were paved are almost worn away. We pull into a gas station and a swarm of dusty-faced, barefoot boys aggressively smear their sad faces against the windows. I can see only one new building: an abstractly-designed and brightly-colored community center.

Before we head out to Darou Mouniaguene forty miles away, one of the caseworkers from ACI has invited me to tag along with him for a day as he makes his rounds visiting clinics, NGOs, and community-based organizations in Kaolack.

Abdoulaye Konate meets Abdou-Karim and me at our hotel and directs us to our first stop, a public health clinic. Abdoulaye, in pressed jeans and shirt, has a well-trimmed goatee and reveals an easy manner and a healthy ambition that has, no doubt, landed him his enviable position with ACI. The clinic is orderly and clean but scarcely equipped. I meet the part-time doctor and the nurses who are the backbone of the clinic. Outside, patients sit under a tree. We are joined by a young man who is a community organizer from a nearby village. Seeing my tape recorder, the doctor has an idea. He invites us into his tiny office, which is so packed with books, boxes, medicines, and cleaning supplies that we can barely fit in. He wants to record us for a community radio program. "People need to hear more from different people, not just me. People don't know about this virus; they think it's somewhere else, someone else's problem," he tells me hurriedly in French. Indeed, according to the doctor and Abdoulaye, Kaolack has a growing problem: as it is a crossroads and a market town, attracting people from Mali, Guinea, and The Gambia where infection rates are much higher. Where there is a transient population of men, there are always sex workers. Together they create the environment for the spread of HIV.[7]

The doctor passes the tape recorder first to Abdoulaye, then to the youth leader, and finally to me, asking us to say a few words about who we are and what we do. A voice comes out of me I do not recognize as I string together Wolof phrases explaining who I am, why I am here, and something that took me years to admit in English—that I am living with

HIV. The doctor nods eagerly, thanks me, and adds a spiel about how the medications work and how important it is to be tested, referring to me as an example.

After a meeting at a community youth center in an old French-colonial building without furniture or lights, we have lunch and then follow Abdoulaye to a meeting with several officials at the regional public health office. Abdoulaye hopes an official will take us to a clandestine bar to talk with sex workers. When Abdoulaye brings this up, the official laughs so hard he begins to choke, doubting I really want to see what I'm asking to see. I wait until his coughing fit subsides to tell him that I am HIV positive. He lights another cigarette and points for us to go into his office. Before he can fully explain how serious the situation is with Kaolack's sex workers, the reason for the meeting arrives by chauffeured car—the Minister of Public Health. Sleekly suited, thin, urbane, fast-talking, cell phone in hand, he is here to make his rounds. He offers a rambling lecture full of ideas from a recent international conference. Everyone dutifully nods. He's upset about diets and how unhealthy they are for people in the country. "Poor diets cause sickness. Why do our people eat imported junk food when we have good food from our own country?" Then his cell phone rings and everyone sits in silence as we listen to him converse loudly for five minutes. This happens two more times before he excuses himself and heads back to his car. But our visit isn't totally for naught—the official we'd talked to earlier agrees to take us later that evening to meet the sex workers.

As it approaches mid afternoon, I feel the intensity of the infamous Kaolack heat, which regularly tops 110 degrees. We take refuge under an awning at a Lebanese-run restaurant. As Abdou-Karim and Abdoulaye, total strangers only a few hours before, converse like old friends, I stare out onto this sun-bleached city of mud-brick and corroded zinc and recall that for ten months it was for me the most romantic city in the world, the city where I spent all day in the markets with Elizabeth haggling with the vegetable ladies for fish and cabbage and drinking tea with her dressmaker and his friends.

After lunch, as the heat subsides, we head past the market and through the old part of the city near the river to find the sex workers. I look this way and that, trying to recognize a building or a landmark. The taxi turns down a tree-lined street, and suddenly, I know exactly where we are: at the road that leads to my village. Abdoulaye tells the driver to stop, and we climb out into the chaos of the taxi station where I used to board the bush taxis that took me to Darou Mouniaguene. There are more cars and buses now, but much remains the same, like the stands where I'd buy oranges and cola nuts for the villagers, and the corpulent women selling sugary café au lait and the mysterious, medicinal *quinqueliba* tea from smoldering pots. Teams of teenagers covered in tattered, oil-stained clothes still pound away on auto carcasses, trying to turn scraps into salvage. The deafening din of the station, with its taxis and buses honking and boys shouting for passengers, creates a mixture of nausea and fear. I walk by these young men, who sleep in the oily sand where they work, living no better than the dogs that slink about the market, and I ask myself: Had it been this bad before and I'd never noticed? Was I that naïve?

The sex workers live in the squatter camp on the salt flats of the Saloum River, across from the taxi station. They must contend with the rising waters and mud in the rainy season and the stench from the trash and human waste. Beyond the huts as far as the eye can see, blue plastic bags dot the landscape—thousands and thousands everywhere. In my day, the shopkeepers used old French newspapers or leaves to wrap purchases, but now, along with plastic bottles, these bags litter the countryside. Across the river, I spot the familiar two mountains of salt and their shadow, a black tanker, docked at the salt processing plant. The "gennkats," as the Senegalese refer to them (literally, women who work outside), live in a compound of primitively-made huts with thatch roofs and corrugated doors, not unlike those of my village.

The skinny public-health worker leads the way, greeting the women and the poor families that live around them. Feces and condoms are everywhere. He enters a hut and motions with his ever-present cigarette to wait. When he emerges, he beckons with a smile, whispering to Abdoulaye that they will expect payment for their time. We pull back the ragged sheet hanging from the door frame and on a bed sit two women, one in her late twenties, another over twice her age. The elder, who seems to be in charge, has a round, copper-colored face. She wears a slip over drooping breasts and a wrap-around piece of cloth for a skirt. Her skin is worn and wrinkled, her face etched in a permanent long frown. Abdoulaye greets them, explaining who we are and why we have come. She solemnly invites us to sit on one of the beds, which are nothing more than burlap bags sewn together and filled with old straw. Two more women enter shyly, one with a baby. Their bodies sag, their shoulders and heads droop. It's late afternoon. They will start working soon—working sometimes all night. The elder woman does the talking. She says they are not proud to do this but have no choice. They can make 1,000 francs, (a little more than a dollar per trick), though it is often less. She pulls a box out from under her bed. She won't take a man unless he uses one, she tells us sternly. "Not even if he gives me 5,000!" "Waaw, waaw! (Yes, yes!)," the others chime in, nodding. Animated, she now pulls out a chart from behind her bed that shows how to put on a condom. As she explains, she rips open one of what must be a hundred condoms in the box and puts her fingers up through one, demonstrating. Abdoulaye leans over and tells me she regularly gives a demonstration at a clinic for women. Through the back door, I see a woman pouring water from a cup onto her arms and chest, washing herself as the sun drops lower in the sky.

I whisper to Abdou-Karim, who whispers to Abdoulaye, who tells the elder woman that I'd like to hear some of the other women's stories. They confer, and the younger woman who had been there from the start drops her head, straightens her shirt, and begins to speak. Behind terribly sad eyes, she appears to be losing the battle to maintain her dignity and health. As she talks, she holds back tears, pulling them in by puckering her face and staring hard at me. She tells us she has two children, and her voice breaks. When her husband died, she came to visit relatives in Kaolack and, with no other support, decided to stay, leaving her children with her family. She doesn't tell them where she gets the money that she brings back on her monthly visits. Describing how hard her work is, she pounds the bed to remind us that they must lie every night with men on top of them. As she pounds, a cloud of dust and flies lift from the threadbare bed sheet. "You hurt; you are sore," she points to her neck and back. Abdou-Karim and Abdoulaye are gripped by her testimony.

"Do they know anyone who has SIDA?" I ask without Abdou-Karim's help.

They shake their heads no, solemnly.

"Are they worried about it?"

The room is suddenly quiet. They nod looking at me and then away.

I want to hear from the four others sitting there. But Abdou-Karim and Abdoulaye both look eager to get going. We get up together. I tell them in Wolof that I'm grateful, and both men relay the same more eloquently. I fish around for the money I have promised to them, 1,000 CFA for each one, and hand it to Abdoulaye who gives it to the older woman to disburse. The exchange is awkward. The women say their goodbyes while eyeing the money. I wasn't going to reveal my status, but suddenly I feel that I must. I want them to know that I didn't just come here as a journalist, as an American with 1,000 franc notes to hand out. My mouth begins to speak almost before I can think of what to say. I turn to them and plead in English: "Protect yourselves. Be careful. Our bodies are sacred." My legs begin to shake, as I hear Abdou-Karim's translation, knowing what I want to say but not sure how to say it in Wolof. "Parce que, SIDA, Am naa Sida." I finally spit it out, pointing to myself with my thumb, "Waaw waaw, man. Am naa. (Yes, me, I have it)" They look at me confused, then turn to Abdou-Karim and Abdoulaye for help. Abdou-Karim explains and Abdoulaye reinforces, they get it: the white man has SIDA.

All at once there is a clamor of responses. By admitting my status, I'm no longer the white man with the pen and paper. I have become the very thing that we have been discussing: I am SIDA. "Dimbalenu, dimbalenu! (Help us, Help us!)" A woman pleads holding my hand, "We don't want to get SIDA, too. We don't want to do this. We want—if we had money, if we had other work." They huddle around me, pushing back Abdou-Karim and Abdoulaye, patting me on my arms, instinctively wanting to touch me. As is Wolof custom, upon learning of sad news, they offer me their pity, "Ndeysaan, ndeysaan," and call out to Allah to protect me from death. The public health official leads us away, laughing at the stunned looks on our faces, offering some jocular expression in French that I don't catch as I struggle to avoid stepping on the trash and the shit.

As we reach the road, I feel a hand on my shoulder and the silence of Abdou-Karim as he walks with me down the road. If we'd been better friends, he would have taken my hand, as Senegalese men often do to express their enduring respect and affection. I turn to look at the sun hanging in the haze over the salt flats and the river, as it makes its way back to the sea. Looking out over that vast plain as it darkens, I feel as if the land itself has a memory, and in it I have been preserved in my innocence of twenty years ago. For it was here, on the outskirts of the city at the taxi station, that Elizabeth and I would meet, waiting for each other to return from working in our villages.

How far away she is from this place and this time that we once shared. Years ago, we lost touch. She got married not long after she came back, moved west, had several children, and never went back to school. I should be sad thinking about her, sadder still that after twenty years I have yet to feel the same way with anyone else. But, strangely, in the deepening company of this land, I feel just the opposite.

When asked "How are you?" Wolofs respond: "Maa ngi fii rek (I am here only)." I have always admired this philosophical response to the basic question we must answer every day, be it good or bad. Today, indeed, I feel that I am here only, in a place I once believed I wouldn't live long enough to see again. And tomorrow, I will return to my village, Darou Mouniaguene—"the place where one learns that patience is better."

On the other side of town, Abdoulaye has set up one more meeting with a youth group. We find the youth leader's house. Young and shy, she meets us outside her family compound, dressed in a beautiful, indigo-dyed skirt and matching blouse, her hair exquisitely styled and braided. She curtsies as we enter. The family is sitting outside in the communal courtyard surrounded by cement buildings daubed in shades of white and light blue. Here children play, women sit, talking softly and braiding hair, and men lounge, slurping tea. It's a scene reminiscent of those evenings in Darou Mouniaguene in the compound of the village chief, where I would lie on similar wood benches with his children asleep at my feet, as I listened to the stories of his wives and the devotional songs spilling from his radio.

But those radio days are numbered, or at least in the cities. This is now the age of television in Senegal as well. There, proudly on a wooden table at the center of the compound stands the prized possession. In the past, we would have gone through a series of greetings, food would have been offered, tea served. But now we exchange just a few nods and mumbled greetings, before everyone hurries to join the neighbors awaiting the evening's TV broadcast from Dakar.

We gather in the sitting room, characteristically crammed with several absurdly large chairs. A young man and woman join us from her youth group. Abdoulaye explains that they volunteer to give talks to other youth groups and families—presenting a video from ACI and leading a discussion afterward on HIV and safe sex. But when I ask if they know anyone with HIV, they admit that they don't. This time there are no second thoughts about declaring my positive status. I turn to Abdou-Karim and whisper, "Well, you do now." He laughs out loud, and I tell them in French that I'm seropositive. As if waiting for this, Abdoulaye respectfully offers a tribute to me, still moved by our visit with the sex workers. The young people are silent, stealing glances at me, then back at Abdoulaye. Then the other young woman, who appears a bit worldlier in her jeans and t-shirt, interrupts Abdoulaye, "Can I ask him a question?"

"Oui," I answer for Abdoulaye.

"You really have SIDA?"

Before I can answer, both women want to know if I'm married.

I shake my head, "I have no wife."

"What do you tell your girlfriends? I want to know," the feisty woman in blue jeans asks, challenging me.

I think about explaining that I'm bisexual, but I have a hard enough time explaining that even to myself in English. Instead, I tell them that I let my partners know when I meet them. The women press for more.

"But they can get it from you? You must use a condom." The tall woman in the jeans reminds me.

"Waaw, waaw," I say.

"Isn't she afraid?" the host asks.

"We have talked about it. She is not afraid."

The young man, who has said nothing, looks like he's about to climb under the table. But the women are sitting up, animated, vying for my attention, asking me things they have obviously not been able to ask before: How do people treat you? Does your family know? How do you keep healthy? Can you get it through kissing? I try to answer, with Abdou-Karim's help. And then to my surprise, the woman who seems to be getting bolder and bolder as we talk, asks: "How do women get this SIDA then, if not from the kissing?"

So there we are, sitting in near darkness with a TV blasting at full volume outside, a white man and two Senegalese men, trying to explain how women can become infected by men. I step back and listen to them, describing in their ancient language how a virus enters the blood through sex. I'm struck as I watch and listen to these young people, trying to make each other understand, trying to free themselves from this fear called SIDA. With Abdou-Karim's help, Abdoulaye is doing his job, just as ACI and Engleberg had hoped, by helping people and their communities evolve faster than the virus.

❋

The road south is no better than the road from Dakar. We pass the weekly markets. We pass the turnoff to Elizabeth's old village. We pass the offices of the sous prefet, where I remember watching my Senegalese boss beat a prisoner until he peed all over himself. We drive through the little town of Nioro du Rip, the administrative center for the region. We pass the little Catholic Church, presided over by the only other white person in the area, the French priest, an arrogant man who refused to speak to me in French, always answering me in Wolof. Looking back, however, I realize that his development work was perhaps the most pragmatic and successful of all the various international organizations in my region. He'd helped me find a well-digger for my garden projects and offered cement and iron to repair the wells. The Senegalese would often confuse us: me a stick-figure, blond American on a cheap Chinese bicycle and him a fifty-something Frenchman with a beard who drove a Peugeot station wagon. It always angered me that they couldn't tell us apart. Now I'm glad they mistook us.

My education as a Peace Corps volunteer began within the first month of my arrival in the village. Fresh from my training, I ventured out to check on the progress of a project left behind by a former volunteer some eight miles from me. I slogged through the sand and heat one morning only to discover that the villagers had abandoned his project three months after the volunteer left. When I tried to ask what happened, arguments broke out over who really owned the gardening tools and who had taken the money they'd saved from selling the vegetables. I was told this project was one of the largest and most successful Peace Corps projects in years. I should have seen the writing on the wall, but I was twenty-two years old, and the Peace Corps had replaced the fears that had chased me out of the theater in New York and Chicago. I desperately needed a new role. And this was it.

I tried to implement the same community-development model, working primarily with the village women on a collective vegetable garden and other idealistic, but impractical, projects. On paper and at dinner parties years later my work always made me look like a junior Albert Schweitzer. But the truth is, I did little more than cause more work for the women I was there to help. How absurd to ask people to grow vegetables in a semi-arid desert during the dry season. But we did it anyway. I supervised as the youngest of the women (the lowest in status in Senegalese society) pulled up bucket after bucket of water, only to watch it evaporate within minutes of touching the sand. Most of what the women managed to grow was eaten by pesky birds and monkeys. But my project kept me occupied.

The village looks nearly the same as when I left, with no electricity or running water. The garden has been abandoned. My old hut has been torn down. But I see the chief's compound and I tell the driver to stop. I grab my traditional gift of cola nuts and tea and get out of the car. A band of children comes running as they always did when a car came into the village. But when they see me, they pull back, afraid. I wave greeting them, Asalaamaalekum! I get no response except cold stares. It has been over eighteen years, and long ago the letters stopped coming when I never responded to their pleas for money and dreams about coming to America. I brace myself for the worst—a lukewarm reception and the discovery of all those who have passed away. But like the prodigal son, I have faith that whatever I will find is what I have come to seek.

"Mustapha Mbaye new na!" I say, announcing my arrival, using my Senegalese name. Abdou-Karim follows behind slowly. On a bench I spot an old woman holding a child. It's the chief's second wife. Her wrinkled face squints as she tries to figure out who this white man is bounding into her compound as if he lives here. I can see her mind working as she tries to register who I am. Then all of a sudden her mouth opens, her eyes brighten and she slowly rises.

"Mustapha Mbaye, Mustapha Mbaye new naa. Asalaamaalekum! (It's me. It's me. I have come back. I greet you in peace!)" She grabs my hand and I can feel her body shaking with emotion, as she holds on to me. She fumbles for words, repeating my name again and again, as if calling me back into her world. Her hand tightens as her eyes glisten. She blurts out what I don't want to hear: "El Hadj [the chief] has died, he died two years ago." She leads me into the compound, calling out to everyone, "Tapha Mbaye, Tapha Mbaye has come!" Children begin to gather around us; faces appear in door-ways and around the corner of huts. Some people I recognize, but many I don't. I am not a stranger after all.

Then the eldest wife of the chief sees us coming. She looks no older than when I left, though she must be in her seventies. "My son has come back," she says clapping over her head. My legs wobble, as one wife passes me on to the next. We go through the greetings. She asks about my family, who'd come for a visit in 1982. The eldest wife asks about my old Peace Corps friends and Elizabeth, remembering her Senegalese name. The crowd gets bigger. "Ana waa Amerique? (How are the people of America?)" she asks, her tone shifting in the middle of the word Amerique—like the rest of the world, she knows about September 11. She looks at me with pity just as those sex workers had the day before.

"They are there only. They thank God," I say, evoking the name of

Allah, as they taught me years ago was the appropriate response for people who have survived some kind of suffering.

I'm so overwhelmed that I have already forgotten that the chief is dead. When I'm led to his hut, I'm shocked to see who steps out. Instead of the old, gray chief, who would be nearly eighty-five years old now, a young man bends his head down and appears through the curtain. It's his son, Mustapha Mbaye, after whom I was named. When I left, he was fourteen years old; now well over six feet tall, he towers over me. He trembles, as his mother did when she first saw me, sucking in his breath as if seeing a ghost.

The compound is now filling with neighbors, and they clap when they see the surprise on his face at seeing me. We then fall into a long series of greetings, where he addresses both Abdou-Karim and me. Inside his hut, he asks me to sit on his bed—the bed of his father, the bed in which he was conceived, the bed in which he has conceived his own children. He stares at me as if he is not sure it is really me, then breaks out again into greetings. "How are your parents and your family, and the people of America . . ." I try to carry out a rudimentary conversation with him in Wolof but simply can't express myself. He laughs: "You can't speak Wolof anymore."

"Yes, I have forgotten everything." It's painful for me to rely on Abdou-Karim, as Mustapha was my first teacher and translator. "I'm a teacher now. I'm writing a book." I open my hands out to form the universal symbol for book. "A book on SIDA."

Then come the difficult questions: "We wrote to you, but you didn't write back," and, "How are your wife and children? You must have many, recalling my conversations about Erin, by now." I sidestep these questions with Abdou-Karim's help, who, recalling my conversations about Erin, simply tells him I have a girlfriend.

The word of my arrival has spread, and a stream of women flow toward Mustapha's hut to offer their greetings. Some scream when they see me, laughing uncontrollably in such emotional outbursts that I don't know what to say. Mustapha picks up right where he left off twenty years before, whispering their names to me as they enter so that I can answer their greetings with their last names as is customary. Each asks, "How is your wife?" Even here, Mustapha proudly chimes in as Abdou-Karim had, "He has a girlfriend. He is a teacher at a university. He is a journalist. He is writing a book."

I'm eager to visit the village and give my respects to the elders, including the women with whom I worked. But lunch arrives with apologies for not having more than a standard mid-day meal of rice and peanut sauce. When I think back on what these women did day after day, I'm still in awe. Every morning they rose before dawn to draw water from the deep wells hundreds of yards away; then they cooked breakfast for up to twenty or thirty people. They never stopped cleaning something or someone—clothes, huts, children, the yard. Then back they went to preparations for lunch and dinner, pounding heavy wooden mortars to crush millet or corn. When they had a chance, they worked in their own fields and gardens. Their day went on and on, until they finally allowed themselves to sit down. Even then they kept their hands busy sewing or braiding a child's hair.

After eating, we head out into the village with a troop of children following. People come out of their compounds, some wondering who I am, others greeting me while cooking or feeding animals, as if I'd only been gone a couple of months rather than two decades. We walk by the small, squat mosque that is indistinguishable from much of the rest of the buildings except for its tarnished, gold-painted crescent at the top of a chimney that serves as a minaret. Like the rest of the village homes and huts, it seems to have deteriorated from the harshness of the weather and the termites. Next to the mosque is the same mango tree, but larger, and underneath it is the same platform of logs where the men would take their siestas and hold village meetings. But today these log platforms are empty.

"Where are all the men?" I ask Mustapha.

"Gone to Kaolack," he tells me. Abdou-Karim whispers more details as we walk by one of the wells that looks completely dry. Apparently, the men have had to go to the regional magistrate's office to vouch for the story of one of the villagers who accidentally killed a village boy with his truck during a holy festival the week before. The men that I do meet are just where I left them twenty years before, sitting in their huts or doing odd jobs around their homes. Despite years of labor in their peanut fields, they seem actually poorer. On the walls hang the same old calendars with a photo of Mecca; in the corners rest the same farm tools and clay jars for drinking water. All just as it was before. They are overjoyed to see me, slapping their hands around mine and looking at me as if I'd come back from the dead. When I ask them how things are, they shake their heads and then ask if I can't do something. "The farmers, we have nothing." Forced by the International Monetary Fund and World Bank, the government has privatized its huge agricultural agency. SONICOS was once responsible for all aspects of the peanut crop: providing seeds, fertilizer, storage, and transportation and, most important of all, assuring a fixed price that farmers could rely on. Certainly, it was not the best system, riddled with corruption, but now it is gone entirely. These farmers must fend for themselves in a world market that will no doubt bury them. Yet they praise me, remembering my meager little projects and thanking me for the three volunteers who have followed me, though I, of course, had nothing to do with their coming.

I ask Mustapha if Osman Loum, the village muezzin, is still alive. Loum was the reason I didn't quit during my first year, as he doggedly defended me from the naysayers and assisted me in all my projects. I am relieved to hear that his is still here. Entering his compound, I can see him in his hut sitting on a tattered straw mat with a baby playing before him. He stares blankly out the door, looking up at us through thick, broken glasses when we call out our greetings, "Asalaamaalekum." He struggles to rise but is too sick; Mustapha demands that he stay seated. He's thin and old, with twisted teeth and a little white beard, but he recognizes me. "Mustapha Mbaye how is America?" He coughs, pointing to his chest. "I'm sick." Then he laughs, as he always did when he became emotional.

As I look at old man Loum, who is breathing with difficulty, I recall one evening working with him in the garden fixing the fence after some monkeys had broken in and destroyed all the eggplants. He stopped abruptly and mumbled something I couldn't understand, but when he picked up a handful of soil and used it to wash his hands and face, I knew he was preparing for prayer. That image of Loum praying in the garden, his forehead touching the earth, his lips whispering the ancient prayers he'd said his whole life, was one of many images that came to symbolize my experience living among the Senegalese. Looking at him now, I can still see the dust pasted on his forehead when he came to help me finish fixing that fence.

It's getting late, and I want to visit a neighboring village where I also worked. But I want to make some kind of speech. I want to tell them how I'd held on so desperately to my memories of them and my time there. I want to tell them how, as I have aged, I've come to appreciate their lessons—of generosity, community, tradition and faith. They knew nothing of my past or why I'd joined the Peace Corps, but they respected me for simply coming and living with them. I never understood that until I left. It was no accident that I'd survived the darkest period of my life by using my memories of them as I tried to become a writer. It was no accident that after my diagnosis I performed humorous stories on stage about the absurdity of my Peace Corps projects while fighting off fantasies of putting a gun in my mouth.

But I have no idea how to tell them this. I can't tell them I'm HIV positive. I won't leave them with that image. I must trust Abdou-Karim will help me find the words for them to understand. "I was sick, very sick," I begin. "When I got better, I told myself I wanted to come here again, because when I was sick, it helped to think of the village. I remembered how faithful you were—faithful to your God. I remembered this." I am afraid to look at them now, fearing I'll start to cry. I tell them my memories of the chief praying in his hut and of Loum bowing down in the dust in the fields. I wait for Abdou-Karim's translation, staring at the ugly cat in the corner next to Loum's ragged gowns that hang on nails protruding from the crumbling wall. Then I hear a muffled yelp, a preternatural sound that I think might be from an animal outside, but it is followed by sobbing. When I raise my head, I see the young chief, the towering Mustapha, sitting on the floor, his shoulders hunched and heaving, his head buried in the folds of his long, light-blue djellaba.

The room is silent as we, and it seems the whole village, absorb his sobbing. It's as if time has collapsed; years compressed into each eerie sob. As he cries, I feel what I never believed I would: the deep pride and affection a father feels for his son, as this teenage boy in my mind has turned into a man. In his tears he proves how the life of the dead animates the life of the living.

Loum breaks the silence, telling Abdou-Karim that my coming and my stories have made them remember the past. Pointing to the new chief, he tells me that I have made a man cry by evoking the spirit of his father. "You have not forgotten us and what you learned here. . . ." As he sings my praises, rattling off the list of my good deeds, as is the Wolof tradition, I steal glances at Mustapha whose head is still bent as if in prayer. Listening to Loum's hypnotic voice, it occurs to me: He is not singing my praises, he is singing God's. For them, it is Allah who has brought me back. All day they have showered me with evocations, calling on Allah again and again, as they greeted and praised my coming, punctuating each greeting with "Alxamdulilay! Thanks be to God!" For two years I'd heard them use this expression praising Allah for every act of good fortune, but today for the first time I feel like I understand why they do so.

We cannot stay any longer, as I must stop at another village where I worked. I assure them I will return in a week's time, as my older sister, who'd always wanted to visit the village, will be coming next week. "I will bring her back, my sister. Yes, in two weeks, we will come back." I give Mustapha and his mother money to slaughter a goat for the meal when I return with my sister.

Rolling through the dry grasses of the savanna, we arrive in the second village, Keur Sett Diakhou, where I am hugged by my old friend Babacar, who was a healer who'd always looked after me. Surrounded by his children and two wives, who smile so broadly at me it hurts my own face, I marvel at the insignificance of time. They plead with us to stay the night, but I am too wiped out and have no extra money for the taxi driver, who is already upset with me for making him drive through the bush. I repeat, again and again, that I'll be back with my sister. But it's painful to see their faces as they try to understand our American ways of traveling across the world to only visit for an hour.

That night, back at our hotel in Kaolack, I lie in bed and cannot sleep. My right arm feels like it is on fire from shaking so many hands. My body feels weightless. When I close my eyes, I see the hands of the villagers reaching out to me. I hear them calling, Mustapha Mbaye! Mustapha Mbaye! Then I awake to find myself, sitting, reaching my hand out from under my sheet, wanting to touch them, wanting to touch them all.

Epilogue

"Performing all actions for my sake, desireless,
absorbed in the Self, indifferent to 'I' and 'Mine,'
let go of your grief, and fight!"
—*Bhagavad Gita*

My journey didn't end in the Senegalese village of Darou Mouniaguene. You might say, that's where it began all over again. They warned us years ago in the Peace Corps that the most difficult part of being a volunteer wasn't adjusting to a different culture but readjusting to America after coming home.

That first week back teaching in Chicago, I sat listening to my students read their written introductions of each other. They usually hated this assignment until they realized how much they had in common. It was the usual collection of students: blacks from the South Side, Puerto Ricans from the West Side, whites from the suburbs, Chinese, Nigerians, Ukrainians, Mexicans, Indians, and just to keep me awake, a Buddhist monk, robe and all, from where else?—Bangkok.

When the class was over, one sassy Puerto Rican woman sitting in the front asked: "What about you? Aren't you gonna tell us who you are, where you're from, and all that?"

I glanced at the clock.

Then a Pakistani student blurted out, "Someone said you didn't teach last year because you went to Africa to write a book."

Their bodies, usually restless for the last ten minutes of class, were poised, their eyes focused: They wanted a story. I'd thought about what I might say. After all, everywhere I'd traveled, I'd spoken to young people.

"We don't have time today, but I'll tell you sometime."

They moaned, picked up their book bags and left. A few weeks passed, they forgot, and I was off the hook. Though I did accept the offer of the Thai monk to visit his temple, and there I mentioned that I'd been to Thailand to write about the AIDS pandemic.

"You go to Lopburi?" He asked.

I nodded. And that was it.

I was back. No different, it appeared, than before I'd left, living cautiously, worried about who could hear my story and who could not. How many times had I been reminded in my travels that telling the truth about myself had made the difference between being invited into the lives of people and being shut out? Hadn't I learned that when people asked questions of me, it often had nothing to do with me, personally, but with what they were seeking through me? Why had I assumed that my own students—refugees, immigrants, and teenagers, black men trying to transcend gang life—weren't asking for the same? I was afraid, of course, that one question would lead to the next; that I would have to either lie about my status or risk telling them that their teacher, who looked healthy and straight, was HIV positive, and liked sleeping with men.

I rationalized by telling myself that I was doing enough by writing a book, though it wasn't lost on me that before me were teenagers and twenty-somethings, the group that accounts for 60 percent of new infections worldwide. I'd traveled thousands of miles hoping to redeem myself by collecting the stories of the faithful and the fearless. Why is it that we must listen to the stories of others before we can realize that the story we need to tell is our own?

Almost everywhere I went around the world, activists had asked me to stay and help them. Their pleas for my involvement revealed to me a very simple truth about political and social change: it begins and is sustained by individuals taking action. Yes, money is needed for food and clinics, to purchase equipment and life-sustaining drugs, but to end this epidemic, it will take the individual efforts of people committed to the long-term welfare of others. Certainly, I rationalized at the time, that it wasn't practical to drop my interviewing and writing, forfeit my health, and jeopardize my job and financial security by staying and working. But nobody was asking me to do that. In Vietnam, Pham Van asked me to stay a few weeks and talk to students at some high schools. In Thailand, EMPOWER asked me to teach English to sex workers for a few months. In South Africa, all I had to do was stay and teach something I love to do—yoga. When I did stay and offer a workshop or give a talk, not only did it energize the activists and those they serve, but I gained what I'd been searching for all along: the chance to belong and embody what I believed.

Often, as I tried to write about the passion and commitment of the activists I interviewed, I'd catch myself romanticizing them—a common practice in our celebrity culture, where it is easier to exaggerate the actions of others rather than to take action ourselves. However, the work of those involved in AIDS activism, prevention and care is anything but romantic, particularly for those who live with HIV themselves. Passing out condoms in bars and back alleys, caring for the sick and dying without medication, finding homes for children who've lost their parents, and running grassroots organizations on shoe-string budgets is grueling work. In many places it's not only demeaning to work with people with HIV, as one doctor in India told me, but dangerous and life-threatening. I talked with peer-educators at Sahodaran who were been beaten by the police. In China, activists are commonly jailed. Gugu Dlamini of South Africa was stoned to death by her own community for admitting her status. An HIV-positive journalist and former lover of mine died broke in New York, unable to handle the escalating costs of health care and living in the city. Many of those I have interviewed in this book will die before they see much change in this escalating pandemic and their country's response to it; some have sadly already passed on.

The work of AIDS activism is not only unromantic, it's neither new nor revolutionary. Well before the age of AIDS, development organizations and religious groups have lived and worked among the poor, tirelessly fighting disease, educating children, training men and women in ways to improve their quality of life. Twenty-five years ago, when I was a clueless Peace Corps volunteer, it was the local French priest who showed me what community development was all about. The model was simple and effective: you live in the community of the people you serve; you learn their languages, traditions, and religious beliefs; you respect their elders and community leaders; you invest your faith and your experience in small-scale economic development that make a difference to their health and welfare; you work without concern for reward or personal achievement. You serve the people as if you were serving God.

The same pragmatic philosophy and faith in upholding the dignity of all human beings guided the work of the most effective activists in the six countries I visited. It made no difference how much money they had or whether they were Muslim, Christian, Buddhist, Hindu, animist, or communist. The mission of the Church of Christ AIDS ministry in northern Thailand was no different than the mission of the largely gay/bisexual run Test Positive Aware Network of Chicago: serve those at-risk and those with HIV, help them find doctors and alternative treatment, give them spiritual and community support, and advocate in the community at large to change attitudes and open hearts. Chantawipa Apisuk, founder of EMPOWER in Bangkok, an impassioned feminist, knew that sex work was dangerous and demeaning to Thai women, but she also knew that the political and social dynamics of Thailand provide few opportunities for poor women. So EMPOWER offers educational programs and job counseling, works to secure better health care and protects the rights of sex workers. Unlike those in the so-called "AIDS business" who seem more concerned with proving a political philosophy or moral belief, people like Dave Jimenez, Gary Engleberg, Sunil Menon, and others have learned to serve without judgment or agendas. More than once, I heard this adage among activists: "Work with people where they are."

Everywhere I traveled, activists worked with a variation of this pragmatic theme, linking HIV prevention with programs that address the basic needs and offer life-skills to those most at risk. Gay/bisexual activists work in the streets, parks, and bars not just to provide condoms but to listen and offer counsel and comfort. Villas Tyeku provides safe haven to other HIV positive women and children cast out by their families in her Cape Flats neighborhood. "Step by step" was how Pham Van described his work with the communities he serves in Ho Chi Minh City. Phra Phonthemp of Friends For Life in Chiang Mai not only offers hospice for the dying but trains them to care for each other, even as they approach death.

Often as I moved from community to community, I felt as if I were no longer in control of where I was headed. Yoga teachers describe the evolution of spiritual practice in a similar way. The intellect alone is not the source of true direction. The body, too, speaks a language, providing wisdom, surprising us by showing us the way. We never know where or when or from whom our next lesson will come. I was so sure that day in Durban five years ago as I stood before that room of people from around the world—doctors, activists, social workers, HIV-positive people—that I was the one imparting the wisdom. That was until the workshop was over and a teenager from Soweto by the name of Precious came up to me, picked up my handouts on how to do headstands, and politely wondered if I had time to come to her church and offer the same workshop for those who were infected in her community. "I think they would really like this yoga. Can you come to Soweto? It's not far." That one voice, that one question came to represent the request that animated this odyssey: for your sake as well as ours, please, we don't need you to talk about the importance of acting or healing, we need you to act and to heal.

People have asked me how, without any affiliation or much financial support, I could possibly make connections to such a diverse group of people across the globe. Remarkably, I had to go no further than my own friends to connect to the vast worldwide network of AIDS activism. All I had to do was ask. From colleagues, writers, and doctors I was led from country to country, from office to office, and from door to door. But networks go both ways. And with each door that was opened for me, I was asked to reciprocate. Many of those I interviewed demanded my vulnerability and honesty. Perhaps, at first, they wanted to test this stranger's sincerity, but then, to my surprise, I found them urging me to share my story more broadly, recognizing that through bearing witness I would give and receive healing. As I embodied their voices and typed them into my computer, I realized that they had become the teachers I had been longing to find. Gathering them around me, putting their photos on the walls of my apartment, emailing letters to them, living with their stories week after week, I found myself speaking more and more honestly about my struggles with shame, desire, depression, and addiction. They demanded that I no longer live separate identities, but define for myself a masculinity that encompassed the fullness of my life experience as a sexually and spiritually active man. From this strength and purpose, they asked me to speak as honestly as I could about the most neglected element in AIDS prevention: teaching people, especially young people, that their physical and spiritual health is directly related to their knowledge of their body and sexuality. Essentially, the spiritual practice of yoga is nothing more than learning that by being objective about the function of the body and the mind one begins to comprehend the presence of the Divine, of God, of whatever you want to define that which animates and connects us to this ecology called Earth. Understanding ourselves in this way, we can experience desire as a transformative energy rather than as a force to separate us from our bodies and that which nourishes us—*shakti*, God's unconditional love manifested in all of creation.

I've heard and seen too much to speak opaquely. I don't have the time. The activists in this book have taught me to be wary of talk and endless circumlocutory rationales of people in power. Their activism teaches us all that the choices we make each day make a difference. We can act and make a difference in the economic lives of millions of people who are begging for a chance to grow food, feed themselves, sell their own goods, and teach the wisdom of their ancestors to their children. In a time of unparalleled prosperity, technological advancement, and medical knowledge, it's not only barbaric and ignorant to willfully hoard that which would uplift and nourish millions of souls eager to enter the markets of trade and knowledge, but it's tantamount to economic and spiritual suicide. The words of Pastor Sanan of the AIDS ministry in Chiang Mai ring with all the clarity and faith of the Gospels he tries to live by: "If we ask these people to change their behavior to prevent AIDS, why can't society change their behavior too, change their attitudes about those who live with this disease?"

We tend to believe that the solutions to complex social problems require great leaders, technological feats, enormous sums of money, and teams of think tank experts, but the causes of suffering and injustice are never ending. They demand another kind of intelligence, an intelligence that does not always follow reason, the correct political ideology, or religious doctrine. In fact, suffering confounds us precisely because we believe we have the will to eliminate it. Every religious tradition reminds us that our only choice is to embrace and learn from suffering. Prince Siddhartha Gautama had to flee the protected confines of his father's royal estate to discover the importance of suffering to enlightenment. Jesus of Nazareth recognized that compassion was not restricted by social custom or law and sought to comfort those on the margins: the poor, the sick, the prostitute, and the thief, and asked all those in awe of his miraculous healing powers to follow his actions. Spiritual activism is nothing new. The evolution of a spiritual practice challenges us to act not only out of our religious beliefs and ethical principals but out of a recognition that God exists in all living things. In the words of the poet and theologian Martin Buber, I hear the same question I heard twenty-two years ago when, haunted by loss and failure, I first discovered him: "You always know in your heart that you need God more than anything; but do you not know, too, that God needs you . . . ?"[8]

Acknowledgements

This book has its roots in six countries and twelve cities. In my research, I interviewed over a hundred people, visiting community organizations, non-governmental organizations, homes, clinics, prisons, temples, colleges, and governmental agencies, not to mention bars, parks, beaches, bathhouses, and cafés. From friends and friends of friends I was led into the network of AIDS activism—the most powerful drug and vaccine at work today in the world to prevent HIV/AIDS. In gratitude and honor for their work and faith, their honesty and compassion, and their dedication to the dignity of all human beings, here follows the chain of people that led me from country to country.

In South Africa: Rob Nixon, Pam McClusky, Anne McClintock, Sue McClintock, Buzo Mgandi, Michael Nixon, Andre Lcvember, Joy Wilson of Joy For Life, Villas Tyeku of Wola Nani, Sister Irene of the Sisters of Nazareth; Maizima Norman, Charles Chan, Peter Busse, Dr. Rebello, Merci Mancy, Credo Mutwa, Romy Mathys, and Mercy Makhalemele of South Africa's National Association for People With AIDS.

In India: Sunil Menon, Anto Paul Benjamin, and all the peer counselors and young men at Sahodaran, Shivananda Khan at the Naz Foundation, Lakshmi Shankaran, yoga teachers at Krishnamacharya Centre, Dr. Yepthorani, Dr. Mandivandan, Dr. Kumarasamy, Dr. Sunita Solimon and all the dedicated staff at the YRG Clinic in Chennai, Dr. Bimal Charles and Dr. Kumar at VHS government hospital, Dr. Pranesh, P. Kousalya and her staff at Woman Positive Network, Ashok Pillai and K.K. Abraham at Indian Network for People Living with HIV, and B. Sekar and his staff at Social Welfare Association for Men.

In Thailand: Paul Toh at UNAIDS, Chumpon Apisuk, Chantawipa Apisuk and the staff of EMPOWER, Greg Carl at the International Red Cross, Julailak Khampeera and Pastor Sanan of the AIDS Ministry of The Church of Christ of Thailand, Dr. Sangrog Pradupkeow, Phra Phongthemp Dhammagaruku of Friends For Life Centre, and Samran Takan and the members of New Life Friends Centre.

In Vietnam: Dr. Dung, the honorable Le Hong Thai at Ben Tre Temple, Mr. Pham Thanh Van and family and Ms. Hong and the staff of Vietnam AIDS Program, Tuong Nguyen and his family, particularly Nguyen Vinh Trung, Le Hoang Phuong, and Nguyen Vinh Tien.

In Chicago: Per Erez, Dr. Malte Shultz, Dr. JR Harris, Howard Spiller, the staff of Luck Care Clinic, Dr. Kirby Cunningham at Cermak Health Facility of Cook County Jail, Chicago Core Center, the staff of Howard Brown Health Center, Fikerte Wagaw and her staff at the Chicago

249

Department of Public Health HIV Program, David Ley, Dave Jimenez, Willy Leeks, Tyson Everett and the staff of Jordan House, Rae Lewis Thornton, Mary Lewis, Jim Pickett of the AIDS Foundation of Chicago, Ida W. Blyther-Smith, Elijah Ward, Father Juan Read of the Episcopal Church of Austin, Kevin Iega Jeff of Deeply Rooted Dance Company, and the late Charles Clifton and the staff of Test Positive Aware Network.

In Senegal: Leigh Swigart at the Center for International Peace and Justice at Brandies University, Charles Becker, Wendy Wilson of West African Resource Center; Gary Engleberg, Dr. Fatim Louise Dia, Ibrahima Bob, Abdoulaye Konate of African Consulates International; El Hadj Demba Thiaw of L'Institute Islamique, Professor Mbake at the University of Dakar, Amadou Diarra Gueye, SIDA Service of Dakar and Kaolack, Peace Corps Senegal, Osman Camara and the Sierra Leonian young men at Baker Collier House in Dakar, Babacar Jeng and the village of Keur Sett Diakhou, El Hadj Mustapha Mbaye, Ousmane Loum, Amina Ba, Issitu Cissay and the people of Darou Mouniaguene. I want to specifically thank my interpreter, assistant and friend Abdou-Karim Sylla, his wife Xady and his family for their care and support throughout my stay in Dakar. Also Ibrahima Top for his sensitive translation of the conversations on the second visit to my village with my sister, Jody Ash.

Numerous people, foundations, and artist residencies assisted me through my travels and writing of this book: The American Pen Center, International AIDS society, MacDowell Colony, Yaddo Corporation, and Ben Strader and the true blue staff of Blue Mountain Center. I'm particularly grateful to Susan Tillet, the friends and staff of Ragdale for their warmth and generous support throughout this entire project. Friends and family also offered generous moral and financial support: Patrick Carew and Kathleen Mullaney, Carol Parnell, Jody and David Ash, Julie and Ted Hill, Mickey and Bill McColly.

For their faith in me and this book, I thank Joy Harris, Alexia Paul, and Cheryl Pientka of Joy Harris Agency.

For their vision and dedication to the literature of spiritual activism and the fight against HIV/AIDS, I'm indebted to Richard Nash and the many hands and hearts at Soft Skull Press for making this possible. Also, I'm grateful to Michael Vasquez and Nicole Lemy of the international journal *Transition*, who first recognized the import of this book.

For lending me his aesthetic brilliance, sensitivity, and courage in portraying the story of AIDS in Africa, I am deeply grateful to photographer and activist, Jide Adeniyi-Jones, whose artwork graces the cover of this book.

A number of writers and friends had a hand in helping me shape and understand what this book was really about: Lauren Brenner, Clayton Luz, Neil Chudgar, Michael Sledge, Gerry Gorman, Barb Ranes, Mike Puican,

Mary Childers, Tony Trigillio, Shelly Hubman, and Mary Lewis. I'm particularly in debt to Caroline Walker, Mira Bartok, and Tim Gray whose careful and sensitive editing came at the right time.

I'm deeply grateful to so many friends and colleagues that kept me sane, healthy, and focused on my goal: my physicians, doctors Malte Schultz, Lee Roberts, Jenny Lee; my colleagues at Northeastern Illinois University and Northwestern University; my friends, Molly Miller, Todd Smith and Sandy Yee, Doug and Kate Moody, Mark and Ann Alderfer, Matt Chotkowski, Tim McMains, Ann Ryan, Ellen Wadey and the board and staff of the Guild Literary Complex of Chicago, Hector Giuffre and Martha Ponzio, Bill Finnegan, David Shields, and Jaci Lyden. All of them and many other friends demanded that I take belief into action.

I am grateful for the support and guidance of the yoga community in Chicago and my spiritual teachers through the years: Mary Jo Weaver, Claude Marie Barbour, Paul Jones, Vern La Plante, Pam McClusky, Julie Hill, Suddha Weixler, Ann Fitzgibbons, Tim Miller, Anna Forrest, Gabriel Halpern, Sri K. Pattahbi Jois, B. K. S. Iyengar, John Friend, Krishna Das, Beth O'Neil, Nelson Peery, Per Erez, David Ley, Erin Love, Gerry Gorman, and the volunteers and men in the Zen Buddhist sangha at the Indiana State Prison in Michigan City.

Through the course of the past five years, several people unselfishly entered into this project, offering their time, energy and most importantly their unwavering belief in me and this book. In particular, I would like to thank: Tuong Nguyen who encouraged me to come to his country and kept me going thereafter; Quinn Kearney, my spiritual brother, who opened his home and heart to me, recognizing what I couldn't about what this journey meant; and Rob Nixon, who not only pulled me out of that freezing lake in New Hampshire but pulled this book out of me as well, making me ask and answer the difficult questions.

Without the love of my sisters, Jody and Julie, their families, my relatives alive and dead, and my parents Mickey and Bill McColly, I would never have set off on this journey nor had the character to chronicle it.

Since I set out on this journey in 2000, 15 million people have died of AIDS and 20 million more have been infected. Several people I interviewed in this book as well as friends, lovers, activists, and healers have passed, too: Forrest Hightower, Charles Clifton, Eunice Odongo, Leroy Whitfield, members of Pham Van's HIV group, and I'm afraid many others with whom I have lost contact. Their work and compassion live on.

Notes

Prologue

1 Thousands of Senegalese fought for the French, often used on the front lines in northern Africa, where they claimed to use their amulets filled with powerful medicine that would protect them from bullets. In reality, many of the Senegalese soldiers were slaughtered.

2 This lynching, the last known above the Mason-Dixon line, was memorialized by a photograph that has subsequently become a symbol of America's tragic racial history, revealing in brutal clarity the hypocrisy of the American legal system and the cowardice of American leaders. Recently, the lone survivor of the lynching, James Cameron, appeared with senators when Congress finally passed a bill apologizing for the hundreds of lynchings in the U.S. which were never prosecuted or investigated.

Chapter 1

1 UNAIDS and the World Health Organization estimate that South Africa has 5.3 million people living with HIV and an adult prevalency rate that ranges from 15 to 21 percent, although perhaps 90 percent are unaware that they are infected.

2 According to figures from 2004 from WHO/UNAIDS, 370,000 people died in South Africa from AIDS, over half under thirty. South Africa's life expectancy rate, once at sixty-three, has dropped to fifty-three, and some predict it will go as low at thirty-eight before the pandemic bottoms out.

3 There is limited information on the infection rate of MSMs (men who have sex with men) in South Africa. UNAIDS figures indicated that in Cape Town roughly 11 percent of MSMs are infected.

4 According to Amnesty International, South African police statistics for 2003-2004 recorded over 52,000 cases of sexual assault on women, a rate of 119 per 100,000, which is the highest rate in the world. For comparison, the U.S. rate is 30 per 100,000. Though the South African judicial system has created more courts specifically for sexual assault, most experts agree that it will do little to encourage more women to file cases. What is more alarming is the rise in reported cases of assault on children by adults and increasing by other children. One cause to this disturbing trend is the persistent superstitious belief that sleeping with a virgin cures a man of HIV infection.

5 Epstein, Helen, "Mozambique: In Search of the Hidden Cause of AIDS," *New York Review of Books*, May 9, 2002.

6 As of 2004, despite international assistance and an increase in government

spending for drug treatments, only some 28,000 people received the anti-retroviral treatment in South Africa's public clinics, only half of the goal set by the government of 53,000. At least 500,000 people are in need of these life-saving drugs. Some 45,000 pay for the cocktail themselves either from insurance or out of pocket.

7 As of 2004, South Africa has 1.1 million orphans. The United Nations AIDS program projects that the numbers of orphans throughout sub-Saharan Africa will climb to 19 million before tapering off.

Chapter 2

1 Nkosi Johnson died the next year in 2001. At his funeral, Nelson Mandela called him "an icon in the struggle for life." A foundation for orphans now bears his name.

2 MSMs (men who have sex with men) is the accepted umbrella term that refers to all men who have sex with other men: men who identify themselves as homosexual, bisexual, transgender, or straight. From country to country, terms such as gay or even bisexual don't adequately describe the complex and fluid sexual preferences of men. It must be remembered, as well, that in many countries men will have sex with other men as a means of barter or for money without any sexual interest in men. I will, where appropriate, use this term, even when referring primarily to gay and bisexual men.

3 According to PROMETRA, the International Organization to Promote Traditional Medicine, Africans are resorting to forms of traditional medicines as they search for options to deal with either symptoms of AIDS-related illnesses or as actual cures for HIV infection.

4 Credo Mutwa is an African storyteller, historian, and traditional healer. His book *Indaba, My Children: African Tribal History, Legends, Customs and Religious Beliefs,* (Blue Crane Books, 1964) is a collection of his retelling of tales and legends of African tribal life.

5 Gugu Dlamini became a martyr for AIDS activists and people living with HIV and AIDS after she was stoned to death by her own village when she'd come out as HIV positive on World AIDS day in 1999.

6 Mandela's speech was an enormous victory both symbolically and politically for South Africa's AIDS movement. Mandela had stepped out from behind Mbeki and embraced the cause and the millions who had suffered since the early nineties when, if more had been done, South Africa might have averted the explosion and the loss of hundreds of thousands of its people. AIDS detracts from the valiant struggles of his people against apartheid, and Mandela understood this as his own failure, knowing that he could have made a difference. In 1990, South Africa had roughly the same rate of infection as Thailand, 2 percent of the adult population. But while South Africa struggled to rid itself of apartheid, Thailand mobilized

and decreased its rate. In South Africa the opposite occurred. Rates doubled to 4 percent and again to 8 percent and once more, reaching over 16 percent of its population. In 2004, Mandela's own son died of AIDS.

Chapter 3

1 In Tamil Nadu state, UNAIDS and the World Health Organization estimates that 1 percent of the adult population is HIV positive, one of the highest rates of any state in India. The virus is passed primarily through heterosexual intercourse. Among female sex workers the rates of infection are estimated at over 50 percent.

2 Exacerbating India's HIV epidemic is the tremendous population shift from rural to urban. Since 1971, the urban population of India has increased by 200 million.

3 As of 2004, UNAIDS/WHO estimates that India has the same number of infected as South Africa, 5.3 million, with an adult prevalence rate of less than 1 percent. The government strongly disputes these figures, saying it is much lower. Still with over a billion people and over a third living in poverty and more and more people living with poor health care in major urban areas, India's epidemic is accelerating at an unpredictable and potentially disastrous rate.

4 Pantanjali (BCE 2000), philosopher and Sanskrit scholar, is generally credited as the father of raja yoga, which emphasizes the use of meditation as the path to spiritual enlightenment. In short aphoristic sutras, Patanjali set down the ancient Vedic teachings of yoga in *The Yoga Sutras*, which explains the practice of the eightfold path toward samadhi (the mystical union of the Self with God).

5 Of the 40 million people living with TB in the world a third of them, 13 million, live in India. Two million people develop active TB each year and over 430, 000 die. TB is also the leading cause of death worldwide for those with AIDS.

6 Khan, Shivananda, "Under the Blanket: Bisexuality and AIDS in India," *Bisexualities and AIDS: International Perspective*, edited by Peter Aggleton, London, Taylor & Francis.

7 YRG now has other clinics in South India and there are others as well outside of Chennai, but when I was there it was the only one serving those with HIV in South India.

8 Recently, Kousalya told me in an email that she and the women of PWN have access to antiretroviral treatment. She also excitedly told me that several more branches of PWN have been started around India.

9 According to UNAIDS, as of 2003, 30,000 HIV-positive Indians received antiretroviral medications of nearly 600,000 who could benefit from treatment.

10 Khan and Sunil told me that by and large most homosexual and bisexual

men in India do not refer to themselves with the Western term "gay," particularly poorer and lower class men. However, among educated and professional men living in the major urban centers of India, the term is being used more and more frequently.

11 This fishing village was severely damaged in the deadly tsunami that struck Indonesia and South Asia in 2004.

12 Sri Aurobindo (1872–1950) believed that the classic concept of karmayoga came from his study of the *Bhagavad Gita*. In several of his principle philosophical writings, he describes the human path toward identity with the Absolute as an evolutionary process that begins with the active pursuit of knowledge and higher consciousness through the disciplined study and practice of yoga. By stages, then, through the practice of yoga, each individual transforms the mind, the body, and their lives, and as a consequence over time, all human beings evolve to higher states of consciousness.

Chapter 4

1 Before the Vietnam War, the estimated number of women working in the sex industry in Thailand was around 20,000. By the end of the war, the numbers had risen to over 200,000. After the War, it took little time before Bangkok businessmen realized that the influx of dollars from GIs needed to be replaced, and the sexual tourism industry was born. Though nearly impossible to calculate, NGOs working to protect the rights of commercial sex workers claim that up to 18 percent of Thailand's GNP can be attributed to the commercial sex industry.

2 The V-1 Immunator was eventually discredited by the Thai government and the Salaam Bannag Foundation dropped its support. Sadly, I have seen reports that the V-1 has popped up in East Africa on the black market and sold as a scientifically proven drug to cure AIDS.

3 At over 2 percent of the adult population, Myanmar has the highest HIV infection rate in Southeast Asia. Most attribute this to the historic use of heroin in this region of the world as well as Myanmar's corrupt military government which supports itself by drug trafficking.

4 Dr. Yves Adaan from Belgium has been working here since 1995. His devotion is exemplified by the fact that he has contracted tuberculosis twice and has often worked alone without proper equipment, treating thousands of patients a year. His memoir, *Echoing Voice from Wat Phra Bat Nam Phu*, (Matichon Publishing) describes his work at the hospice in Lopburi.

5 This teenager became a poster child for AIDS activism when he was denied the right to return to his junior high school after he was diagnosed. Eventually, his mother obtained a court order allowing him to return. Congress would go on to enact this historic legislation to ensure the rights and health care for people living with HIV and AIDS, now known as the Ryan White Act.

Chapter 5

1 This term defines those Vietnamese who left Vietnam for the U.S., or for any foreign country.

2 UNAIDS estimates that less than 1 percent of Vietnam's adult population is infected with HIV with some 200,000 people living with the virus.

3 Vietnam's per capita income is $392, five times lower than that of Thailand.

4 Since 2001, Vietnam has provided more antiretroviral drugs to those with HIV. The U.S. has chosen Vietnam as one of the countries to receive antiretrovirals from the Bush administration's $15 billion drug-assistance plan. Yet, as of 2005, no drugs have made it to the thousands who desperately need them.

5 As of 2005, according to UNAIDS figures, the number of people living with HIV in Ho Chi Minh City (Saigon) is now four times higher, or roughly 20,000.

Chapter 6

1 At the urging of Nelson Mandela, Achmat, after becoming very ill, eventually realized he had made his point and began to take medications again.

2 The Thai government is slowly offering more generics as they become available. However, U.S. trade policies keep Thailand from purchasing life-saving generic HIV drugs from other countries and have contributed to the deaths of many Thais over the past several years who might have been saved had these trade barriers been lifted.

3 Viral load tests can cost from $100 to $150. CD4 counts cost $40. This is an enormous amount considering that the minimum wage (in Bangkok) is 175 Bt, or about $5 per day. The average income for Thais is on the rise, but it's still less than $2,000 per year.

Chapter 8

1 Uganda's remarkable drop in infection from 15 percent in 1991 to 5 percent in 2002 is now in jeopardy due to the political and religious beliefs of the Ugandan President Museveni and his wife who, under pressure from the Bush administration and conservative evangelical churches, have now become promoters of abstinence as the single most important element in Uganda's successful prevention programs. The Musevenis have downplayed the overwhelming evidence of the critical role that condom use and faithfulness to a single partner have played in prevention.

2 Baldwin, James, "Letter From A Region In My Mind," From *The Fire Next Time,* The Dial Press, 1963.

3 After years of neglect, the city finally has began to tear them down. Some would say concern over the social and financial costs of these poorly-maintained buildings was far less important than the interest in cashing in on the real estate boom across Chicago, particularly in areas close to the Loop. To date, however, there's been a fraction of the new, low-rise public housing the city promised CHA residents. Like everywhere in urban America, Chicago has a severe shortage of affordable housing, and the city is dragging its heels, and, in effect, forcing the poor out of the city altogether.

4 The Tuskegee Syphilis Study is one of the most blatant examples of racism, ethical misconduct, and governmental abuse in American medical history. In the longest recorded non-therapeutic study on human beings (1932-1972), doctors knowingly did not treat half of the 400 poor, black share-croppers in their study of syphilis in Macon County, Alabama.

5 Fears, Daryl, "Study: Many Blacks Cite AIDS Conspiracy Hurts Prevention Efforts," *Washington Post*, January 25, 2005.

6 In line with national figures, Jimenez tells me, in Chicago 17 percent of those living with HIV are Latino/Hispanic, with Mexican-American men being the largest group. In the Puerto Rican community, HIV has disproportionately affected both men and women; it is the leading cause of death for women and second leading cause after murder for men between the ages of twenty-five and forty-four.

7 D'Eramo, Marco, *The Pig and the Skyscraper: Chicago: A History Of Our Future*, Verso, 2002.

8 Though it's nearly impossible to determine the prevalence of sexual assault in prisons, various studies, based on interviews with former inmates, suggest that it could be as high as 30 percent in the U.S. penal system.

9 The Illinois General Assembly recently passed a bill to increase such funding for HIV programs in Illinois prisons in a sweeping HIV prevention measure in response to the alarming rise of HIV in the state's black population.

10 A recent study by the Centers for Disease Control interviewed and tested gay and bisexual men in five major U.S. cities. Among the black men they tested, 46 percent tested positive and more than two-thirds did not know of their status.

11 Tragically, those who died were mostly elderly people of color found alone in bedrooms or apartments without air-conditioning or fans. The highest rates of death were in Chicago's poorest and most crime-ridden neighborhoods on the South and West Sides. Many of the dead were found in rooms with windows bolted shut because of the fear of crime. Klinkenborg, Eric, *Heat Wave: A Social Autopsy of Disaster In Chicago*, University of Chicago Press, 2002.

12 Chicago's murder rate has gone down. In 2004, Los Angles edged ahead of Chicago as the murder capital of America.

13 The UN estimates that Ethiopia has 1.5 million people living with HIV, or 4.4 percent of its adult population, and the epidemic is growing rapidly. Only 4,500 people are being treated with antiretroviral drugs. Chicago, in comparison, has over 11,000 people living with HIV, of which almost all have access to antiretroviral drugs.

14 Lewis, Mary C., "Welfare and Remedy," (reading from book-in-progress, symposium Writing AIDS, Center For The Humanities, University of Wisconsin-Madison, October 29, 2004).

Chapter 9

1 A third of Senegal's population can afford only one decent meal a day.

2 Islam's influence on West Africa dates back to the 9th century when Berber and Arab merchants carried their beliefs along with salt and other goods south across the Sahara to exchange for gold and slaves. For several centuries, the converted African noblemen and royalty blended Islam, particularly the mystical and devotional practices of Sufism, with indigenous traditional beliefs, creating what would become the hybridized Islam that is practiced across the continent.

3 The Mouride brotherhood has gained enormous power over the years, so much so that there are growing communities among the Senegalese who live in Europe and America. The Mbacke family holds considerable influence over the current president, Abdoulaye Wade, who is also a follower. The people in the village where I lived are deeply devoted followers of the Mbacke family and this sect. In fact, two miles from my village, there is a major Mouride shrine, the tomb of Amadou Bamba's mother.

4 I discovered toward the end of my stay in Senegal in the resort area of Mbour that finding a willing partner, female or male, to have sex is not a problem. In Mbour at a luxury French-owned hotel, I was hit on within minutes of walking onto the beach by a fast-talking English-speaking Senegalese in a Speedo. These men are not necessarily sex workers or gay, they are opportunists. Though he simply wanted to accompany me as I went jogging, it was pretty obvious what he was willing to offer. Homosexuality or bisexuality is completely hidden in Senegal, and many Senegalese are sure it is virtually nonexistent except for Westerners or those influenced by them.

5 Pikine is now Senegal's most populous city, quadrupling in size since I left in the early eighties.

6 Over 50 percent of Senegal's population is under the age of twenty-five.

7 From 1986 to 2002, the infection rates in Kaolack for female sex workers went from 0 to 20 percent.

8 Buber, Martin. *I and Thou*, Charles Scribner and Sons, New York, 1958.

South Africa

NGOs and HIV/AIDS Organizations referred to in this book.

Treatment Action Campaign
34 Main Road
Muizenberg 7945
South Africa
www.tac.org.za
To Donate: South African
Development Fund
555 Amory St.
Boston, MA 02130
freesa@igc.org

NAPWA National Association for
People with AIDS/HIV (South Africa)
P.O Box 66
Germiston 1400
South Africa
www.napwa.org.za
napwadir@sn.apc.org

Sisters of Nazareth (Nazareth House
Children's Home)
P.O. Box 12116
Mill Street
Cape Town 8010
South Africa
www.nazhouse.org.za

Joy For Life
1 Moltono Road
Oranjezicht, Cape Town 8002
Joy4life@wn.apc.org

Wola Nani
P.O. Box 16082
8018 Vlaeberg
South Africa
wolanani@iafrica.com

WOFAK (Women's Organization For
AIDS in Kenya)
P.O. Box 35168
Nairobi, Kenya
www.wofak.or.ke

India

YR Gaitonde Centre
www.yrgcare.org

Naz Foundation
Palingswick House
241 King Street
London W6 9LP, UK
www.nazfoundation.org

Sahodaran
25, Sterling Road First Cross Street
Nungambakkam
Chennai 600 034
Email: sunilSuniloc@yahoo.com
PH. 044-28252859

Positive Woman Network
9/5 Shanthi Apt.
Nungambakkam,
Chennai 600034
www.pwnplus.org
India Network for People Living with
HIV (INP plus)
Inpplus@vsnl.com

Social Welfare Association for Men
5 Natarajan St. Balakrishnan Nagar,
Jafferkhanpet
Chennai 600 083
Email: siaap@satyam.net.in

Thailand

Kenya

Wat Phra Bhat Nam Phu (AIDS
Temple) Lopburi

Thai Red Cross AIDS Research Centre
1871 Rama 4 Road,
Bangkok, Thailand 10330
Tel/fax: 66-2 256-4107/66-2254-
7577

Thai Red Cross provides medicines
for women and children as well.
To donate: **Thai Red Cross Society,
(Save A child's Life Project)**
ACCT. # 045-2-004236 Siam
Commercial Bank's Thai Red Cross
Branch

EMPOWER
P.O. Box 1065
Silom Post Office
Bangkok 10504, Thailand
Tel/fax 66-2 236-972
www.empowerfoundation.org

New Life Friends Centre
9/57 Moo 3 Suthep Road
Tumbon Suthep
A. Muang, Chiang Mai, 50200
Tel/fax: 053-808-233

Friends For Life Centre
Klung Cholarpratan Road
Chiang Mai, Thailand

**Church of Christ of Thailand AIDS
Ministry**
1/100 Rattanakosin Road
Chiang Mai 50000

Vietnam

Chuong Trinh AIDS (AIDS Program)
54/32 Le Quang Dinh, Q. Binh
Thanh
Ho Chi Minh City, Vietnam
Phamthanhvan@cinet.vnnews.com

Chicago

AIDS Foundation
411 S. Wells St Suite 300
Chicago, IL 60607
www.aidschicago.org

Test Positive Aware
5537 N. Broadway
Chicago, IL 60640
www.tapn.com

Vida/Sida
2703 W. Division
Chicago, IL
773-278-6737

Howard Brown Health Center
4025 N. Sheridan
Chicago, IL 60640
773-338-8936
www.howardbrown.org

**NAPWA (National Association For
People With AIDS) USA**
1413 K. Street NW Seventh Floor
Washington, D.C. 20005-3442
www.napwa.org

AIDS Treatment Activists Coalition
Old Chelsea Station
PO Box 1514
New York, NY 10113

Trinity United Church Of Christ
400 West 95th Street
Chicago, Ill. 60628
www.tucc.org

Core Center
2020 W. Harrison St.
Chicago, IL 60612
www.corecenter.org

Luck Care Clinic
1701 W. Monterey Ave.
Chicago, IL
312-233-5850

Jordan House
7431 South Chicago Blvd
Chicago, IL

Senegal

ACI Africa Consultants International
http://www.acibaobab.org
ACI Sante – Baobab III
Villa 4346, Sicap Amitie III
BP 5270, Dakar-Fann
Senegal

FARE (Fund for African Relief and
Education)

SWAA (Society for Women and AIDS
in Africa)
6, Avenue Bourguiba
BP 16425 Dakar-Fann
Senegal
www.swaainternational.org
contact@swaainternational.org or
swaa@telecomplus.sn

Catholic Relief Services (Programs in
Senegal)
Sida Service
BP 15314
Fann-Dakar
Senegal

ANP+ (Organization for HIV Positive
People)
BP 7388
Medina-Dakar
Senegal

To Donate to CRS:
CRS
209 W. Fayette St.
Baltimore, MD 21201-3443
donorservice@catholicrelief.org

To assist the refugees from Sierra
Leone at Baker Collier House:
FARE (Fund For African Relief and
Education)
P.O. Box 7265
Silver Springs, MD 20907
www.fundforafricaneducation.org

JAMRA (Islamic non governmental
organization working with HIV preven-
tion)
C/o Bamar Gueye
10 Avenue Bourguiba
SICAP Darabis
B.P. 5716
Dakar, Senegal
Ongjamra78@hotmail.com or ong-
jamra78@yahoo.fr

PROMETRA (Association for
Promotion of Traditional Medicine)
International Headquarters
BP 6134
Dakar-Etoile, Senegal
Prometra@prometra.org
www.prometra.org

WARC (West African Research
Center)
www.warc-croa.org

For more current information about
the international AIDS pandemic and
these organizations see:
www.unaids.org
HIV-AIDS@who.int
www.thebody.org
http://mccoly.ecorp.net

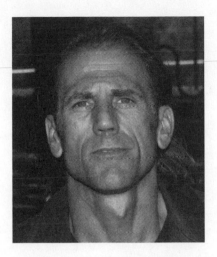

Michael McColly teaches creative writing at Northwestern University. His work has appeared in the *New York Times, Chicago Tribune, Salon, The Sun, Ascent,* and other publications. He is a former Peace Corps Volunteer in Senegal (1981–83). He is featured speaker on college campuses on spiritual activism and the AIDS pandemic.